Law for Nurses and Midwives

Law for Nurses and Midwives

Tenth Edition

HON PATRICIA J STAUNTON, AM, RN, CM, LLB, MCrim

Barrister-at-Law of the Inner Temple, London, United Kingdom

PROFESSOR MARY CHIARELLA, AM, RN, LLB (Hons), PhD (UNSW), FACN, FRSM

Professor Emerita, Susan Wakil School of Nursing and Midwifery, University of Sydney, NSW, Australia

ELSEVIER

ELSEVIER

Elsevier Australia. ACN 001 002 357
(a division of Reed International Books Australia Pty Ltd)
475 Victoria Avenue, Chatswood, NSW 2067

ISBN: 978-0-729-54470-2

National Library of Australia Cataloguing-in-Publication Data

A catalogue record for this book is available from the National Library of Australia

Content Strategist: Melinda McEvoy
Content Project Manager: Abdus Salam Mazumder
Edited by Laura Davies
Proofread by Tim Learner
Copyrights Coordinator: Vengatesh T
Cover Designer: Gopalakrishnan Venkatraman
Index by Innodata
Typeset by GW Tech
Printed in China

Last digit is the print number: 9 8 7 6 5 4 3 2 1

TABLE OF CONTENTS

DEDICATION

To my parents with love and affection. Patricia Staunton

For my beloved family and my grandchildren, at home and abroad. Mary Chiarella

PREFACE

It has always been our goal to provide nursing and midwifery students as well as practising registered and enrolled nurses and midwives throughout Australia with an introduction to the legal issues relevant to the delivery of their professional services, and to do so in a practical and readily understandable text with a clear, concise and readable exposition of the law.

With the recent updates to regulation for nurses and midwives under national registration, we have updated the tenth edition of *Law for Nurses and Midwives* with the aim of reflecting these standards, and incorporated legislation relevant to midwifery practice.

All chapters have been revised and updated to reflect recent changes in legislation and regulations relating to nursing and midwifery practice, as have references to relevant court decisions. Special attention has been given to areas where legislative provisions apply, such as professional standard of care, workplace health and safety, coroners' jurisdiction and mental health, to ensure that a nationwide perspective is provided.

Chapter 4 'Professional regulation of nurses and midwives' has been updated to further examine the standards and regulations established by the Nursing and Midwifery Board of Australia for national registration, and includes a specific section on maternity services law to address the standards and guidelines for endorsed midwives. In light of the NMBA's adoption of two international Codes of Ethics for Midwives and Nurses respectively, we have updated the chapter that looks specifically at these Codes and explores how they might influence the practices of midwives and nurses by their introduction. Chapter 6 has been updated to address the introduction of voluntary assisted dying into each of the states in Australia.

As always, we are extremely grateful for the comments and feedback we have received from readers and professional critics of our text to ensure it remains relevant to those who use it.

Again, we thank the staff who have provided us with assistance in undertaking our task as well as our publishers for their support and patience during the writing of the tenth edition.

We trust this most recent edition of our text continues to provide assistance to all who use it and we thank them for their encouragement and interest in the ongoing editions of this text.

ABOUT THE AUTHORS

Hon Patricia J Staunton AM, RN, CM, LLB, MCrim; Barrister-at-Law of the Inner Temple, London, United Kingdom

Patricia Staunton has had a professional career encompassing both the health and legal systems. She has qualified and worked as a registered nurse and midwife both in Australia and overseas. She is legally qualified and has practised as a barrister in Australia, during which time she represented nurses and midwives in matters relating to their professional activities as well as industrial matters relating to their professional career structure, wage rates and conditions of employment.

Patricia was the elected General Secretary of the NSW Nurses and Midwives Association for eight years and was instrumental in introducing the professional career structure and wage rates into industrial awards for nurses and midwives in both the public and private sectors. She was also the elected Federal President of the Australian Nursing and Midwifery Federation.

Subsequently Patricia was appointed a Magistrate of the Local Courts of NSW and ultimately the Chief Magistrate of NSW. She was then appointed a Judge and Deputy President of the Industrial Court of NSW. Since retiring from that position, Patricia spent a number of years as a part-time Deputy President on the NSW Mental Health Review Tribunal.

Patricia has lectured extensively for many years to nurses and midwives throughout Australia addressing legal issues relating to their professional practice. She continues to do so.

In 1995, Patricia was appointed a Member of the Order of Australia for her services to nursing.

Professor Mary Chiarella AM, RN, LLB (Hons), PhD (UNSW), FACN, FRSM
Professor Emerita, Susan Wakil School of Nursing and Midwifery, University of Sydney, NSW, Australia

Mary's career spans 40 years in both the United Kingdom and Australia across a variety of nursing services. Mary is Professor Emerita, Susan Wakil School of Nursing at the University of Sydney. In 2003–04 she was the Chief Nursing Officer, NSW Health Department and prior to that was the Foundation Professor of Nursing in Corrections Health, with the University of Technology, Sydney.

Mary has provided her professional expertise to health services, organisations and governments over the years. She is Deputy Chair of Northern Sydney LHD and currently chairs its Health Care Quality Committee. She also serves on the Clinical Ethics Advisory Panel to the NSW Minister for Health and the Australian Health Ethics Committee of the NHMRC.

Mary's particular research interests focus on legal, policy and ethical issues in nursing, midwifery and healthcare delivery. She publishes and speaks nationally and internationally on her work

She was awarded an AM for significant contributions to nursing and midwifery education and healthcare standards in June 2019 and was made an Honorary Fellow of the Australian College of Nurse Practitioners in 2022.

REVIEWERS

DARREN CONLON BN, BCL(HONS), GCUT, GDLP, LLM, PHD CANDIDATE
Lecturer in Law, Ethics and Professional Practice,
School of Nursing and Midwifery
Faculty of Medicine, Nursing and Midwifery and
  Health Sciences,
The University of Notre Dame, Sydney, Australia

DR. TONIA CRAWFORD RN, BAPPSC(NURSING), MHSC(ED), PHD
Senior lecturer and Director, Pre-registration
  programmes
Susan Wakil School of Nursing and Midwifery
Faculty of Medicine and Health
The University of Sydney, Sydney, Australia

DR. SOPHIA DYWILI PHD, RM, RN
Lecturer in Nursing
School of Nursing, Paramedicine and Healthcare
  Sciences
Faculty of Science and Health
Charles Sturt University, Wagga Wagga, Australia

JO SOUTHERN RN, BHLTHSCNR, LLB, GCERTACUTECARE, MNCED, PHD CANDIDATE
Lecturer in Nursing
School of Nursing and Midwifery
University of Southern Queensland, Ipswich,
  Australia

ROZ WILLIAMSON RN BBUS BED BSC(HONS) MNPRAC MACN
Lecturer and Bachelor of Nursing Deputy Course
  Director
Faculty of Medicine, Nursing and Health Sciences
School of Nursing and Midwifery
Monash University, Melbourne, Australia

TABLE OF ABBREVIATIONS

A

AC	appeal cases
ACAT	ACT Civil and Administrative Tribunal
ACFI	Aged Care Funding Instrument
ACM	Australian College of Midwives
ACMI	Australian College of Midwives Inc
ACN	Australian College of Nursing
ACORN	Australian College of Operating Room Nurses
ACSQHC	Australian Commission on Safety and Quality in Health Care
ADHA	Australian Digital Health Agency
AHEC	Australian Health Ethics Committee
AHMAC	Australian Health Ministers' Advisory Council
Ahpra	Australian Health Practitioner Regulation Agency
AIMS	Advanced Incident Management System
AIN	assistant in nursing
AIRC	Australian Industrial Relations Commission
ALJ	Australian Law Journal
All ER	All England Law Reports
ALR	Australian Law Reports
ALRC	Australian Law Reform Commission
ANCI	Australian Nursing Council Inc.
ANF	Australian Nursing Federation
ANMAC	Australian Nursing and Midwifery Accreditation Council
ANMC	Australian Nursing and Midwifery Council
ANMF	Australian Nursing and Midwifery Federation
APAC	Australian Pharmaceutical Advisory Council
APSF	Australian Patient Safety Foundation
ART	assisted reproductive technology
AVM	arterio-venous malformation

C

CCO	continuing care order
CCP	Chief Civil Psychiatrist
CFP	Chief Forensic Psychiatrist
CHF	Consumer Health Forum
CHRE	Council for Healthcare Regulatory Excellence
CLR	Commonwealth Law Reports

CMO	community management order
COAG	Council of Australian Governments
CPD	continuing professional development
CRM	crew resource management
CRPD	Convention on the Rights of Persons with Disabilities
CTO	community treatment order

D

DET	Department of Education and Training
DPP	Director of Public Prosecutions
DST	deep sleep therapy

E

ECT	electroconvulsive therapy
ECV	external cephalic version
EHR	electronic health record
ELS	English language skills
EM	eligible midwife
EMM	electronic medication management
EN	enrolled nurse
ETP	electronic transfer of prescriptions

F

FAQ	frequently asked questions
FCTO	forensic community treatment order

G

GIFT	gamete intrafallopian transfer

H

HCCC	Health Care Complaints Commission
HCE	health complaints entity
HDU	high-dependency unit
HIM	health information management
HPCA	Health Professional Councils Authority
HSR	health and safety representative

I

ICM	International Council of Midwives
ICN	International Council of Nurses
ICSI	intracytoplasmic sperm injection
IDRS	Intellectual Disability Rights Service
IELTS	international English language testing system
IIMS	Incident Information Management System
IPO	involuntary patient order
IQNM	internationally qualified nurses and midwives
ISR	Incident Severity Rating
ITO	involuntary treatment order
IV	intravenous
IVF	in vitro fertilisation

J

J   Judge

L

LQR   The Law Quarterly Review
LRC   Law Reform Commission

M

MBS   Medicare Benefits Scheme
MHIPU   Mental Health Inpatient Unit
MHR   My Health Record

N

NEHTA   National E-Health Transition Authority
NGMI   not guilty on the grounds of mental illness
NHMRC   National Health and Medical Research Council
NMBA   Nursing and Midwifery Board of Australia
NP   nurse practitioner
NRAS   National Registration and Accreditation Scheme
NSQHS   National Safety and Quality Health Service
NSWLRC   New South Wales Law Reform Commission
NSWR   New South Wales Reports

O

OAIC   Office of the Australian Information Commissioner
OD   open disclosure
OH&S   occupational health and safety
OTA   Organ and Tissue Authority

P

P   President
PBS   Pharmaceutical Benefits Scheme
PCA   patient-controlled analgesia
PCBU   person conducting a business or undertaking
PCEHR   Personally Controlled Electronic Health Record
PEP   Professional Education Package
PII   professional indemnity insurance
PIN   Provisional Improvement Notice
PPM   privately practising midwife
PPTP   Prescribed Psychiatric Treatment Panel

Q

QAHCS   Quality in Australian Health Care Study
QB   Queen's Bench
QC   Queen's Counsel
QPD   Queensland parliamentary debates

R

RCA   root cause analysis
RCNA   Royal College of Nursing Australia
RIPN   rural and isolated practice nurses

RM	registered midwife
RN	registered nurse
RoP	recency of practice
RTAC	Reproductive Technology Accreditation Committee
S	
SAC	severity assessment code
SASR	South Australian State Reports
SAU	sub-acute unit
SMHU	secure mental health unit
SOP	standard of practice
SQF	Safety and Quality Framework
SQGs	safety and quality guidelines
SUSMP	Standard for the Uniform Scheduling of Medicines and Poisons
T	
TEN	trainee enrolled nurse
TO	treatment order
TTO	temporary treatment order
V	
VCAT	Victorian Civil and Administrative Tribunal
VHIMS	Victorian Health Incident Management System
W	
WHS	Work Health and Safety
WLR	Weekly Law Reports
Z	
ZIFT	zygote intrafallopian transfer

Section 1

INTRODUCTION

1 AN INTRODUCTION TO THE LAW AND AUSTRALIA'S LEGAL SYSTEM

INTRODUCTION

To practise as a registered nurse, enrolled nurse or midwife in Australia requires registration with the Nursing and Midwifery Board of Australia. Once gained, that registration incorporates adherence to a *Code of conduct*[1] and a *Code of ethics*[2] as well as a *Standards for practice*[3] that sets out in broad principle-based terms the professional, ethical and legal responsibilities expected of nurses (both registered and enrolled) and midwives in the delivery of healthcare and health services.

More specifically, requirements within the *Standards for practice* make provision for such responsibilities in specific terms. For example, Standard 1.4 relating to a registered nurse states that, when practising, a registered nurse should comply 'with legislation, regulation, policies, guidelines and other standards or requirements relevant to the context of practice when making decisions'.[4] Similar such provisions apply in relation to the specific Standards for enrolled nurses[5] (Standard 1.1) and in relation to midwives[6] in Standard 3.2.

For a nurse (registered or enrolled) or midwife to attain the standard expected requires, in the first instance, a rudimentary understanding of what the law is, where it comes from and how it operates relevant to your professional practice. Such an understanding is essential to enable you to extract from a seemingly complex system sufficient practical information to be of benefit to you in your professional life.

The Development of the Law and Its Role in Society

Rather than seek to precisely define what the law is, it is more important to understand the rationale behind the development of the law and its role in society.

The sophisticated and complex legal system that exists in Australia today represents the development of many centuries of Western civilisation. The discovery and colonisation of Australia by England over 200 years ago saw the adoption in this country of the legal system and principles that existed in England at that time. The English legal system, as it then was, originated in primitive community or village systems and its historical development can be traced back over centuries of invasions. These primitive communities recognised the need for rules of behaviour which encompassed respect for each other and each other's property to ensure a degree of order in the community.

Hand in hand with such recognition was the inevitable desire for dominance and power over others, which has played such a major role in the development and subsequent decline of civilisations over the centuries.

Inevitably, what started as a crude system for rules of behaviour, operating on an individual community or village basis, was forced to develop and change over the centuries with the growth of the population and the diversity and sophistication of community systems, as well as the rapid growth of industry and technology.

As earlier stated, the laws of a community essentially comprise rules of behaviour as well as the recognition of personal and property rights. Within that process, certain philosophies have influenced, and continue to influence, the development of such rules. Primarily these are referred to as natural law and positive law philosophies.

Natural law philosophies, as a general rule, saw the origins of law as arising from a higher or divine being, which encompassed the notion of divine retribution operating in human affairs. Such a philosophy embraced the concept of sin as a transgression against the divine will, or contrary to certain principles of morality.

The development of the Greek civilisation, and to a lesser extent the Roman civilisation, was influenced by such natural law philosophies (in the shape of their gods), which stressed individual worth, moral duty and universal brotherhood. Such philosophies were developed further during the medieval period in Europe by the increasing influence of the Catholic Church, which set the tone and pattern of all speculative thought at that time. The Catholic Church pursued this natural law view as law derived from God with one faith, one church, one empire — not created by human societies but conceived as part of the universe.

In summary, natural law philosophies view situations as they might or ought to be, as opposed to how they are. It is an idealist notion with strong moral overtones. As an example, the United Nations Declaration of Human Rights is essentially a natural law document.

Positive law philosophies view law in a totally secular cast without regard for divine prescriptions or intervention. Such views emerged during the Renaissance period of European history (fourteenth to sixteenth centuries), which saw the rise of independent national states and an emphasis on the individual. Further development occurred during the nineteenth century, when states were established with absolute sovereignty not subject to an external natural law. The industrial revolution and the development of science supported this imperative theory of law, which saw the key concepts of law as being:

1. the command;
2. of a sovereign (used in this context, sovereign means the government of the state or country);
3. backed by a sanction (i.e. the penalty imposed for non-compliance with the command of the sovereign).

Such a view of the law takes no account of morality, and indeed positive law is most evidenced in the rigid separation of law and morals.

The Influence of Natural and Positive Law Philosophies on the Development of Legal Systems

Natural law philosophies have had their greatest impact on the development of the legal systems of Western civilisation in shaping statements of ideal intent. Apart from the United Nations Declaration of Human Rights, another example of the incorporation of natural law philosophies into a legal document can be found in the United States Constitution that provides for the individual right to certain fundamental freedoms — two of which are the freedom of speech and freedom of the press. Although such rights are guaranteed in the Constitution, such rights are not absolute in practice, as they are subject to constraints that prohibit that freedom in certain circumstances. As an example, the freedom of the press is subject to the laws of defamation, which will prevent the publication of material in particular circumstances and provide for the courts to award monetary compensation if defamatory material is disseminated. Nevertheless, it is the *intent* of the United States Constitution to guarantee absolute freedom of speech and of the press, so that every citizen and the press should be able to speak their mind and state their views freely, without fear of reprisal.

Natural law philosophies have also been responsible for the continuing influence of morality in shaping some of our present laws, much to the disapproval of positivist lawyers who believe morality should play no part in such an activity. As an example, areas of law-making where morality and/or religious influences have played a significant role in influencing our present laws have been the contentious areas of abortion, same-sex marriage and voluntary euthanasia.[7]

The positive law view that law is a command of a sovereign backed by a sanction means that no regard should be paid as to whether the command of the sovereign may be considered immoral by general community standards or a particular group in the community. The mere fact that the sovereign (the parliament) has the power to command and, where necessary, impose a sanction for non-compliance legitimises such a command. An example of such a situation is the international legal recognition that is given to governments of various countries whose government regimes would be considered by any moral standards to be odious and repressive. At a more local level, an example would be where parliament has approved laws to permit same-sex marriage, abortion and voluntary euthanasia that some sectors of the community would not support because of their religious or moral beliefs.

Both philosophies have had an impact on the laws that we have today and will have in the future.

WHERE DOES OUR LAW COME FROM?

As a legacy of our colonisation by England, Australia as a nation inherited many of England's laws — certainly its legal principles — and in doing so the historical development of its legal system. Therefore, let's examine briefly the history of the English legal system in order to understand ours.

The development of the English legal system saw the emergence of two major sources of law:

1. common law;
2. parliamentary or statute law.

The Development of the Common Law

To understand how the common law principles developed, appreciate that the land mass known to us as England and Wales[8] was not always the densely populated modern community that it now is. The development of English common law principles that were established on a central unified basis goes back

to the time of Henry II, who ruled England from 1154 to 1189.

At that time Henry's kingdom consisted of a large number of feudal villages, each presided over by the feudal lord or chief of the village. Communication as we know it today did not exist, battles between warring factions were not uncommon, and Henry was having the usual problem of maintaining power and control over his kingdom that English monarchs were wont to have in those times.

The law, as then understood and applied, consisted of the rules of the individual villages, generally based on custom and practice, which were administered and interpreted by the feudal lord of the village. Such rules were generally arbitrary and subjective, were changed frequently and varied from village to village.

In an attempt to unify his kingdom and as an alternative to the capricious and variable nature of the individual village laws, Henry offered his subjects access to his law, known as the King's law. This law was also based on custom but had the great advantage of universal application. Henry arranged for his knights to visit each village in his kingdom on a regular basis to deal with disputes that had arisen. The villagers had the choice of being dealt with by the feudal lord according to the laws of the village, or they could wait and be dealt with by the King's knight according to the King's law. The King's emissary was usually fairer, as he was able to be more objective and his decisions were more certain and predictable. In due course more and more people chose to have disputes dealt with in this way and gradually the King's law supplanted the village law system completely.

In offering an alternative system of development and administration of law to his subjects, Henry II was also responsible for commencing the first central unified system of law reporting. In travelling from village to village, not only did his knights attempt to administer the law fairly and objectively but, having applied certain principles to a particular set of facts in one village, they would do so in all future situations where the same facts arose. To be able to do that, they kept notes of the cases they had dealt with and referred to them as required. The recording of previous decisions and the facts on which they were based saw the emergence of certain principles concerning personal and property rights, which became established and were known as **common law principles**.

The writing down of facts and decisions of decided cases also saw the development of what became known as the doctrine of precedent. That is, when a similar case came before the King's judges (knights) they would refer to the notes of previously decided cases based on similar facts to use as a precedent in determining the matter before them. Over the centuries this convenient practice became well established and developed into a rule of law known as the doctrine of precedent where a previous judgment of a court is used as an authority for determining a case based on similar facts. By the early twentieth century the doctrine of binding precedent had been established.

As communities developed and society became more complex and sophisticated, the common law principles as well as the doctrine of precedent were expanded and developed by the courts and judges who had long replaced Henry's knights of old.

It is interesting to consider that the present-day court structure, where magistrates or judges preside in our cities and towns in each state and territory to administer the law, owes its origins to the primitive system of the King's knights travelling on horseback from village to village administering the King's law.

Clearly, the centuries that have passed since Henry II's time have seen the continued development by the courts of the common law principles. Such principles are well enunciated and recorded in the present sophisticated system of law reporting, which represents the history of such development through decisions of the courts. The principles enunciated in the recording of cases in the law reports are the authorities relied on by lawyers to support a legal argument based on common law principles. This is sometimes referred to as **case law**.

As the court system applied the common law principles and recorded them, certain power struggles were developing, centred on the perceived divine right of the monarchy and the right of the people to have a say in the affairs of government. This struggle culminated in the establishment of the second major source of our law — parliament.

Parliamentary Law or Legislation

The institution of parliament as we know it today, with the power to make and unmake laws, was the result of many years of turmoil and struggle in English history.

The long-established divine right of the monarchy, with the power to make and unmake laws and to tax the people at will without accountability, was gradually eroded by increasing demands for representation and participation in government. Out of the demands for representation and participation came the early beginnings of a parliament representative of the people. One of the powers that the early parliaments soon took upon themselves and away from the monarchy was the power to make laws. Although parliaments have also changed in complexity and sophistication, their fundamental right to make laws has remained unchallenged. In the last century particularly, parliaments have increased their law-making role significantly, to keep pace with social, industrial and technological changes in the community. Today many of the well-established common law principles have been extended or replaced by parliamentary-made law to take account of such changes.

Laws created by a parliament are embodied in documents known as **Acts** of that parliament and commonly referred to as **legislation**. When a document concerning a particular matter is placed before a parliament with the intention of creating legislation, it is known as a **Bill**. Once it has been passed by both houses of parliament (with the exception of Queensland, which has only a lower house) and subject to any amendments on the way, it then receives the Royal Assent from the King's representative and is formally proclaimed an Act of parliament. The provisions of an Act are known as **legislation** or **statutory law** (or statutory authority).

Acts of parliament often have a separate document known as **Regulations**, which accompany the Act and should be read in conjunction with it. The Regulations generally give precise directions that must be followed to comply with the intent of the Act; for example, the Regulations relating to the New South Wales (NSW) *Poisons and Therapeutic Goods Act 1966* provide considerable detail as to how drugs of addiction are to be stored and the steps that must be observed by registered nurses and midwives in administering such substances. This topic is covered in detail in **Chapter 8**.

Apart from their role in expounding and applying the common law principles, the courts are now increasingly occupied with interpreting the legislation passed by the relevant parliaments.

The Application of English Legal Principles to Australia's Laws and Legal System

The inheritance of the principles and sources of law arising from our colonisation by England laid the groundwork for the development of our legal system.

The English common law principles have been universally adopted throughout the states and territories of the Commonwealth as the basis for future development of the law.

The Impact of the Federation of the Commonwealth of Australia on Australia's Parliamentary Law-making Powers

Prior to Federation, the land mass known as Australia consisted of a number of self-governing and independent colonies of the United Kingdom with no Commonwealth Government as we know it today. However, the creation of the Federation in 1901 with a Commonwealth Parliament together with the existing concurrent parliamentary systems in each state, with their inherent law-making powers, posed significant challenges as to what power to make laws would remain with the state parliaments and what powers would be transferred to the newly created Parliament of the Commonwealth of Australia.

The creation of the Federation pursuant to the *Commonwealth of Australia Constitution Act* (Cth) established a Commonwealth Parliament, and the former self-governing colonies became states of the Commonwealth of Australia. In the same Act, exclusive powers to make laws in relation to certain areas were given to the Commonwealth Parliament. Those areas are set out in section 51 of the Act, and include such common policy matters as customs, currency, overseas trade, defence, invalid and old age pensions as well as divorce and matrimonial causes (amongst others). At the same time, section 51 allowed certain powers to be shared between the Commonwealth and the states and territories. Such powers are known as **concurrent powers**. By implication, matters not mentioned in section 51 or elsewhere in the Constitution comprise the powers that can be exercised exclusively by the state or territory parliaments.

The outcome of such a sharing of powers with the right to make laws in relation to them means that all Australian citizens are subject to the laws of two parliaments — the Commonwealth Parliament and the parliament of the state or territory in which they reside. Understandably it can sometimes be confusing.

The power to make laws in relation to health is a concurrent power shared between the Commonwealth and the states and territories. For example, the Commonwealth is responsible for the legislation underpinning the funding of Medicare and general health insurance. Consequently, the Commonwealth has control over the level and extent of financial rebate that is paid by Medicare for general practice fees and medical specialist consultation fees. It also controls the level of fees able to be charged by health insurance companies, and administers and subsidises the Pharmaceutical Benefits Scheme available to all Australians in relation to the cost of approved and prescribed medications. However, it is the state and territory governments that have control of and responsibility for the delivery of hospital and public health services as well as a broad range of community-based health services. In 2012, the Commonwealth introduced a number of sweeping changes to the funding arrangements for the public hospital system in Australia that saw the Commonwealth have a much more direct say in the delivery of public hospital services.

A further example of where the Commonwealth Parliament has extended its powers in relation to healthcare matters has been in relation to the registration and regulation of health professionals. Prior to 2010, in order to practise, health professionals (including registered and enrolled nurses and midwives) were required to be registered in the state and/or territory in which they wished to practise and registration in one state or territory did not automatically confer a licence to practise in any other state or territory of the Commonwealth. Since 2010, however, Australia has had a national registration and regulation scheme for healthcare professionals, including registered and enrolled nurses and midwives. The system is known as the National Registration and Accreditation Scheme (NRAS). Under the *Health Practitioner Regulation (Consequential Amendments) Act 2010* (Cth), nurses (registered and enrolled) and midwives now need to hold only one licence to practise as a nurse or midwife in any state or territory of the Commonwealth.

The national Nursing and Midwifery Board of Australia (NMBA) is charged with overseeing national registration and regulatory provisions for nurses (registered and enrolled) and midwives. See **Chapter 4** for full details of those provisions and the implications for nurses and midwives in relation to their professional responsibilities.

Apart from Commonwealth legislation regarding the regulation and registration of health professionals, there are also specific provisions of individual state or territory legislation regarding the delivery of health services that can, and do, vary. For example, although generally consistent in their respective approaches, each state and territory has its own version of a *Mental Health Act*. The same applies to the legislation relating to the control and supply of poisons and prohibited substances which governs the administration of dangerous drugs and drugs of addiction in each state and territory.

Nurses and midwives quite often move freely between the states and territories seeking employment or to practise independently. Accordingly, when such a shift is made, it is important that differences in legislative provisions which are relevant to one's professional practice are known and emphasised.

THE DIFFERENCE BETWEEN CRIMINAL LAW AND CIVIL LAW

The law is divided into two distinct areas:

1. criminal law;
2. civil law.

It is essential that such a distinction is grasped from the very beginning, as otherwise it makes it difficult to understand and follow the legal process.

Criminal Law

The best way to think of the criminal law is that it is essentially rules of behaviour (laws), backed by the sanction of punishment, that govern our conduct in the community, particularly in relation to other people and their property. Most of us are aware of the more common rules of behaviour — for example, not taking another person's property without their consent, not assaulting another person, or not exceeding the speed limit when driving a motor vehicle. The parliament's power enables it to set the rules by passing legislation (laws) stating what actions are deemed unlawful and generally determining the punishment (sanction) that will apply if a person is found to have committed the particular unlawful act.

The government monitors our behaviour in the community to ensure we obey the laws or face the sanction of punishment, by way of delegated authority to the police force. Their task, in the first instance, is to adopt a preventive role and, in the second instance, to 'catch' us when we do break the law. Having done that, the police must, via the relevant prosecuting authority, charge the person (the accused) with a breach of the law (a criminal offence) and then the prosecuting authority must prove that the accused committed the offence charged.

The task of having to prove an offence has been committed is known as having the **burden of proof** or **onus of proof**. In satisfying the burden of proof, the prosecution must prove the offence according to the criminal law **standard of proof** — that is, beyond reasonable doubt — by producing evidence from a number of different sources, for example:

■ evidence of identification and relevant events from the victim (if possible);
■ direct evidence of eyewitnesses who saw the offence being committed;
■ medical or scientific evidence by experts;
■ written or verbal admissions made by the accused.

A criminal charge will generally be dealt with before a judge and jury or before a magistrate sitting alone. More serious matters are generally always dealt with by a judge and jury, with the jury having the task of deciding the guilt or innocence of the accused based on the evidence presented. The role of the judge in such trials is to determine points of law and ultimately sentence the accused if he or she is found guilty. In some states, it is possible for the accused to elect to be tried by a judge alone without a jury. In such cases, the judge determines the guilt or innocence of the accused and, if found guilty, proceeds to impose a sentence. In less serious criminal matters a magistrate will hear and determine the matter without a jury and, where found guilty, sentence the accused. The degree of the punishment will depend on the nature and seriousness of the offence and can range from fines, bonds, community-based supervision or intensive correction orders, periodic detention and home detention, to imprisonment.

In addition to the criminal offences that most people think of when they think of the criminal law — that is, murder, assault, robbery, theft, fraud and so on — there are other categories of criminal offences that individuals or companies can commit. For example, companies and/or individuals can be prosecuted for environmental, occupational health and safety, or corporate law offences.

Unless the accused is acquitted of the offence, the outcome of the criminal law process is punishment.

What Constitutes a Crime?

If a person is charged with a criminal offence, the prosecution must prove that two essential elements existed at the time the offence was committed:

1. the activity that constitutes the offence; and
2. the intention to carry out the particular activity or a high degree of reckless indifference as to the probable outcome of a particular activity.

The first element is often referred to as the *actus reus* of the offence. For example, in a charge of theft, the 'activity' of the offence would be the dishonest appropriation of property belonging to another person without that person's consent.

The second element is often referred to as the *mens rea* of the offence — that is, the guilty mind, where there is the intention to carry out the offence, or in some instances a high degree of reckless indifference as to the probable outcome of a particular activity.

As a general rule, if the activity is carried out without intention there can be no crime. So, using the example of the offence of theft again, the 'activity' and 'intent' elements of that offence, when expressed together, would be the taking of property belonging to another without their consent with the intention of permanently depriving them of the property. The presence or otherwise of an intention to harm is particularly relevant in the healthcare environment. That is, a health professional may, by their actions or a failure to act, cause harm to a patient but almost invariably they do not intend to harm the patient.

Nurses and Midwives and the Criminal Law

It is hoped that a detailed knowledge of the criminal law does not arise for consideration in your day-to-day professional practice. However, regrettably, there have been instances where registered nurses have been charged with serious criminal offences relating to their professional activities.[9]

Remember, for the actions of a nurse or midwife to constitute a criminal offence it is necessary for the prosecution to prove not only that the nurse or midwife did the act that constitutes the crime but also that he or she intended to do the act. Most actions of a nurse or midwife that do cause harm to a patient are never intended to do so. They are almost invariably a negligent act without any intent to harm. However, the negligent act may create a **civil** liability on the part of the nurse or midwife or his or her employer.

Criminal Negligence and the Significance of Intent

On occasions, incidents may occur in hospitals or healthcare centres that, at first glance, suggest a criminal offence has been committed. For example, if a patient died as a result of the administration of a wrong drug, it might be thought that whoever administered the drug was guilty of murder or manslaughter. However, as far as the criminal law is concerned, the most significant factor to be established would be the presence or otherwise of any intent to cause harm or a high degree of recklessness or inadvertence such as to amount to criminal negligence. If the wrong drug were administered intentionally, with the deliberate intent to kill the patient, this would clearly amount to murder. If the drug were given in the belief that it was the right drug but with an attitude or degree of recklessness as to the amount to be given or the contraindications to be observed in the administration of the drug and the patient died as a result, this may amount to the offence of manslaughter on the basis of criminal negligence.

In most situations in hospitals where mistakes are made, a degree of carelessness or error of judgment is usually present such as to amount to civil negligence. For a nurse or midwife to be found guilty of criminal negligence as a result of their activities at work, there has to be a much higher degree of negligence, which would demonstrate an attitude of recklessness or inadvertence to the possibility of harm occurring.

It follows that it is important to distinguish between civil negligence and criminal negligence. One of the earliest cases that clearly made that distinction concerned the actions of a doctor in attending a woman during delivery. **Case example 1.1** sets out the relevant facts; then consider **Clinical study 1.1**, which follows.

R v Bateman[10]

Dr Bateman attended a woman at home during labour. The labour was prolonged, and the child's presentation was unusual and difficult. The doctor attempted to turn the child by the procedure known as 'version'. In doing so, he used considerable force over a period of an hour and delivered the child, which was dead. In delivering the placenta he also removed, by mistake, a portion of the patient's uterus. After the delivery the doctor left the patient at home. Five days later the patient was so ill that the doctor then transferred her to hospital where she died 2 days later. The post-mortem examination revealed the following:

> …the bladder was found to be ruptured, the colon was crushed against the sacral promontory, there was a rupture of the rectum and the uterus was almost entirely gone.[11]

Comment and Relevant Considerations Relating to R v Bateman and Later Judicial Decisions

Dr Bateman was charged with manslaughter on the grounds of criminal negligence in that he had:

- caused the internal ruptures in performing the operation of version;
- removed part of the uterus along with the placenta;
- delayed sending the patient to hospital.

Dr Bateman was initially found guilty of the charge, but successfully appealed that decision. His conviction was quashed. In handing down their decision the appeal court judges said:

> To support an indictment for manslaughter the prosecution … must satisfy the jury that the negligence or incompetence of the accused went beyond a mere matter of compensation and showed such disregard for the life and safety of others as to amount to a crime against the State and conduct deserving of punishment … there is a difference in kind between negligence which gives a right

to compensation and the negligence which is a crime.[12] *[emphasis added]*

While the appeal court judges may have considered Dr Bateman had been less than professionally competent in carrying out the surgery, they did not accept that his actions amounted to a 'disregard for the life and safety' of his patient such as to amount to criminal negligence.

Although Dr Bateman's case was some considerable time ago, the test to be applied when considering manslaughter by criminal negligence has remained fundamentally unchanged. In 1992, the High Court of Australia approved the following formulation of the elements of manslaughter by criminal negligence in the following terms:

> In order to establish manslaughter by criminal negligence, it is sufficient if the prosecution shows that the act which caused the death was done by the accused consciously and voluntarily, without any intention of causing death or grievous bodily harm but in circumstances which involved such a great falling short of the standard of care which a reasonable man would have exercised and which involved such a high risk that death or grievous bodily harm would follow (and) that the doing of the act merited criminal punishment.[13]

Where, as in the case of Dr Bateman, a specific duty of care is owed to the victim, the elements of the offence that must be established beyond reasonable doubt were expressed in 2019 in the South Australian Supreme Court decision[14] involving a midwife charged with two counts of manslaughter by criminal negligence as follows:

- The accused owed the victim a duty of care.
- The objective standard of conduct required of her was that of a reasonably competent midwife.
- The accused's act and omissions caused the death of the victim (in the sense of being a substantial cause of death).
- The accused's acts and omissions were deliberate.
- The accused's acts and omissions fell so far short of the applicable standard as to amount to gross or criminal negligence and thereby to warrant criminal punishment.

In the above case, after considering all the evidence and the legal elements required to be established, the court determined the midwife not guilty on both charges. The matter involved two homebirth deliveries, one in 2011 and another in 2012 involving two different women. The evidence was that in both situations and given the risk factors present, both women should have delivered in hospital. In the first homebirth the cause of death was determined to be hypoxia due to placental abruption. In the second homebirth in 2012 the cause of death was determined to be total occlusion of the umbilical cord. In both cases, the judge determined that while 'the accused's conduct did not reach the standards of a reasonable competent midwife, I am not satisfied that … the accused was criminally negligent' and further that her actions did not 'answer the quite demanding requirements of the concept of criminal negligence'.

Having regard to the above elements that must be established to satisfy a charge of criminal negligence, consider the hypothetical example set out in **Clinical study 1.1**.

CLINICAL STUDY 1.1

A patient, Mr Smith, was ordered to have a number of units of blood following major surgery. The appropriate cross-matching had been done and the cross-match slip was received in the ward. When one of Mr Smith's units was complete, Ms Jones, a registered nurse, went out to the refrigerator where cross-matched blood for all of the patients in the hospital was kept. Ms Jones picked up the first bag of blood she saw and did not bother to check it against any slip or with any other person. She came back to the ward and then proceeded to administer it to Mr Smith. The blood was incompatible; Mr Smith had an extremely adverse reaction to the incompatible blood; he nearly died and was extremely ill for many months. When questioned about her actions, Ms Jones admitted that she was aware of the dangers of incompatible blood transfusions and the need for checking but thought that on this one occasion it would be 'all right', and that nothing would happen. She also said she was sorry about what had happened and had not really meant to hurt Mr Smith.

Comment and Relevant Considerations Relating to Clinical Study 1.1

Ask yourself these questions:

- Did Nurse Jones owe Mr Smith a duty of care?
- What was the standard of care expected of Nurse Jones in administering the blood transfusion?
- Did Nurse Jones's acts and omissions cause the injury and damage to Mr Jones?
- Were Nurse Jones's act and omissions deliberate?
- Did Nurse Jones's acts and omissions fall so far short of the applicable standard as to amount to gross or criminal negligence and thereby warrant criminal punishment?
- If so, in what way?
- What should Nurse Jones have done?

On the facts provided, it is highly likely the prosecuting authorities would consider Nurse Jones's actions did warrant charging her with criminal negligence. Obviously the example is extreme, but it illustrates the degree of negligence that must be present to constitute the requisite intent in a charge of criminal negligence occasioning grievous bodily harm. If Mr Smith had died as a result of the incorrect blood transfusion, again on the basis of the facts given, Nurse Jones would probably face a charge of manslaughter by criminal negligence.

In considering what Nurse Jones should have done, it would be said that, as a registered nurse, Nurse Jones owed Mr Smith a duty of care. Further, Nurse Jones was well aware of the significant dangers of administering incompatible blood to a patient. As well, there would be a clear policy and checking procedure required to be followed when administering a blood transfusion to a patient. Knowing that, the actions of Nurse Jones would, we submit, be considered as showing a reckless disregard for, or indifference towards, the safety of Mr Smith.

As a general rule (thankfully) the type of professional activity that would constitute criminal behaviour falls outside the scope of practice of most nurses and midwives. However, it is the element of either direct intent or 'reckless indifference' to the possible outcomes of one's actions that can render a harmful act a crime, and it is important to bear this in mind in going about your day-to-day work as a nurse or midwife.

How does the above process differ from the civil law?

Civil Law

The first thing to remember about civil law is that, generally speaking, it has nothing whatsoever to do with the police force and punishment. The best way to think of civil law is that it exists to enable us, individually and collectively, to resolve the disputes and differences of a personal and property nature that arise between us as members of the community and which we are unable or unwilling to resolve ourselves. Usually in resolving such disputes, monetary compensation (damages) will be sought by the person or party alleging personal and/or property loss and damage. There are many divisions of the civil law — for example, family, industrial, land and environment, and workers compensation, to name just a few. There is also what is known in civil law as a common law division and into that division are allocated those matters whose origins are the well-established common law principles, such as contract law, negligence, defamation or nuisance.

The person who initiates an action in civil law is known as the **plaintiff** and the person against whom the action is taken is known as the **defendant**. There are exceptions to this; for example, in family law the person seeking a divorce is the **applicant** and the spouse from whom the divorce is sought is the **respondent**.

Similar to the requirement in criminal law, the person who brings an action in one of the areas of civil law (the plaintiff) bears the burden of proving the matter in dispute. The significant difference here is that, although the plaintiff has that onus, the standard of proof in civil matters is not the same as in criminal matters. In a civil action the plaintiff has to prove his or her case only on the balance of probabilities. What this means is that the evidence would disclose that, on balance, the allegation made by the plaintiff, when considered against the evidence produced, and in light of the law as currently applying, is the most probable cause of the matter in dispute. Proving an allegation on the balance of probabilities is a much lower standard of proof than that required in criminal law.

When the plaintiff succeeds in proving the matter in dispute, the final and most important issue to be determined by the court will be the amount of monetary compensation (damages) to be awarded to the plaintiff. In most circumstances, the outcome of the civil law process is compensation. There are some exceptions to this and civil law does provide for other remedies that may compensate the plaintiff. For example, the court could order that the defendant do a certain thing (specific performance) or refrain from doing a certain thing (an injunction). In family law the court may make a decision about access to or custody of children or the division of the assets of the marriage. However, as a general rule, the awarding of a sum of money to the plaintiff is seen as the most appropriate way of resolving the dispute between the parties.

In the awarding of damages by a court, the court itself does not actually give the money awarded to the plaintiff. The court hands down a judgment identifying the amount of compensation it determines the plaintiff is entitled to. The plaintiff must then recover that money from the defendant. In most civil litigation that means recovering the money from the defendant's insurance company. However, if there is no relevant insurance company standing behind the defendant and the defendant is impecunious, then the plaintiff may well be left without compensation. It is a salutary reminder of one of the pitfalls of civil litigation.

Civil and Criminal Consequences Arising from One Action

Having taken pains to distinguish between the civil and criminal law processes, we must now muddy the waters somewhat and point out that one incident can lead to both civil and criminal law proceedings. For example, while driving your motor vehicle one day you wrongfully fail to give way to traffic on your right at an intersection and, as a result, an accident occurs and a number of people in the other vehicle are badly injured. The police will be called, and you, as the driver of the vehicle that caused the accident, will be charged with a number of offences such as negligent driving and failing to give way. Your action and the charge that follows is deemed to be a criminal act pursuant to the legislation covering motor traffic offences in your state or territory, and in due course you will be dealt with before the appropriate court. Assuming your guilt, you will then be punished — you will probably be fined, your licence may be taken away or an even more severe penalty may be imposed, depending on the culpability of your action.

However, the people that you have left badly damaged at the scene of the accident may be more concerned with seeking some money from you to compensate them for the pain, injury, loss and suffering you have caused them as a result of your negligent act — that is, your **civil wrong**. Those people will commence an action against you and allege that, on the basis of certain facts, you drove your car negligently, as a result of which they suffered certain damage. They will have to prove, on the balance of probabilities, the facts and damage they are alleging. Assuming they are successful, they will be awarded damages as compensation for their injuries and the subsequent losses that flow from those injuries.

It will be seen from the above example that the major distinction to be drawn between the civil and criminal act *resides not in the nature of the wrongful act but in the legal consequences that may follow it*.[15] That is, if the wrongful act is capable of being followed by what are called **criminal proceedings**, that means that it is regarded as a **crime** (otherwise called an offence). If it is capable of being followed by **civil proceedings**, it is regarded as a civil wrong. If it is capable of being followed by both, it is both a crime and a civil wrong.[16]

Civil and criminal proceedings are (usually) easily distinguishable; the procedure is different, the outcome is different and the terminology is different.

ADMINISTRATIVE STRUCTURE OF AUSTRALIA'S LEGAL AND COURT SYSTEM

The administrative structure of Australia's legal and court system encompasses the Commonwealth and the states and territories. In its day-to-day operation the administration of the law is also divided along criminal and civil lines. In addition, there is a hierarchical structure that determines:

- what matters can be dealt with by particular courts;
- the powers that are vested in the different courts to deal with matters that come before them;
- if a right of appeal exists from a particular court, how and in what circumstances it is to operate.

All the states and territories have a similar basic hierarchical structure of the administration of the law. The titles of the courts may vary from state to state or territory, but not to any significant degree. The following summary of the roles of the various courts should be read in conjunction with **Figure 1.1**, which illustrates the basic hierarchical structure of courts in Australia.

State and Territory Courts
Local or Magistrates' Courts

The *Local Courts Act 1982* (NSW) formally changed the title of magistrates' courts from Courts of Petty Sessions to the Local Courts of New South Wales. The Northern Territory did likewise in 2016. In the other states and territories, such courts continue to be known as Magistrates' Courts.

These courts are at the bottom of the legal hierarchy, but undoubtedly deal with the greatest number of matters. They are presided over by magistrates, who are legally trained and qualified. Even tiny country towns have sittings of the Local or Magistrates' Court and, in big cities, Local or Magistrates' Courts are located in many suburbs.

In carrying out their task, magistrates sit without a jury and can deal with criminal and civil matters, including some family law matters. However, magistrates can deal only with those matters they have the power (jurisdiction) to deal with. In general terms, magistrates can deal with civil matters where the amount claimed in damages does not exceed the amount determined by the relevant legislation. In most states that amount is generally $100 000, up to $150 000, with some provision for extending that for money claims excluding personal injury cases, except in Tasmania where it is expressed to be 'more than $50 000 if all parties agree'.[17] In the Northern Territory and the Australian Capital Territory, the jurisdictional limit is $250 000.

In criminal matters, magistrates deal with a wide range of criminal offences as well as applications for apprehended violence orders and alleged breaches of such orders. Not surprisingly, such offences constitute the bulk of crimes committed in the community. Magistrates have the power to impose a custodial sentence limited generally to between two and five years, and are also able to impose a range of other sentencing orders such as fines and community service orders.

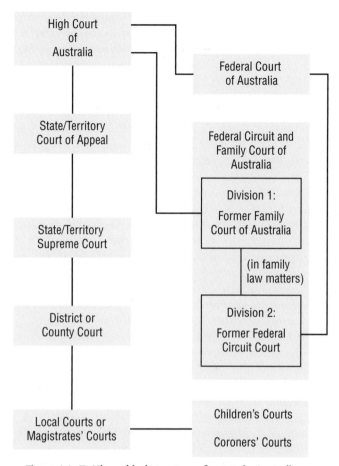

Figure 1.1 ▪ **Hierarchical structure of courts in Australia.**

One extension of a magistrate's role in criminal matters is that, in relation to serious criminal offences which they do not have the power to deal with to finality, they do have the job of deciding whether there is sufficient evidence to establish a *prima facie* case against the accused — that is, based on first impressions and from a consideration of the evidence, whether there is sufficient evidence to show that a jury is likely to find the accused guilty. If they so decide, the accused is then sent for trial before a higher court. Such proceedings are known as **committal proceedings**. In some states now, the initial committal process has been significantly truncated: instead of having an extensive preliminary hearing at the committal stage, the prosecution simply tenders the statements from those persons they wish to call at trial. Witnesses may or may not be called at that stage. Whatever procedure is observed from state to state and territory, the magistrate is still required to formally commit the accused to stand trial.

Magistrates also deal with the bulk of bail applications. Granting bail to a person arises when the person is charged with a criminal offence and is remanded in custody before they come before a court in the first instance. Very often, when they do appear before the court, an application is made that the person be granted bail — that is, released into the community subject to certain conditions while waiting for their matter to be heard by the court.

In some states, Magistrates may also preside over a range of other courts — for example, Coroners' Courts and Children's Courts. Of all of those subsidiary courts, the Coroner's Court is most relevant to nurses and midwives. **Chapter 11** outlines the role of the Coroner's Court in more detail.

District or County Courts

The next tier in the hierarchy of the court and judicial system is the District or County Court, depending on the state or territory. In New South Wales, Queensland, South Australia and Western Australia it is known as the District Court, whereas in Victoria it is called the County Court.

Because of their relatively small size or population, the Australian Capital Territory, the Northern Territory and Tasmania do not have an equivalent intermediate court, and rely on the Magistrates' Court and Supreme Court to cover their criminal and civil jurisdictions.

Sittings of the District or County Court are presided over by a judge appointed from the legal profession. The judge sits with a jury in criminal matters, but generally sits alone in civil matters. The role of the jury in criminal matters is to decide on the guilt or innocence of the accused. The role of the judge in criminal matters is to decide questions of law, direct the jury on relevant points of law that arise, and punish the accused when, and if, he or she is found guilty of the offence. Juries are not routinely used in all civil matters. When they are, their role is to decide the issue in dispute and, if decided in favour of the plaintiff, to generally determine the amount of compensation to be awarded.

The role of the District or County Court judge is divided into civil and criminal sections and, like the Local and Magistrates' Courts, there is a limit placed on the jurisdiction of these courts to deal with such matters. There are variations between the states; in New South Wales, for example, the jurisdiction of the District Court to deal with civil matters is limited to those matters where the amount claimed in damages does not exceed $750 000 and is unlimited in relation to motor vehicle injury claims.

In criminal matters the District or County Court deals with all major criminal offences except murder, piracy and treason. In other states and territories the civil and criminal jurisdiction of this court does vary. The power of this court to punish extends to the penalties provided for the offences it has to deal with. Judges of this court sit daily in the capital cities and large country towns and travel on circuit to smaller country towns for a week or two at regular intervals.

Judges of this court can also hear appeals from a decision of a magistrate and, where provided for, in certain other matters.

Supreme Courts

All states and territories have a Supreme Court. It is the highest or most senior court in the judicial system within state and territory boundaries. Sittings of this court are presided over by judges appointed from the legal profession and, in carrying out their task, they sit with a jury in the same circumstances as judges in the District or County Court. The role of this court is divided into civil and criminal sections. This court has unlimited financial jurisdiction in civil matters and its criminal role is generally confined, as a matter of practice, to dealing with the capital offences of murder and serious sexual offences.

Like the District or County Court judges, judges of the Supreme Court sit daily in the capital cities. There are regular sittings of the court in major country towns, which are presided over by the judges travelling on circuit in the same way as the District or County Court judges do.

One of the additional tasks of the Supreme Court is to hear appeals from the lower courts and from decisions of a single judge of the Supreme Court. To do this, a Court of Appeal has been established within the Supreme Court and is presided over by at least three judges of appeal. Once again the appellate role of the Supreme Court is divided into civil and criminal sections.

Commonwealth Courts

Federal Circuit and Family Court of Australia

The Federal Circuit Court was created in 2013 replacing the old Federal Magistrates Court. In September 2021, the Federal Circuit Court was merged administratively with the Family Court of Australia and the new structure is now known as the Federal Circuit and Family Court of Australia (FCFCA). The intention was to create a consistent framework and case management approach in relation to family law matters.

The new court entity (FCFCA) has two Divisions. Essentially Division 1 replicates the existing Family

Court of Australia and Division 2 replicates the existing Federal Circuit Court. All family law cases now start in Division 2 of the new court structure and will be dealt with by that Division unless they are transferred to Division 1 of the new court structure. Judges of Division 1 will hear appeals from decisions of judges in Division 2.

In addition to being the starting point for all family law matters, judges in Division 2 of the new FCFCA will, as allocated, also continue to share concurrent jurisdiction with the Federal Court of Australia on the following matters:

- administrative law;
- bankruptcy;
- unlawful discrimination;
- consumer protection and trade practices;
- privacy law;
- migration;
- copyright;
- industrial law;
- admiralty law.

Judges of Division 2 of the new FCFCA do not deal with criminal matters.

Appeals from decisions of judges of Division 2 of the FCFCA can be made as of right either to a judge of Division 1 of the FCFCA or to the Full Court of the Federal Court of Australia depending on the jurisdiction exercised by a judge of Division 2 of the FCFCA.

Federal Court

The Federal Court was created by the Commonwealth Parliament in 1976 by the enactment of the *Federal Court of Australia Act 1976*. The main reason for its creation was to relieve the High Court of its workload that arises from some of the exclusive constitutional powers of the Commonwealth — for example, trade practices, bankruptcy, immigration and federal industrial issues. Within the Federal Court structure, there is provision for an appeal court of three judges known as the Full Court of the Federal Court. That court hears and determines appeals from decisions of single judges of the Federal court and, where appropriate, from judges of Division 2 of the FCFCA. There is also an appeal right with leave from the Federal Court to the High Court.

High Court

The High Court was created by the *Commonwealth of Australia Constitution Act*, which has been previously referred to. The initial intent in creating the High Court was that it would deal with constitutional disputes that arose between the Commonwealth and the states and territories.

In addition to dealing with constitutional matters, the role of the High Court as a senior and final court of appeal from the Supreme Courts, as well as the Federal and Family Courts of Australia, has increased considerably to embrace civil and criminal matters. An appeal in such circumstances is not automatic, as the High Court must grant leave to appeal and will do so only if the matter to be appealed constitutes a point of law of general public importance.

For many years there was a right to seek leave to appeal from a decision of the High Court to the Privy Council in the United Kingdom, but this was abolished in 1975.

The High Court is the final Court of Appeal in Australia on all matters.

Other Court Systems and Tribunals Including Professional Disciplinary Tribunals for Nurses and Midwives

Coexisting with Australia's courts, and feeding into them at various points, generally for appeal purposes, is a wide range of courts and tribunals dealing with specific matters — for example, industrial courts, workers compensation courts, land and environment courts, anti-discrimination and administrative appeals tribunals as well as professional disciplinary tribunals. **Chapter 4** outlines in more detail the role of the nurses' and midwives' professional disciplinary procedures and administrative tribunals that deal with such matters.

The Appeal Process

Provision is made within the court structure for an appeals process. Generally speaking, there is nothing to prevent a person or party who so wishes from appealing against a decision of a magistrate to a higher court. Such an appeal may be based on a number of points — for example, that the magistrate erred on a point of law or that the punishment imposed was too severe or too lenient. Likewise, the decision of a District or County Court judge or a single Supreme Court judge may also be appealed against to the appeal court of the Supreme Court of the state on similar grounds. From there, an appeal may be made to the High Court, subject of course to leave being granted.

CONCLUSION

Understanding Australia's legal system and court structure is an important first step that should assist nurses and midwives to readily and correctly incorporate their professional and legal responsibilities into the appropriate legal context.

CHAPTER 1 REVIEW QUESTIONS

Following your reading of **Chapter 1**, consider these questions in reaching the objectives of this chapter. Guidance on which part of the chapter will assist you in answering the questions can be found at http://evolve.elsevier.com/AU/Staunton/law/. You may, of course, consider other sources as part of your considerations.

1. What are the two major sources of law in Australia's legal system and from what events did they develop?

2. Both the Commonwealth and the state and territory parliaments have the power to make laws in relation to the delivery of health services including the registration and regulation of health professionals. Name two areas of healthcare where laws have been made by the Commonwealth Parliament and two that have been made by a state or territory parliament in which you currently practise as a nurse or midwife.

3. Is it possible to have a civil law action and a criminal law action arising out of one action? If so, give an example where such a situation may arise.

4. If a nurse or midwife were negligent in the course of their professional practice and a patient suffered harm as a result, what circumstances and legal principles would need to be considered to warrant the nurse or midwife being charged with criminal negligence as distinct from civil negligence?

ENDNOTES

1. A new Code of conduct for registered nurses and a Code of conduct for midwives were issued by the Nursing and Midwifery Board of Australia, effective from 1 March 2018.
2. In March 2018 the Nursing and Midwifery Board of Australia, the Australian College of Midwives, the Australian College of Nursing and the Australian Nursing and Midwifery Federation jointly adopted the International Council of Nurses (ICN) and the International Council of Midwives (ICM) Code of ethics.
3. The Nursing and Midwifery Board of Australia: Registered nurse standards for practice: June 2016. See Chapter 4 for more information.
4. Ibid, Standard 1.
5. The Nursing and Midwifery Board of Australia: *Enrolled nurse standards for practice*: June 2016.
6. The Nursing and Midwifery Board of Australia: *Midwife standards for practice*: October 2018.

7. It is worthwhile reflecting on recent developments in Australia where parliaments have passed laws in relation to each of these areas, all of which were subject to diverse community views. For example:
    (i) in December 2017, the Commonwealth Parliament approved an amendment to the *Marriage Act* permitting same-sex marriage in Australia;
    (ii) in October 2018, the Queensland Parliament decriminalised and approved the availability of abortion on request in the first 22 weeks of pregnancy: Qld *Termination of Pregnancy Act 2018*;
    (iii) in November 2017, the Victorian Parliament approved the *Voluntary Assisted Dying Act* permitting a person to voluntarily request medical assistance to end their life in circumstances where the person had a terminal illness together with a life expectancy of less than 12 months;
    (iv) in 2019, the NSW Parliament decriminalised abortion by removing it as an offence under the current NSW *Crimes Act*.

8. Scotland has developed a slightly different legal system from England, Wales and Northern Ireland, based on a combination of common law and Roman law principles.

9. For example:
   (i) in May 2013 a registered nurse, Roger Deans, pleaded guilty to 11 counts of murder and eight counts of causing grievous bodily harm arising from his actions in starting a fire in a nursing home in NSW. He started the fire to cover up his theft of prescription drugs particularly drugs of addiction. He was sentenced to 11 life sentences;
   (ii) in 2016 a registered nurse, Megan Hains, was sentenced to 36 years imprisonment with a non-parole period of 27 years for the murder of two elderly patients in a nursing home in NSW. It is alleged she injected them with insulin. She has appealed her conviction and sentence;
   (iii) in March 2019 a midwife, Lisa Jane Barrett, went on trial for manslaughter over the deaths of two babies in South Australia delivered in October 2011 and December 2012. On 4 June 2019, following a trial in the Supreme Court of South Australia, she was found not guilty on two counts of manslaughter. See *R v Barrett* (No 3) [2019] SASC 93.

10. R v Bateman (1925) All ER 45.

11. Ibid, at 47.11.

12. Ibid, at 49, 51.

13. Wilson v The Queen (1992) 174 CLR 313 at 333 approving the formulation as established in Nydam v The Queen (1977) VR 430 at 445.

14. R v Barrett (No 3) [2019] SASC 93, Vanstone J, at 110.

15. Williams G, Learning the law, 10th ed, Stevens, London, 1979, p 2.

16. Ibid, p 62.

17. Section 11 *Magistrates Court (Civil Division) Act 1992* (Tas).

2

THE RELATIONSHIP BETWEEN LAW AND ETHICS

LEARNING OBJECTIVES

In this chapter, you will:

- consider differences and similarities between law and ethics
- examine well-known ethical theories and principles
- identify and explore a practical model for ethical decision-making
- apply ethical theories and principles and an ethical decision-making model to an ethical dilemma.

INTRODUCTION

This chapter provides a basic overview of the relationship between law and ethics and an example of how the two both interlink and diverge. It explains ethical theories and principles, offers a practical model for ethical decision-making and, perhaps most importantly for the reader, provides excellent references in the endnotes for those who wish to explore ethical decision-making in greater depth. In keeping with the objectives of this book, the chapter has a practical, rather than theoretical, focus.

THE APPLICATION OF LAW AND ETHICS TO PRACTICE

To use a personal example to explain the relationship between law and ethics, if you were told you needed to have an operation, there would be a number of concerns you would wish to have addressed:

- You would want to be informed adequately about the nature and consequences of the surgery so that you would be able to make a wise choice.
- You would want to know that the surgeon and anaesthetist are competent, that the nursing staff are competent and will care for you in a compassionate manner, and that the private information you choose to share with the nursing and medical staff will be treated confidentially and not discussed inappropriately.

For each of these concerns to be addressed properly, the nursing and medical staff who care for you will be required to behave in a professional manner. In the majority of cases, this is indeed how nursing and medical staff do behave.

All of the above professional behaviours are ethical behaviours — they comply with established ethical principles and theories. Nurses, midwives and doctors normally behave in these ways because they are professional and they wish to give the best possible care to their patients. However, in Australia all of the above behaviours are also legal requirements. This is because these behaviours are so fundamental to people's expectations of health professionals that they have been either incorporated into the common law or enshrined in legislation. **Chapter 1** discussed this need to provide for orderly and good conduct through the development of legal systems.

From a legal perspective, if these expectations are breached, there will be some form of redress, sanction or adverse consequence, in some instances for the health professional concerned.

However, sometimes the relationship between legal and ethical requirements is not as clear as in the above example. Not all laws are necessarily ethical — for historical examples, consider the laws governing slavery in America, the laws allowing persecution of the Jews in Nazi Germany, or the apartheid laws in South Africa. Throughout history many people, believing strongly that certain laws were unethical, did not comply with them and as a consequence put themselves at considerable personal risk. These are obviously extreme examples, but there are other scenarios where two or more possible courses of action are available, each of which may be perfectly legal, but over which there may be disagreement as to the best, or most ethical, course of action. Such situations may offer a range of alternative solutions, none of which will offer an ideal outcome. Consequently, these will create ethical quandaries or dilemmas, often described as 'moral distress' for the people involved. A moral or ethical dilemma is inevitably a choice between two or more unacceptable alternatives. Villa and colleagues describe this as a common phenomenon for health professionals.

The concept of moral distress … [describes] the psychological distress of being in a situation in which a healthcare professional is constrained from acting on what he/she knows to be right. Conflicting emotions are common in those professions based on the permanent contact with people, as many types of environmental constraints (from prudential reasons to physical barriers) can prevent the operators from acting and reacting as they would.[1]

However, there is more to making ethical decisions than simply adopting a stance on what someone 'knows to be right', for example, according to strong religious or moral beliefs. Ethical decision-making is a complex and rigorous process, whereas our morality is what propels us to adopt a particular stance based on a particular set of beliefs, many of which have been inculcated into us since childhood. Johnstone, who argues that linguistically there is no significant difference between ethics and morality, provides an example of a scenario where holding a moral viewpoint is different from justifying it ethically:

For example, a nurse may make an 'ordinary' moral judgment that abortion is wrong and conscientiously object to assisting with an abortion procedure. Whether her conscientious objection ought to be respected, however, requires a critical examination of the bases on which the nurse has made that judgment and a consideration of the justifications (moral reasons) she has put forward to support the position she has taken.[2]

Ethics requires a consideration not only of morality but also of many other factors, as will be discussed further later in this chapter.

Because of the human and complex nature of healthcare, ethical dilemmas are not uncommon in clinical practice and have received much attention in both academic and media circles over the past three decades. The study of ethical dilemmas in healthcare is often called *bioethics*. There are many comprehensive texts available on the subject, a number of which are used as references in this chapter.

Some of these ethical dilemmas have been major issues for society as a whole to ponder, such as resource allocation, euthanasia and gene technology; but other, more individual clinical dilemmas, such as telling patients the truth, challenging doctors about choices of treatment and prioritisation of care, have also been reported by nurses and midwives as causing considerable angst.[3] This has been particularly distressing during the recent COVID-19 pandemic, where health professionals have been forced to address old and new ethical dilemmas as this unprecedented global situation unfolded.[4]

Making decisions about any ethical dilemma is complex. Usually there are no simple answers; otherwise there would be no dilemma. However, it is possible to become skilled at ethical decision-making by developing and refining those decision-making processes and by being aware of the motives and values with which they are undertaken. Justice Michael Kirby made the observation that 'good law and good ethics must be grounded in good data'.[5]

In analysing ethical dilemmas, the legal parameters of the situation are inevitably important aspects, but are unlikely to be the only considerations. While it is far beyond the scope of this chapter to provide a sound grounding in ethical decision-making or reasoning, it does set out some basic ideas about ethics and provide a range of sources, some practical, some more theoretical, to enable you to research the issues in more depth. To begin, the next section attempts to define ethics and differentiate it from other concepts with which it is commonly confused.

ETHICS: WHAT IT IS

Johnstone defines ethics as 'a generic term that is used for various ways of thinking about, understanding and examining how best to live a "moral life"'.[6] Words like 'should' and 'ought' are often used in ethical discussion, but, although they are helpful as a starting point, they are sometimes limiting, as such terms can also be applied to school rules and table manners. Johnstone goes on to provide a helpful amplification to this introduction by introducing bioethics and nursing ethics and differentiating between the two.[7] Allan explains that:

> The study of ethics has hence developed such that it is not only a question of what should be done but it also requires individuals to critically examine the reasons and justifications for why they consider a particular act to be right or wrong or the reason for holding particular values.[8]

It is this systematic approach to addressing problems that is probably the most important aspect of ethics for nurses and midwives who are commencing on a path of ethical inquiry and study. It is for this reason that the need to understand ethics is as important as the need to understand clinical practice. Maeckelberghe and Schröder-Bäck make the point that:

> Ethical reflection is not done in splendid isolation but thrives on the collaboration between the parties involved, in this case … researchers, professionals, and practitioners alongside ethicists.[9]

Perhaps it would be fair to say that ethical decision-making is as much about asking questions as it is about finding answers. Clearly, the process of making careful ethical decisions takes time, yet often nurses and midwives are confronted with ethical dilemmas in the course of their working day and may have little opportunity to consider their immediate response. That is why the academic study of ethics is so helpful to nurses and midwives, as it enables them to explore in advance key issues that might arise regularly and to develop at least some rudimentary decision-making skills. However, junior clinicians are always advised to discuss ethical dilemmas with more senior, experienced colleagues or other clinicians who may have more expertise in this area.

Singer, in his seminal text *Practical ethics*, makes the point that ethics is fundamentally a practical concern.[10] It is concerned with making decisions and taking (or not taking) actions. Allan suggests that the point of bioethics is to 'intentionally and critically evaluate the basis for such [moral] judgements in order to find reasons that support one decision over another, and that may be applied in future sitations'.[11] Both undergraduate and some specialist postgraduate programs now contain the study of ethics within their curricula, which provide nurses and midwives with opportunities to hone and practise these skills away from the immediacy of the clinical environment.

ETHICS: WHAT IT IS NOT

Charlesworth points out a major problem — that ethical discussions often take place:

> … between people with widely differing interpretations of what the terms of the discussion mean, how the facts may be interpreted or described, and also with differing ethical stances.[12]

For this reason, it is helpful to differentiate ethics from other issues with which it is often confused. This enables nurses and midwives to look at what other value systems and ideas they might bring to any ethical decision-making process and to be explicit about identifying them. In differentiating ethics, it also needs to be recognised that all of these factors are likely to be involved in and inform ethical decision-making. Although the famous bioethicist Peter Singer[13] was probably one of the first to embrace this differentiation approach, a number of other authors on health law and ethics have adopted it in recent times. These other issues are listed below and then a case study is given that explores each issue.

- Ethics is not law.
- Ethics is not a professional code of ethics or a code of conduct.
- Ethics is not hospital or professional etiquette.
- Ethics is not hospital or institutional policy.
- Ethics is not ideology (including religion or morality).

- Ethics is not public opinion, populism or the view of the majority.
- Ethics is not following the orders of a supervisor or manager.[14]

In addition to Johnstone's list above, it should be added that ethics is not gut feeling or intuition (although this can feel compelling) and is not simply a collection of empirical data (although facts are clearly of great value).

An example of an ethical problem is explored in **Case study 2.1**. Although this example is a nursing example, the questions it raises and the way that it is worked through are of equal value to students and practitioners of midwifery and could equally be applied to an ethical dilemma experienced by a midwife.

How Might a Nurse Respond to an Ethical Problem?

Case study 2.1 outlines a difficult situation, which requires skilful and careful ethical decision-making. It may well be that you have already had an immediate reaction to this scenario — a *gut feeling* as to what *ought* to be done. You may have strong *religious* or *moral* convictions and believe that, as you consider truth-telling to be a critical moral issue, your only option would be to answer Mr X truthfully that he is dying. You may already have found yourself taking sides in this situation, believing that the *view of the majority* taken by the surgeon and the sons was 'wrong'. Conversely, you may feel that the surgeon is in charge;

he has made the decision and *professional etiquette* demands that you do not challenge him.

The *law* here is clear. Mr X has a legal right to be informed of all material risks relating to his treatment options (see *Rogers v Whitaker*, which is discussed in detail in **Chapter 7**).[15] Such a right would require him to be aware of his diagnosis in order to evaluate the treatment options before him. The *hospital policy*, particularly in relation to consent for surgical treatment, would mirror the law and would undoubtedly state that Mr X must be informed of his diagnosis and treatment options. Your immediate response might be to comply with the law and hospital policy, in disregard of the family's wishes, and advise Mr X of his diagnosis. Only 'therapeutic privilege' would permit the surgeon not to inform Mr X fully about his surgery, and this limited defence can be exercised if either the patient expressly states that he or she does not wish to know (in which case it would be the patient's choice), or if the surgeon believed the information would be likely to cause serious physical or psychological harm to the patient. Therapeutic privilege is discussed in **Chapter 6**. The surgeon has conceded 'reluctantly' to the family's request and even he might consider the scenario does stretch the ambit of therapeutic privilege. However, a decision not to advise the patient may cause significant ethical distress for you, even if you decide to *follow the orders of your manager* and not provide information to the patient. Thus it can be seen that in some clinical situations, decisions may be made for a range of reasons, not all of which may conform to

---

CASE STUDY 2.1

AN ETHICAL DILEMMA

Mr X, an 89-year-old man, has been admitted in extreme pain with urinary retention. He has prostate cancer with multiple secondaries throughout his abdomen. He is middle European in origin and has limited English. His distraught wife and two sons are with him — both sons speak fluent English. Effective analgesia has been provided and he is sleeping when the surgeon arrives to see him.

The surgeon speaks with the sons and explains that the situation is terminal and that only palliative surgical measures will be undertaken to relieve his symptoms. The sons request that their father not be given his diagnosis. They

explain that culturally it is the role of the family to be the decision-makers during illness and that their father would not expect to be involved. Furthermore, they all believe it would be detrimental to their father's wellbeing for him to be given a terminal diagnosis.

The surgeon reluctantly accedes to this request because the sons are so adamant about their cultural practices. He simply tells Mr X that they will insert a supra-pubic catheter later that day 'to bypass your blockage and sort out your pain'. However, when you are caring for Mr X during that day, he constantly asks you, in his limited English, whether or not he is dying. How would you deal with this situation?

the health professional's sense of what is ethically appropriate.[16]

If you were to consult the (updated) International Council of Nurses (ICN) *Code of ethics for nurses*,[17] adopted by the Nursing and Midwifery Board of Australia (NMBA), you would find some relevant (if potentially conflicting) advice. For example, Element 1 of the code states that '[n]urses promote an environment in which the human rights, values, customs, religious and spiritual beliefs of the individual, family and communities are acknowledged and respected by everyone'. So perhaps you might think that, in withholding the information as requested by the sons, you are respecting the patient and his family's cultural beliefs. However, it also stipulates that '[n]urses ensure that the individual and family receive understandable, accurate, sufficient and timely information in a manner appropriate to the patient's culture, linguistic, cognitive and physical needs and psychological state on which to base consent for care and related treatment'. Here you may feel that, given the patient is asking about his prognosis,

he does not have enough information on which to base his consent to treatment. Element 1 of the code is outlined in full in **Box 2.1**. (There is a separate *Code of ethics for midwives*, also adopted by the NMBA.[18])

You might wonder if it is possible in the circumstances under consideration to provide 'understandable, accurate, sufficient and timely information to the patient in a manner appropriate to the patient's culture, linguistic, cognitive and physical needs and psychological state'. Further, you might question how you can reconcile respect for 'values, customs, religious and spiritual beliefs' with the patient's right for information. This conundrum does not negate the value of a code of ethics, even though it clearly demonstrates why a code of ethics cannot be a manual for ethical behaviour. Rather, the code will help you identify the ethical issues involved in your dilemma so that you can then address them and, if necessary, make a choice between them.

You will remember that Michael Kirby stated that 'good ethics must be grounded in good data'.[19] All the responses and pieces of information discussed above

---

BOX 2.1
THE ICN CODE OF ETHICS FOR NURSES, ELEMENT 1. NURSES AND PATIENTS OR OTHER PEOPLE REQUIRING CARE OR SERVICES[20]

1. Nurses and Patients or Other People Requiring Care or Services

1.1 Nurses' primary professional responsibility is to people requiring nursing care and services now or in the future, whether individuals, families, communities or populations (hereinafter referred to as either 'patients' or 'people requiring care').

1.2 Nurses promote an environment in which the human rights, values, customs, religious and spiritual beliefs of the individual, families and communities are acknowledged and respected by everyone. Nurses' rights are included under human rights and should be upheld and protected.

1.3 Nurses ensure that the individual and family receive understandable, accurate, sufficient and timely information in a manner appropriate to the patient's culture, linguistic, cognitive and physical needs, and psychological state on which to base consent for care and related treatment.

1.4 Nurses hold in confidence personal information and respect the privacy, confidentiality and interests of patients in the lawful collection, use, access, transmission, storage and disclosure of personal information.

1.5 Nurses respect the privacy and confidentiality of colleagues and people requiring care and uphold the integrity of the nursing profession in person and in all media, including social media.

1.6 Nurses share with society the responsibility for initiating and supporting action to meet the health and social needs of all people.

1.7 Nurses advocate for equity and social justice in resource allocation, access to health care and other social and economic services.

1.8 Nurses demonstrate professional values such as respect, justice, responsiveness, caring, compassion, empathy, trustworthiness and integrity. They support and respect the dignity and universal rights of all people, including patients, colleagues and families.

1.9 Nurses facilitate a culture of safety in health care environments, recognising and addressing threats to people and safe care in health practices, services and settings.

1.10 Nurses provide evidence-informed, person-centred care, recognising and using the values and principles of primary health care and health promotion across the lifespan.

1.11 Nurses ensure that the use of technology and scientific advances are compatible with the safety, dignity and rights of people. In the case of artificial intelligence or devices, such as care robots or drones, nurses ensure that care remains person-centred and that such devices support and do not replace human relationships.

will form part of your ethical decision-making process. However, having all the *empirical data* before you will not ultimately provide you with the reason to make this decision. For example, there may be pieces of information you choose to reject — possibly you may decide that the family will suffer immeasurably if the father is told the truth, despite the fact that you discover he really wants to know. But you still need to recognise that the family members are present in your thought processes and acknowledge the influence they will have on your decision. Whatever decision you come to, you have to be able to justify it in terms of both the purpose of the decision itself and the process employed in making it.[21] Thus the questions you ask and the discussions you have with the key participants in such a scenario will determine the quality of the decision you eventually make.

What Resources are Available to Assist Nurses and Midwives to Address Such Dilemmas?

All of the information discussed above as part of the nurse's immediate response is critical to the decision-making process and will inform the final decision. The nurse needs to know what the law says and what the hospital policy states. The nurse will be assisted greatly by being familiar with the elements of *The ICN code of ethics* and any other codes of ethics or conduct which might bear upon nurses' practice (e.g. some health departments also have codes of ethics and/or conduct). The nurse's own religious or moral convictions may influence the way he or she feels about whatever decision is finally made, even if the outcome is that the nurse opts not to be involved in the management of this problem. However, to obtain 'good data' and to 'justify the decision' the nurse does need to ask more questions and have further discussions with all parties involved in the situation. Furthermore, even a basic understanding of ethical theories and principles will assist the nurse to make better decisions.

However, people don't usually make ethical decisions based on theories alone. Some very useful practical skills that are essential for ethical decision-making are listening skills, communication skills and the ability to trust ourselves and to value our own experiences, although not to the exclusion of those of our peers. We also need to be aware of the influence of power

relationships on our ethical decisions. As nurses, we often imagine that we are powerless in clinical situations, but frequently it is the patient who is the least powerful participant. The risk of privileging such an important process as ethical decision-making to the sole domain of health professionals is that it can disempower the very group it had set out to assist.

The remainder of this chapter highlights major ethical theories, principles and models for ethical decision-making, and recommends useful resources for further reading.

MAJOR ETHICAL THEORIES

The study of ethics, of determining 'what ought to be done', has been around since the time of the Ancient Greeks, and their ways of examining ethical behaviour provide the foundations for the two main branches of study of ethical theory: deontology and teleology. Other theories have developed over time, such as feminist moral theories and virtue ethics, and these are considered by some ethicists to be more appropriate to the caring professions. Both Johnstone and Allan provide readable discussions on the different schools of thought in relation to these theories and their relevance to healthcare.[22] All of these theories in their most extreme application can be controversial, and Allan highlights some of the difficulties with their application in her discussion.[23] However, one of the most useful aspects of learning about ethical theories for ethical decision-making is that nurses are able to identify the sources of the differing arguments being put forward by key players — it helps nurses to work out 'where (ethically) a person is coming from'.

Deontological or Intrinsicalist Theories

Deontological theories are sometimes known as intrinsicalist theories because they propose the view that actions are intrinsically right or wrong in themselves, and thus the way to determine what one ought to do is guided by the action itself. For example, if a nurse believed that telling the truth was intrinsically right, then that nurse's view of the correct action in our scenario would be determined according to that belief. Similarly, if a nurse believed that taking a person's life was intrinsically wrong, then that nurse's position in any debate about euthanasia would be clear.

Allan points out:

Deontologists tell us we must examine the duties and responsibilities of the person performing the action and the rights of those affected by that action.[24]

Indeed, deontological positions are more likely to be held by people with strong religious beliefs.

Teleological or Consequentialist Theories

Teleological theories are sometimes known as consequentialist theories because an action is not necessarily considered to be morally right or wrong in and of itself, but rather is judged to be morally appropriate because of the consequences its position produces. The best-known branch of the teleological theories is known as utilitarianism, which is popularly described as an attempt to obtain 'the greatest good for the greatest number'.[25] Taken to extremes, of course these theories can have bizarre outcomes. Nurses will find that such theories are often invoked in discussions about resource allocation.[26] However, they usually arrive at an individual level for health professionals when faced with a particular patient who would be disadvantaged by resource restrictions.
Allan states that:

Consequentialism is very influential in medicine given the focus on patient outcomes — in general, we think that we should do whatever achieves a good outcome.[27]

Other ethical theories and concepts include rights-based theories, virtue ethics, discourse ethics and narrative ethics, all of which are accessibly covered to varying depths in either Johnstone or Allan. Johnstone also makes a particularly strong case for nursing ethics, which she describes as:

… the examination of all kinds of ethical and bioethical issues from the perspective of nursing theory and practice, which, in turn, rests on the agreed core concepts of nursing, namely person, culture, care, health, healing, environment and nursing itself (or more to the point its ultimate purpose).

She goes on to say:

Unlike other approaches to ethics, nursing ethics recognises the 'distinctive voices' that are nurses and emphasises the importance of collecting and recording nursing narratives and 'stories from the field'.[28]

Most bioethics texts recognise the inadequacy of ethical theories in their application to practical bioethics. However, these inconsistencies and differences probably reflect the real difficulties nurses have in ethical debate in clinical practice, where many competing imperatives will shape the dilemma, as seen in **Case study 2.1**. Notwithstanding these criticisms of ethical theories, using theories, concepts and principles to inform our ethical thinking is of great importance if we are to improve our ethical practice as clinicians. Johnstone argues that one of the major moral problems nurses (and other health professionals) encounter is that of 'moral unpreparedness'. She argues that this is analogous to and as unacceptable as clinical unpreparedness — for example, putting a clinically unprepared nurse in charge of a ventilated patient in intensive care.[29]

Perhaps more recognisable to clinicians than ethical theories are the four ethical principles identified by Beauchamp and Childress. These are widely accepted as valuable in bioethical decision-making.[30]

The Four Major Ethical Principles

The notion of a principle is that it is a rule or standard to be applied in any given situation. There is a sense in a principle that it is the right thing to do, that it will guide one's behaviour. The four ethical principles commonly used in bioethics are:

1. autonomy;
2. beneficence;
3. non-maleficence; and
4. justice.

Just as with ethical theories, these principles are not without controversy and, as will be seen in the ensuing discussion, can also be in competition with one another in any given situation. But their usefulness as a means of examining ethical dilemmas is apparent from their popularity in models of bioethical decision-making. Johnstone states that 'ethical principlism has become widely regarded as a reliable and practical framework for identifying and resolving moral problems in health care contexts.'[31]

Autonomy

Autonomy is commonly described as the right to self-determination, the ability to control what happens to us and how we behave. This exercise of our own free will is acceptable only if it does not adversely affect the rights of others. It is an important ethical principle as it involves respect for individuals and their personal space. This principle is also reflected in a number of areas of health law, particularly in relation to one's right to consent to treatment and to receive information about one's treatment; however, this ethical principle is not upheld in law in every situation. For example, there are still some groups of people in Australia who do not have the right to exercise autonomy in relation to voluntary euthanasia, as although it is now legalised in all states in Australia, the eligibility criteria are very narrow. For further discussion on this see **Chapter 6**.

Nurses and midwives need to remember that, to exercise autonomy, it is often necessary to be assertive. It is not always easy for a patient to be assertive when they are 'at the mercy' of the nursing and medical staff, particularly if their exercise of autonomy would bring them into confrontation with those staff. Nor has it always been easy for nurses to be assertive, schooled as they have been in the past in the need for absolute obedience, particularly to the doctor.[32] Furthermore, the principle of autonomy is, as seen in **Case study 2.1**, culturally a Western concept. Some other cultures do not think primarily in terms of autonomy and individualism, but rather in terms of interdependence and community, and yet the laws in Australia usually uphold the principle of autonomy.[33]

Beneficence

Beneficence is often described as the principle of 'above all, do good'. This desire to do good is undoubtedly what motivates most health professionals. However, it is valuable to recognise that there are times when people's idea of what constitutes 'doing good' may go against the wishes of an individual — for example, when a patient is terminally ill and may be prepared to die, but the doctors and nurses cannot bear to cease treatment. One of the important questions to ask in situations relating to beneficence is: 'Whose good are we trying to serve?' If a patient's autonomy is overruled on grounds of beneficence, this is known as paternalism.[34] Beneficence and non-maleficence are often two sides of the same coin — but often the difficulty in practice is to work out where one ends and the other begins. For example, if a nurse is debriding burns or

performing some other painful dressing for a patient, the nurse may well be causing the patient some discomfort (at least) which could be construed as 'doing harm' and yet the nurse's motives for undertaking the dressing or debridement are to 'do good'. In such a situation, it is clear that the nurse must debride the wound, yet the principles could be construed as being in conflict with one another.

Non-Maleficence

Non-maleficence is the principle of 'above all, do no harm'. This is a very strong principle in healthcare and forms the basis of nurses' and midwives' duty to take care in the way in which they look after their patients. It can also be recognised in the 'duty of care', which is one of the elements of the tort of negligence. This obligation to do no harm is argued to override the principle of beneficence ('above all, do good'). Beauchamp and Childress argue that our duty to do no harm is greater than our duty to do good, particularly where our duty to do good may put others or ourselves at risk.[35]

Justice

Justice has two meanings in ethics: justice as fairness, and justice as an equal distribution of burdens and benefits. Justice as fairness also has two interpretations: that of treating people equally and that of 'getting one's just deserts' — deserving what happened.

The principle of justice as fairness implies and expects a level of impartiality and neutrality in dealings with others. However, treating people equally does not necessarily equate with treating people in the same way. Patients are not the same in terms of their social, educational and cultural backgrounds, and nurses may need to adopt widely differing strategies to achieve equal treatment for two patients. For example, providing adequate information about a laparoscopic cholecystectomy for an elderly man from a non-English-speaking background may require very different strategies than providing the same information to a university-educated, English-speaking 45-year-old woman. With these considerations in mind, justice as fairness is the basis for the requirement to avoid discrimination against people who are different for whatever reason.

The second meaning of justice as an equal distribution of burdens and benefits is sometimes known as distributive justice. This principle is often used to address questions relating to resource allocation. The central tenet is that whoever we may be in society, the benefits and burdens would be equally shared between us. It is clear to see that this is not the case in modern society. This concept creates huge ethical difficulties for health professionals when they are required to apply the principle in practice. Questions arise such as: Which patients should receive treatment? If we close our mental institutions, how do we fund care in the community adequately? Such questions pose real dilemmas for health professionals, who have traditionally tended to operate in terms of individual patient relationships.

Models for Ethical Decision-Making in Healthcare

With these theories and principles in mind, a number of authors have suggested models to assist in ethical decision-making, some of which are more complex than others. All adopt a problem-oriented approach to ethical decision-making and involve a number of steps which include assessment, information-gathering, planning or goal-setting (including weighing options) and implementing and evaluating the chosen plan. However, it may be that the issue is not so clear-cut, in which case a decision-making model may help the individual work through the ethical dilemma. One of the more comprehensive decision-making models, by Allan,[36] is reproduced in **Box 2.2** with permission. It involves seven steps, to which I would add an eighth, which would be to evaluate the outcome of the decision to determine whether you can learn from your decision-making process on reflection.

BOX 2.2
A MODEL FOR ETHICAL
DECISION-MAKING

1. Identify what the ethical issue is (or ethical issues are)
2. Identify personal reaction to the case
3. Gather any relevant facts regarding the situation
4. Identify the values at stake in the scenario
5. Identify the options in the case
6. Consider what you should do and relevant justification for doing so (i.e. why)
7. Consider if the ethical problem could have been prevented

Source: Reproduced from Allan S, *Law and ethics for health practitioners*, Elsevier, Sydney, 2020, pp 29–30.

If this model were used to address the dilemma in **Case study 2.1**, it would clearly provide useful pointers as to how to deal with the issue.

1. Identify What the Ethical Issue Is (or Ethical Issues Are). How one frames this ethical issue will depend on one's own value systems. But, in anyone's language, there seems to be a discrepancy between what Mr X has been told about his condition and what he has a legal right to be told. Furthermore, what he has been told is not complete and he seems to be asking for more information. However, it will be important to ascertain linguistically that this is exactly what he is asking, as he has limited English and may be requiring a different outcome, such as reassurance, or even denial. We also know that the surgeon is not happy about the situation but has reluctantly agreed to the family's request on cultural grounds. However, little conversation has taken place between Mr X and the surgeon. It will also be necessary to factor in the impact on the family if a decision were made to inform Mr X of his diagnosis in contravention of the family's wishes. This problem raises cultural and legal issues as well as ethical issues, and there are a number of people already involved in **Case study 2.1** — Mr X, his wife and sons, the surgeon, and you, at the very least.

2. Identify Personal Reaction to the Case. As previously explored, when describing this case in relation to what ethics is not, it may well be that you have already had a *gut reaction* as to what *ought* to be done. This may be based on strong *religious* or *moral* convictions — for example, that you consider truth-telling to be a critical moral issue and are appalled that Mr X is not being told the truth. You may already have found yourself taking sides in this situation, believing that the view of the majority taken by the surgeon and the sons was 'wrong' because the patient seems to be asking for more information. Conversely, you may feel that the family know the patient better and this is a cultural issue about which you should be respectful. What is important is not that you have these personal views, but that you acknowledge them and recognise them for what they are.

3. Gather Any Relevant Facts Regarding the Situation. There is much work to be done to find all the facts in **Case study 2.1**. Further discussions are required with the surgeon, the family and the other health professionals involved in caring for Mr X, even including community carers, such as his GP, his community nurse or his religious adviser. This is a critical time in the lives of Mr X and his family, and the hospital staff who are currently caring for him probably know him least well. Discussion is especially required with Mr X to ascertain what information he really wants to know. It may be advisable to use an interpreter rather than a family member to assist the surgeon and you in having these conversations with Mr X. However, at this stage you will need to be particularly aware that you and the interpreter are trying to find out all the facts, not institute solutions. Each conversation may lead to more information being required. It is most important to have all the information you need before you determine what ought to be done.

4. Identify the Values at Stake in the Scenario. Think about the ethical theories that are in play here. What duties are in conflict here? The duty to tell the truth? The duty to respect cultural norms? The duty to provide Mr X with more information? If we adopt a utilitarian approach, what is the best outcome? Are we concerned with the best outcome for Mr X or the best outcome for his family? Are those optimal outcomes different or the same?

Let us consider each of the ethical principles:

- Autonomy: What is the patient's approach to the problem?
- Beneficence: What benefits can be obtained for the patient?
- Non-maleficence: What are the risks to the patient, and how can they be avoided?
- Justice: How are the interests of different parties to be balanced?
- Confidentiality/privacy: What information is private, and does confidentiality need to be limited or breached?
- Veracity: Has the patient and their family been honestly informed, and is there any reason the patient cannot know the truth?

Your consideration of these principles will depend on what facts and information you have found. However, it seems clear that Mr X's wishes must be balanced against the family's desire to 'do good' according to their culture and the surgeon's desire to 'do no harm'.

The question of veracity, particularly from the patient's perspective, is highly significant here.

Questions about the key stakeholders are critical here, particularly as they will undoubtedly become clearer as further information emerges. You will also need to consider questions of power in this decision-making process. This will be particularly important if your preferred ethical decision is in conflict with that of other members of the healthcare team, especially if you are not in a position of authority. Rights-based ethics may move the decision in favour of advising Mr X but, conversely, if you determine that his relationship with his family is more important than his need to know his prognosis, an ethic of care may prevail.

5. Identify the Options in the Case. From a legal perspective, the law is fairly clear in this situation. One question that has framed this ethical dilemma in the first place is whether the legal requirement to give information and consent can be overridden because of either therapeutic privilege or cultural norms.

At first glance there do appear to be ethical conflicts between the need to enable Mr X to exercise autonomy by providing the information he seems to be seeking and the desire to do good by respecting his and his family's cultural norms. However, the need to do no harm through avoiding any disharmony with the family dynamics is also critical. Other conflicts may also arise as you discover more information. On the other hand, it may transpire that, when you have gathered all the information, these conflicts will resolve.

6. Consider What You Should Do and Relevant Justification for Doing So (i.e. Why). When you are exploring the options that are available to you, be clear about them and then make yourself justify them. For example, specify how you came to your decision and why you chose the guiding principles and theories that you did. Whatever decision you finally make will be determined by the facts you discover in your decision-making process and the value you place on the differing pieces of information. Before you implement the decision, step once again through your justification, ensuring that your rationale is considered and robust. It may be that there is no consensus on the best way forward, in which case a decision will have to be made and any differing views ought to be documented. Make sure you document all this information and leave a clear decision-making trail.

7. Consider if the Ethical Problem Could Have Been Prevented. It is helpful to examine an ethical situation post-hoc and think about how the situation might possibly have been avoided. Often in clinical ethics the problems appear "on the run" and we are forced to respond to a situation quickly. Thinking through how you managed a situation and whether it might have been avoided is an important process in learning from issues and potential errors.

8. Reflect on and Evaluate the Process and Outcome. If your preferred decision is the one to be implemented, then it is critical that you take responsibility for the decision and manage the consequences of the decision, following through on both positive and negative outcomes. Any difficult decision will not produce perfect outcomes, and it is vital that the impact of the decision is handled with care and compassion. Evaluating the process as well as the outcome is essential, as otherwise you will have learned little from the experience.

The opportunity to reflect on our most difficult dilemmas and the choices we made about them is always to be welcomed. However, it is important to recognise that real reflection, as opposed to post-hoc justification, can sometimes be painful. We may honestly feel on reflection that we could have managed the situation better or made better decisions. But clinical–ethical decision-making is often made 'on the run' and, with the best will in the world, we will not always get it right. It is important to welcome the evaluation as a learning opportunity and to recognise the potential for improvement.

CONCLUSION

Law and ethics are not the same, although ethical decision-making will always involve a consideration of the law. In addition, good laws should arguably also be ethical laws but, as seen from the ethical theories and principles presented above, there may be disagreement about their morality, depending on which ethical theory or principle is being promulgated. However, there are a number of desirable healthcare practices, such as the requirements for confidentiality and consent, respect for persons, and care, in terms of both compassion and rigour, which are both ethically sound and legally required. Olejarczyk and Young make the point that 'establishing clearly defined patient rights helps standardise care across healthcare fields and enables patients to have uniform expectations during their treatment'.[37] In addition, when the courts are presented with issues they have not previously dealt with, such as withdrawal of life support (e.g. *Airedale NHS Trust v Bland*), or the harvesting of spermatozoa from a posthumous donor (e.g. *R v Human Fertilisation and Embryology Authority, ex parte Blood*), they draw on ethical principles and theories to assist them in their deliberations.[38] This will become clear in some of the cases discussed later in this book, and the reader might find it interesting to examine the case law with a view to ascertaining which principles were being upheld.

As this chapter has highlighted, ethical theories and principles are not without difficulty in relation to their application to practice. However, using an ethical decision-making model can provide a clear structure to addressing the complex and often difficult dilemmas that nurses and midwives meet in clinical practice. Yet it is also important for nurses and midwives to recognise that, even after they believe they have reached an appropriate ethical decision, the power differentials in healthcare may mean that their decision is not the decision of choice. This can be extremely frustrating for nurses and midwives and has been the subject of much discussion, particularly in relation to recruitment and retention.

CHAPTER 2 REVIEW QUESTIONS

Following your reading of **Chapter 2**, consider these questions in reaching the objectives of this chapter. Guidance on which part of the chapter will assist you in answering the questions can be found at http://evolve.elsevier.com/AU/Staunton/law/.

You may, of course, consider other sources as part of your considerations.

1. Think of an ethical dilemma you have encountered in practice. Would using an ethical decision-making model have assisted you?

2. Apply it to your dilemma now and work through both what you actually did and what you might have done differently had you had such a model available.

3. Consider the ethical principles. How are they applied on an almost daily basis in clinical practice? Give examples of each principle being applied in your own practice.

ENDNOTES

1. Villa G, Pennestri F, Giannetta N, Sala R, Mordacci R and Firoenzo Manara D, 'Moral distress in community and hospital settings for the care of elderly people: a grounded theory qualitative study', (2021) *Healthcare (Basel)* 9(10):1307, https://www.ncbi.nlm.nih.gov/pmc/articles/PMC8544437/.

2. Johnstone M-J, *Bioethics: a nursing perspective*, 7th ed, Churchill Livingstone Elsevier, Sydney, 2019, p 14.

3. Haahr A, Norlyk A, Martinsen B and Dreyer P, 'Nurses experiences of ethical dilemmas: a review' (2020) *Nursing Ethics* 27(1):258–272, https://journals.sagepub.com/doi/pdf/10.1177/0969733019832941; Chiarella E M, *The legal and professional status of nursing*, Churchill Livingstone, Edinburgh, 2002.

4. Gebreheat G and Teame H, 'Ethical challenges of nurses in COVID-19 pandemic: integrative review' (2021) *Journal of Multidisciplinary Healthcare* 14:1029–1035, doi: 10.2147/JMDH.S308758.

5. Kirby M, 'Bioethics and democracy — a fundamental question' in Charlesworth M, *Life, death, genes and ethics — the 1989 Boyer lectures*, ABC Books, Sydney, 1989, p 3.

6. Johnstone, 2019, op. cit., p 14.

7. Ibid pp 15–18.

8. Allan S, *Law and ethics for health practitioners*, Elsevier, Sydney, 2020, p 25.

9. Maeckelberghe E and Schröder-Bäck P, 'Ethics in public health: call for shared moral public health literacy' (2017) *European Journal of Public Health* 27(suppl 4):49–51.

10. Singer P, *Practical ethics*, Cambridge University Press, Cambridge, 2011.

11. Allan S, 2020, op. cit., p 25.

12. Charlesworth M, *Life, death, genes and ethics — the 1989 Boyer lectures*, ABC Books, Sydney, 1989, p 23.

13. Singer P, 2011, op. cit., pp 3–4.

14. Johnstone, 2019, op. cit., pp 18–31.

15. *Rogers v Whitaker* (1992) 109 ALR 625.

16. Johnstone, 2019, op. cit., p 20.

17. *The ICN code of ethics for nurses*, International Council of Nurses (ICN), 2021, https://www.icn.ch/system/files/2021-10/ICN_Code-of-Ethics_EN_Web_0.pdffiles/2012_ICN_Codeofethicsfornurses_%20eng.pdf.

18. A separate code of ethics exists for midwives, *International code of ethics for midwives*, International Confederation for Midwives (ICM), https://www.internationalmidwives.org/assets/files/general-files/2019/10/eng-international-code-of-ethics-for-midwives.pdf

19. Kirby, 1989, op. cit., p 3.

20. *The ICN code of ethics for nurses*, International Council of Nurses (ICN), 2021, https://www.icn.ch/sites/default/files/2023-06/ICN_Code-of-Ethics_EN_Web.pdf.

21. Xafis V, Schaefer, O, Labude M, Brassington I, Lim H, Lipworth W, Lysaght T, Stewart C, Sun S, Laurie G and Tai S. 'An ethics framework for big data in health and research' (2019) *Asian Bioethics Review* 11:227–54, https://link.springer.com/article/10.1007/s41649-019-00099-x

22. Johnstone, 2019, op. cit., p 37 et seq. Allan, 2020, op.cit p 24 et seq.

23. Allan, 2020, op. cit., p 28.

24. Ibid. pp 27–28.

25. Johnstone, 2019, op. cit., p 64.

26. Allan, 2020, op. cit., p 27.

27. Ibid.

28. Johnstone, 2019, op. cit., p 17.

29. Johnstone, 2019, op. cit., pp 96–8.

30. Beauchamp T L and Childress J F, *Principles of bioethics*, 7th ed, Oxford University Press, New York, 2013. For an interesting discussion on the history of the development of the principles see Beauchamp T and Childress J, 'Principles of Biomedical ethics: marking its 40th anniversary'(2019) *American Journal of Bioethics* 19(11), https://www.tandfonline.com/doi/full/10.1080/15265161.2019.1665402.

31. Johnstone, 2019, op. cit., p 41.

32. Chiarella, 2002, op. cit. See specifically Ch 6 and the discussion of the nurse as the doctor's handmaiden.

33. For an excellent discussion on cross-cultural ethics see Johnstone, 2019, op. cit., Ch 4, p 71 et seq.

34. Johnstone, 2019, op. cit., p 187.

35. Beauchamp and Childress, 2013, op. cit.

36. Allan, 2020, op. cit., p 29.

37. Olejarczyk JP, Young M. Patient Rights And Ethics. [Updated 2022 Jun 15]. In: StatPearls [Internet]. Treasure Island (FL): StatPearls Publishing; 2022 Jan-. Available from: https://www.ncbi.nlm.nih.gov/books/NBK538279/.

38. *Airedale NHS Trust v Bland* [1993] 2 WLR 316; *R v Human Fertilisation and Embryology Authority, ex parte Blood* [1997] 2 WLR 806.

3

THE INTERNATIONAL CONFEDERATION OF MIDWIVES CODE OF ETHICS FOR MIDWIVES AND THE INTERNATIONAL COUNCIL OF NURSES CODE OF ETHICS FOR NURSES

LEARNING OBJECTIVES

In this chapter, you will:

- review the history of codes of ethics in nursing and midwifery
- explore the difference between codes of ethics and codes of conduct
- examine the content of both the International Confederation of Midwives *International code of ethics for midwives* (the ICM Code) and the International Council of Nurses *The ICN code of ethics for nurses* (the ICN Code)
- compare the content of the ICM Code and the ICN Code with the NMBA *Code of conduct*
- consider how codes of ethics might provide assistance to midwives and nurses in their practice.

INTRODUCTION

In 2018, the Nursing and Midwifery Board of Australia made the decision to adopt the International Council of Nurses (ICN) *The ICN code of ethics for nurses* (the ICN Code) (recently updated)[1] and the International Confederation of Midwives (ICM) *International code of ethics for midwives* (the ICM Code)[2] (updated 2014) respectively. As the aim of this textbook is to provide practical guidance for nurses and midwives on how the law and documents produced by government and regulatory bodies impact on their professional practice, this chapter will examine the ICM and ICN codes of ethics from that perspective.

The concept of nursing as an ethical endeavour has been promulgated since the days of Florence Nightingale, and this was later initially codified in the Nightingale Pledge in 1893.[3,4] However, although the ICN first began working on a code of ethics in 1923, it was not until 1953 that the first *Code of ethics for nurses* was published by the ICN and it has been argued that this was as a result of the intense scrutiny that the medical and nursing professions came under following the atrocities of the Second World War.[5] Certainly, following the publication of the *Nuremberg code* of 1947 and the *Universal declaration of human rights* in 1949, there was a significant focus on both medical and nursing ethics.[6] The ICN Code for nurses 'provides ethical guidance in relation to nurses' roles, duties, responsibilities, behaviours, professional judgment and relationships with patients, other people who are receiving nursing care or services, co-workers and allied professionals.'[7]

For some time, and despite midwifery being recognised as a separate profession in many countries, in Australia midwifery became subsumed as a branch of nursing with the passing of the first *Nurses Registration Act*, which was finally passed in New South Wales in 1924, and provided for the registration of general, midwifery, mental health and paediatric nurses. Interestingly, this Act received unanimous support from the medical profession, who were particularly concerned about maternal and infant mortality rates and wanted the practice of midwifery regulated.[8] What this meant in practice was that, when the Australian Nursing Council Inc. (ANCI) in collaboration with the (then) Royal College of Nursing Australia (RCNA) and the (then) Australian Nursing Federation (ANF) published the first *Code of ethics for nurses in Australia* in 1993 (revised in 2002), the advice in the Code was taken to be applicable to midwifery as well as nursing, despite the fact that the Code did not include the word 'midwife' at all.[9] In fact, the Code specifically stated that '*nurses* provide care and support before and during birth'[10] (emphasis added). The (then) Australian College of Midwives Inc. (ACMI) published its first *Code of ethics for midwives in Australia*, which was adapted from the 1993 ICM *Code of ethics*, and made specific reference to midwifery-related issues, such as relationships with the women for whom midwives care.[11] When midwifery was eventually recognised as a separate and discrete profession in Australia, the professional regulatory bodies worked together under the auspices of the Australian Nursing and Midwifery Council (ANMC), formerly the ANCI, until the establishment of the National Registration and Accreditation Scheme (NRAS), which will be discussed in detail in the next chapter. The ANMC commissioned research to develop separate codes of conduct for nurses and for midwives in Australia and continued its relationships with the (now) Australian College of Nursing (ACN), the (now) Australian Nursing and Midwifery Federation (ANMF) and the (now) Australian College of Midwives (ACM) to publish separate codes of ethics for nurses and midwives in Australia.[12] After the NRAS was introduced and the Nursing and Midwifery Board of Australia (NMBA) was established in 2009, the NMBA initially adopted all four of the codes: the codes of conduct for nurses and midwives in Australia and the codes of ethics for nurses and midwives in Australia, in 2010.[13] However, on revision in 2018 the NMBA determined to develop new codes of conduct for nurses and midwives, but (as mentioned at the beginning of the chapter) to replace their own codes of ethics for nurses and midwives with the ICN Code[14] and the ICM Code[15] respectively. The new codes of conduct for nurses[16] and midwives[17] are virtually identical in content, with the key differences being the use of 'nurse' and 'person' in the NMBA nurses' Code and 'midwife' and 'woman' in the NMBA midwives' Code.

HOW DOES A CODE OF ETHICS DIFFER FROM A CODE OF CONDUCT?

Although the ICN Code intends to explicate the international ethical standards of the profession, in 1977 the ICN also encouraged its member states to develop national codes of ethics to ensure that it remains relevant to the cultural, social and historical contexts from which ethical dilemmas arise.[18] This has been interpreted such that codes of ethics and conduct are often combined in the single document. Because ethical standards and principles are often implied or even explicitly stated in the legislation and codes of conduct that regulate professional standards,[19] these documents have been argued to fulfil the same or at least a similar role to a code of ethics.[20]

On the other side, it is also argued that codes of ethics and conduct are significantly different from one another in form and function.[21] The rationale is that codes of ethics are aspirational and virtue centred (defining the 'good' nurse), whereas codes of conduct are prescriptive and duty centred (defining the 'just-good-enough' nurse).[22] The analogy of a 'floor and ceiling' has also been used to illustrate this distinction between minimum and ideal standards of practice.[23] Accordingly, codes of ethics tend to be the domain of professional bodies that do not have regulatory powers such as the ICN.[24] Codes of conduct, on the other hand (as discussed in **Chapter 4**), seek to protect the public by establishing minimum standards of professional conduct. Although some ethical behaviours are subject to the individual's discretion, breaches of conduct rules are legal matters that can be investigated or sanctioned by regulatory bodies, such as the NMBA in Australia.

However, rather than having a disciplinary function, the parameters established by the ICN Code are intended to compensate for discrepancies in individual value systems and provide a tool for self-evaluation or peer review of professional ethical competence. It has been argued that:

> In the case of the nursing profession, owing to the complexity of nursing work and the complexity of the contexts in which nurses work, codes of ethics may be inadequate to the task of guiding ethical decision-making and conduct.[25]

Because codes of ethics are intended to be aspirational rather than prescriptive, a deviation from ethical norms cannot necessarily be deemed to be misconduct and the consequences of transgression should therefore not carry the possibility of sanction, unless it simultaneously involves a transgression of a conduct-rule.[26]

In contrast to these aspirational functions, it has been argued that codes of ethics have come to represent mechanisms of control or levers of social recognition, rather than instruments that promote ethical nursing care. In doing so, it is argued, 'codes transgress the boundaries between ethics and politics', whereby a distorted focus on the external functions of codes has detracted from their objective of guiding ethical nursing practice.[27] So the purpose of ethical codes is here argued to be to inspire nurses to provide the best level of care, and not to ensure that they adhere to the minimum professional standards. Therefore, if codes of ethics are to be effective in providing practical guidance for the implementation of ethical service delivery, the focus needs to move away from the external functions of ethical codes (such as professional advancement) so that their moral objective can be emphasised.[28]

HOW DO THE ICM CODE AND THE ICN CODE COMPARE WITH THE NMBA CODES OF CONDUCT FOR MIDWIVES AND NURSES RESPECTIVELY (2018)?

The following discussion offers a direct comparison between the style and content of the four documents, recognising that the NMBA nurses' Code and the NMBA midwives' Code are well-nigh identical. The discussion begins by noting the language styles of the respective codes, in terms of both the degree of compliance required and the status of the functions of the codes. It then goes on to compare and contrast the various provisions of the codes. Finally, an exploration of the more aspirational and unenforceable elements of the ICM Code and the ICN Code is offered.

A key difference between the two documents is the language with which the standards are expressed. Snelling[29] emphasises the significance of the language used when differentiating specific rules of conduct from general moral principles (in this case, codes of ethics), particularly use of the modal verbs 'must' and 'should'. The glossary at the beginning of the Irish *Code of professional conduct and ethics*[30] is effective in clarifying the difference between the two, stating that 'must' 'commands the action a nurse or midwife is obliged to take, from which no deviation whatsoever is allowed' (p 5), whereas 'should' 'indicates a strong recommendation to perform a particular action from which deviation in particular circumstances must be justified' (p 5). Although neither the NMBA Codes of conduct nor the ICN or ICM Codes offer a similar differentiation, the documents still differ somewhat in the style of language in which the standards are expressed. For example, the new *ICN code of ethics for nurses* quite specifically states that it 'is not a code of conduct but can serve as a framework for ethical nursing practice and decision-making to meet professional standards set by regulatory bodies'.[31]

The NMBA Codes use directive language, stipulating that nurses 'must' comply with all of the standards listed in each of the domains. They also use various interdictions such as 'must not', 'must never' and 'must avoid' to articulate those actions that are not permitted. In contrast, the ICN and ICM Codes use more descriptive and positive language that describes what nurses and midwives 'do' as opposed to what they 'shouldn't do'. In doing so, they encourage the adoption of ethical behaviours, as opposed to prohibiting those behaviours that are considered unprofessional or unethical.

Notwithstanding the fact that the ICM describes the sections of its Code as 'mandates', it goes on to state that its purpose is to '*guide* the education, practice and research of the midwife' (emphasis added).[32] Similarly, the ICN Code describes itself as a statement of ethical values, responsibilities and professional accountabilities of nurses and nursing students that defines and '*guides* ethical nursing practice within the different roles nurses assume' (emphasis added),[33] yet it identifies four 'principal elements' that provide a framework for ethical nursing practice, being 'nurses and patients or other people requiring care or services, nurses and practice, nurses and the profession, and nurses and global health'.[34] So although these elements are described as mandates and principal elements that provide a framework, they cannot be enforced by the ICM or ICN, as these are not regulatory authorities. However, what is clear is that many of the mandates and principal elements are also codified by regulatory authorities all over the world. Certainly, in Australia, many of them would be recognised as legal responsibilities as well as ethical responsibilities.

The ICN and the ICM point out they produced their codes of ethics to provide guidance and education and to elucidate the ethical stances these organisations take in relation to the care of people and women respectively. The ICN Code even suggests ways in which the elements of the Code might be applied. These are set out in **Box 3.1**.

Furthermore, the Code makes suggestions as to the way the elements might be applied by three discrete groups within the nursing profession: practitioners and managers, educators and researchers, and national nursing organisations.[35] The NMBA also sets out a list of ways in which the Code will be used (note, these are not suggestions but statements). These are set out in **Box 3.2**.

Note how the purpose of the NMBA *Code of conduct for nurses* is far more outward facing. Although it is envisaged it will be used 'to support individual nurses in the delivery of safe practice', the other uses relate to the expectations of consumers, the protection of the public, and its use in disciplinary matters and

the culture of professionalism in Australian health services. As with the ICN Code, there is reference to the different domains of nursing practice, such as education and management, but also to broader audiences such as administration and policy development in health services.[37] The NMBA *Code of conduct for midwives* is very similar in its exhortations to the NMBA *Code of conduct for nurses*, whereas the ICM Code is also more clinically focused throughout, discussing midwifery relationships, the practice of midwifery and the professional responsibilities of midwives, most of which relate to clinical practice. There is a brief section on the advancement of midwifery knowledge and practice, but as with the *ICN Code of ethics*, it is a more internally facing document.[38]

It can be seen from **Tables 3.1** and **3.2** that, although there are a number of similarities between codes of ethics and codes of conduct, there are also significant differences. In 1995, codes of conduct were differentiated from codes of ethics by describing them

---

BOX 3.1

ICN SUGGESTIONS FOR THE USE OF THE CODE OF ETHICS FOR NURSES[36]

Nurses can therefore:

- Study the standards under each element of the Code
- Personally reflect on what each standard means
- Think about ways to apply ethics to the personal domain of nursing practice, education, research, management, leadership or policy development
- Discuss the Code with co-workers and others
- Use a specific example from experience to identify ethical dilemmas and standards of conduct as outlined in the Code. Identify ways in which the Code guides in the resolution of dilemmas
- Work in groups to clarify ethical decision-making and reach a consensus on standards of ethical conduct
- Collaborate with the National Nurses Association co-workers and others in the continuous application of ethical standards in nursing practice, education, management, research and policy.

BOX 3.2

NMBA STATEMENTS ABOUT HOW THE CODE WILL BE USED[39]

The Code will be used:

- to support individual nurses in the delivery of safe practice and fulfilling their professional roles
- as a guide for the public and consumers of health services about the standard of conduct and behaviour they should expect from nurses
- to help the NMBA protect the public, in setting and maintaining the standards set out in the code and to ensure safe and effective nursing practice
- when evaluating the professional conduct of nurses. If professional conduct varies significantly from the values outlined in the code, nurses should be prepared to explain and justify their decisions and actions. Serious or repeated failure to abide by this code may have consequences for nurses' registration and may be considered as unsatisfactory professional performance, unprofessional conduct or professional misconduct, and
- as a resource for activities which aim to enhance the culture of professionalism in the Australian health system. These include use, for example, in administration and policy development by health services and other institutions; in nursing education, in management and for the orientation, induction and supervision of nurses and students.

TABLE 3.1

The Mandates in the ICM Code and Their Corresponding Principles in the NMBA Code for Midwives

Mandates of the ICM Code (abbreviated)	Corresponding principles in the NMBA Code	Mandates or principles that are unmatched
1. Midwifery Relationships		
1.a Information sharing	Principle 2, Woman-centred practice; VS 2.2 and 2.3 Informed consent	Mandatory reporting Adverse events and open disclosure End-of-life care Professional boundaries Advertising and professional representation Legal, insurance and other assessments Conflict of interest Financial arrangements and gifts
1.b Active participation for women in decision-making	Principle 2, Woman-centred practice; VS 2.2 Decision-making	
1.c Empowering women to speak for themselves	Not specifically addressed	
1.d Fair allocation of resources in policy and funding	Not specifically addressed	
1.e Support for each other	Principle 7, Health and wellbeing; VS 7.1c Your and your colleagues' health requires nurses to 'encourage and support colleagues to seek help if they are concerned that their colleague's health may be affecting their ability to practise safely, utilising services such as Nurse and Midwife Support, the national health support service for nurses, midwives and students'	
1.f Respectful co-relationships	Principle 3, Cultural practice and respectful relationships; VS 3.4 prohibits bullying and harassment and exhorts nurses to 'never engage in, ignore or excuse such behaviour'	
1.g Conflict resolution	Principle 3, Cultural practice and respectful relationships; VS 3.3 Effective communication touches on disagreements in relation to women, not colleagues	
1.h Respect for themselves and their moral worth	Not addressed	

TABLE 3.1		
The Mandates in the ICM Code and Their Corresponding Principles in the NMBA Code for Midwives *(Continued)*		
Mandates of the ICM Code (abbreviated)	Corresponding principles in the NMBA Code	Mandates or principles that are unmatched
2. Practice of Midwifery		
2.a Respect for cultural diversity plus elimination of harm	Principle 3, Cultural practice and respectful relationships, VS 3.2 Culturally safe and respectful practice	
2.b No woman or girl should be harmed by conception or childbearing	Not specifically addressed	
2.c Evidence-based practice	Principle 2, Woman-centred practice, VS 2.1 Midwifery practice	
2.d Non-discrimination	Principle 3, Cultural practice and respectful relationships, VS 3.2 Culturally safe and respectful practice	
2.e Act as effective role models	Principle 3, Cultural practice and respectful relationships, VS 3.2f Create a positive, culturally safe work environment through role modelling ...	
2.f Seek personal intellectual and professional growth	1.1.c Obligations re CPD	
3. Professional Responsibilities		
3.a Confidentiality and privacy	Principle 3, Cultural practice and respectful relationships; VS 3.5 Confidentiality and privacy	
3.b Accountability	Addressed in the introduction and also Principle 1, Legal compliance	
3.c Conscientious objection	Not specifically addressed, but implicit within 4.4.b	
3.d Need to refer on in conscientious objection	Not specifically addressed, but implicit within 4.4.b	
3.e Work to eliminate human rights violations	Not addressed specifically although Principle 7, Health and wellbeing, VS 7.2 Health advocacy, does address 'significant disparities in the health status of various groups in the Australian community'	
3.f Involvement in health policy	Not addressed	
4. Advancement of Midwifery Knowledge and Practice		
4.a All advancement to be based on activities that protect human rights	Not addressed	
4.b Development and sharing of knowledge through peer review and research	Principle 5, Teaching, supervising and assessing, and Principle 6, Research in health	
4.c Contribution to formal education of midwives	Principle 5, Teaching, supervising and assessing	

TABLE 3.2		
The Elements of the ICN Code and Their Corresponding Principles in the NMBA Code for Nurses		
Elements of the ICN Code (abbreviated)	Corresponding principles in the NMBA Code	Elements or principles that are unmatched
Element 1. Nurses and Patients or Other People Requiring Care or Services		
1.1 Primary responsibility to people needing nursing care and services	Not specifically identified, but implicit throughout	Adverse events and open disclosure End-of-life care Professional boundaries Advertising and professional representation Legal, insurance and other assessments Conflict of interest Financial arrangements and gifts
1.2 Respect for human rights, values, customs and spiritual beliefs	Principle 3, Cultural practice and respectful relationships, VS 3.2 Culturally safe and respectful practice	
1.3 Informed consent	Principle 2, Person-centred practice, VS 2.3 Informed consent	
1.4 Confidentiality for patients	Principle 3, Cultural practice and respectful relationships, VS 3.5 Confidentiality and privacy	
1.5 Privacy and confidentiality for colleagues and through social media	3.4.c Bullying and harassment and social media 3.5.c Social media policy	
1.6 Responsible for initiating and supporting action to meet health and social needs, esp. for vulnerable populations	Principle 3, Cultural practice and respectful relationships, VS 3.2c In culturally safe and respectful practice	
1.7 Advocacy for equity and social justice in resource allocation; access to health care and social and economic services	7.2 Health advocacy	
1.8 Demonstration of professional values — respect, responsiveness, trust, compassion and integrity	Not specifically identified in one principle but inherent in several value statements	
Element 2. Nurses and Practice		
2.1 Personally responsible and accountable for maintaining competence	Principle 2, Person-centred practice; VS 1a — names the NMBA standards codes and guidelines	
2.2 Maintains fitness to practise	Principle 7, Health and wellbeing, VS 7.1b and 7.1d	
2.3 Uses judgment regarding competence in accepting and making delegations	See delegation in the glossary for reference to the NMBA decision-making framework	
2.4 Valuing of own dignity, wellbeing and health	Principle 7	
2.5 Maintains personal standards that promote confidence in the profession	Alluded to in the introduction	

TABLE 3.2

The Elements of the ICN Code and Their Corresponding Principles in the NMBA Code for Nurses *(Continued)*

Elements of the ICN Code (abbreviated)	Corresponding principles in the NMBA Code	Elements or principles that are unmatched
Element 2. Nurses and Practice *(Continued)*		
2.6 Share knowledge and expertise and provide feedback to support learning	Principle 5	
2.7 Are patient advocates	2.2.b In general 3.1.b Specifically to Aboriginal and Torres Strait Islander peoples	
2.8 May conscientiously object but must still facilitate access to care for patients	4.4 Broadly addresses this issue	
2.9 Specific support for giving and withdrawing consent to access personal, health and genetic information	Not addressed	
2.10 Taking appropriate actions when health is endangered	Not specifically addressed, but protection of the public addressed throughout	
2.11 Promotion of patient safety	See 2.1 but addressed throughout in different sections	
2.12 Accountability for data integrity	Not specifically stated but implicit in Principle 1	
Element 3. Nurses and the Profession		
3.1 Leads in determining and implementing standards for evidence-informed clinical nursing, management, research and education	See 2.1	
3.2 Develops core of research that supports evidence-based practice	Principle 6, Research in health	
3.3 Active in developing and sustaining a core of professional values	Not specifically addressed, but implicit	
3.4 Active through professional organisation in creating positive practice environment	Principle 7 VS 7.2	
3.5 Contributes to an ethical organisational environment and challenges unethical practices and settings	Not addressed from an ethical perspective, but Principle 1, Legal compliance, VS 1.3 Mandatory reporting does address the challenge in part	
3.6 Engage in research that improves outcomes	Principle 6	
3.7 Nurses prepare for and respond to emergencies, disasters, conflicts, epidemics, pandemics, social crises and conditions of scarce resources	Not addressed	

Continued on following page

TABLE 3.2		
The Elements of the ICN Code and Their Corresponding Principles in the NMBA Code for Nurses *(Continued)*		
Elements of the ICN Code (abbreviated)	Corresponding principles in the NMBA Code	Elements or principles that are unmatched
Element 4. Nurses and Global Health		
4.1 Value health care as a human right	Not addressed	
4.2 Uphold dignity, freedom and worth of all human beings and oppose all forms of exploitation, such as human trafficking and child labour	Not specifically addressed but 1.3 mandatory reporting mentions exploitation	
4.3 Lead or contribute to policy development	Principle 6	
4.4 Contribute to population health and SDGs	Principle 7	
4.5 Advocate for social determinants of health	Also referred to in Principle 7	
4.6 Environmental advocacy	7.2	
4.7 Collaboration to uphold principles of social justice	Principle 7	
4.8 International collaboration of global health	Broadly addressed in Principal 7	

as 'floors and ceilings'.[40] This analysis confirms that analogy. Many of the fundamental requirements for both safe and ethical practice are evident in both codes of conduct and codes of ethics. These include requirements such as confidentiality, privacy, informed consent, research, person (or woman)-centred care, legal compliance and compliance with professional standards. As discussed in **Chapter 2**, although these requirements can be viewed as moral or ethical mandates, they are so fundamental to professional practice that most of them are also enshrined in law and most of them are discussed as legal issues in this book.

However, it is encouraging to see some other commonalities emerging, particularly culturally sensitive practice and self-care. These are no longer seen as aspirational issues in a code of ethics but have now become so fundamental to nursing and midwifery practice that they are also enshrined in the codes of conduct.

A number of other key issues, not identified in the codes of ethics, are also set out as being baseline expectations in the codes of conduct. These include: adverse events and open disclosure; end-of-life care; the prohibition of bullying and harassment; the management of professional boundaries; advertising and professional representation; legal, insurance and other assessments; conflicts of interest; and financial arrangements and gifts. Some of these may seem to be quite commercial concerns for nurses and midwives, most of whom are employees in either the public or the private sectors.[41] However, under the National Registration and Accreditation Scheme, there has been an attempt to have similar principles contained in all codes of conduct across the 16 professions registered under the scheme[42] and, of course, other professions in the scheme operate far more in the commercial spectrum than do the majority of nurses and midwives. Having said that, privately practising midwives provide important services in Australia, particularly in relation to homebirth,[43] and privately practising nurse practitioners are on the increase.[44]

Some of the issues identified in the codes of ethics are clearly more aspirational and arguably it is desirable that midwives and nurses ought, not only to know what the minimum standards of professional behaviour entail, but also to aspire to be the best professionals they can be. For example, in the ICM Code the exhortation that 'no woman or girl should be harmed by conception or childbearing'[45] is incredibly important but may not always be within the control of a midwife to achieve and, unless it were within the midwife's control, could not justly be the subject of disciplinary proceedings. Similarly, in the ICN Code, there is the exhortation to 'preserve, sustain and protect the natural environment and [be] aware of the health consequences of environmental degradation, e.g. climate change',[46] an activity that all nurses ought to take on board as a matter of personal principle, but may yet find challenging in their professional role in terms of influencing the way this is played out (for example, in procurement of equipment). Many of the mandates and elements of the ICM and ICN Codes respectively lift the debate from what must be achieved in practical terms on a daily basis as a midwife or nurse to what it is desirable to achieve in the longer term as active participating members of professions that pride themselves on fostering and embodying social justice and compassion.

CONCLUSION

This chapter has set out to examine the two new codes of ethics adopted by the NMBA: the ICM Code and the ICN Code. It has explored the history of the development of codes of ethics and examined the ways in which they differ from codes of conduct, specifically, in this case, the NMBA codes of conduct for nurses and midwives. Finally, it has discussed why both are important and how both can be used.

CHAPTER 3 REVIEW QUESTIONS

Following your reading of **Chapter 3**, consider these questions in reaching the objectives of this chapter. Guidance on which part of the chapter will assist you in answering the questions can be found at http://evolve.elsevier.com/AU/Staunton/law/. You may, of course, consider other sources as part of your considerations.

1. Reflect on what each element or mandate from the codes discussed in this chapter means to you.

2. How could you use the relevant code of ethics in your practice domain: practice, education, research or management?

3. Discuss the ICM or ICN Code with co-workers and others.

4. Imagine a specific example from your own experience to identify an ethical dilemma and explore whether any of the codes — the ICM, ICN or NMBA Codes — would assist you to resolve the dilemma.

ENDNOTES

1. International Council of Nurses (ICN), *The ICN code of ethics for nurses*, 2021, https://www.icn.ch/system/files/2021-10/ICN_Code-of-Ethics_EN_Web_0.pdf.
2. International Confederation of Midwives (ICM), *International code of ethics for midwives*, 2008, https://www.internationalmidwives.org/assets/files/general-files/2019/10/eng-international-code-of-ethics-for-midwives.pdf Code reviewed 2014.
3. Numminen O, van der Arend A and Leino-Kilpi H, 'Nurses' codes of ethics in practice and education: a review of the literature', (2009) *Scandinavian Journal of Caring Sciences* 23(2):380–94. doi: 10.1111/j.1471-6712.2008.00608.x.
4. Meulenbergs T, Verpeet E, Schotsmans P and Gastmans C, 'Professional codes in a changing nursing context: literature review', (2004) *Journal of Advanced Nursing* 46(3):331–6. doi: 10.1111/j.1365-2648.2004.02992.x.
5. Oguisso T, Takashi M, de Freitas G, Bonini B and de Silva T, 'First international code of ethics for nurses', (2019) *Texto & Contexto — Enfermagem* 28, e20180140. https://www.redalyc.org/journal/714/71465278045/html/.
6. See Copeland D, 'Nurses' participation in the Holocaust: a call to nursing educators', (2021) *Journal of Professional Nursing* 37(2):426–428 for a challenging account.
7. International Council of Nurses (ICN), *The ICN code of ethics for nurses*, 2021, https://www.icn.ch/system/files/2021-10/ICN_Code-of-Ethics_EN_Web_0.pdf, p 2.
8. Chiarella M, *The legal and professional status of nursing*, Churchill Livingstone, Edinburgh, 2002.
9. ANCI, RCNA and ANF, *Code of ethics for nurses in Australia*, 2002, http://www.health.sapanta.com.au/srcn/code.pdf.
10. Ibid, p 1.
11. ACM, RCNA, ANF, *Code of ethics for midwives in Australia*, 2008, http://www.health.sapanta.com.au/srcn/code.pdf.
12. For detailed accounts of these publications see Staunton P and Chiarella M, *Nursing and the law*, 10th ed, Elsevier, Sydney, 2024, Chapter 4.

13. Johnstone M-J, 'Key milestones in the operationalisation of professional nursing ethics in Australia: a brief historical overview', (2016) *Australian Journal of Advanced Nursing* 33(4):35–45.

14. ICN, 2021, op. cit.

15. ICM, 2008, op. cit.

16. NMBA, *Code of conduct for nurses*, 2018 (updated June 2022), https://www.nursingmidwiferyboard.gov.au/Codes-Guidelines-Statements/Professional-standards.aspx.

17. NMBA, *Code of conduct for midwives*, 2018 (updated June 2022), https://www.nursingmidwiferyboard.gov.au/Codes-Guidelines-Statements/Professional-standards.aspx.

18. Johnstone M-J, 2016, op. cit.

19. Staunton P and Chiarella M, *Law for nurses and midwives*, 10th ed, Elsevier, Sydney, 2024, Chapter 2.

20. Verpeet E, de Casterlé B D, Lemiengre J and Gastmans C, 'Belgian nurses' views on codes of ethics: development, dissemination, implementation', (2006) *Nursing Ethics* 13(5):531–45. doi: 10.1191/0969733006nej896oa.

21. Snelling P C, 'The metaethics of nursing codes of ethics and conduct', (2016) *Nursing Philosophy* 17(4):229–49. doi: 10.1111/nup.12122.

22. Ibid.

23. Chiarella M, 'Regulatory standards: nurses' friend or foe?', in Gray G and Pratt R (eds), *Issues in Australian nursing*, Pearson Press, Melbourne, 1995, p 4.

24. Snelling P C, 2016, op. cit.

25. Johnstone M-J, *Bioethics: a nursing perspective*, Elsevier, Sydney, 2019, p 18. https://books.google.com.au/books?hl=en&lr=&id=PsWHEAAAQBAJ&oi=fnd&pg=PP1&dq=Johnstone+M-J+ethics+in+nursing&ots=QclTX_xyX4&sig=ikOg5uIpecSX_cRN4vj9GT8EDYc#v=onepage&q=Johnstone%20M-J%20ethics%20in%20nursing&f=false.

26. Chiarella M, 1995, op. cit.

27. Meulenbergs et al, 2004, op. cit., p 334.

28. Meulenbergs et al, 2004, op. cit.

29. Snelling P C, 2016, op. cit.

30. Nursing and Midwifery Board of Ireland, *Code of professional conduct and ethics for registered nurses and registered midwives*. Nursing and Midwifery Board of Ireland, Dublin, 2021.

31. ICN Code of Ethics for Nurses, op. cit., p 2.

32. ICM, 2008, op. cit., p 1.

33. ICN, 2021, op. cit., p 2.

34. Ibid, p 3.

35. Chiarella M, 1995, op. cit.

36. Ibid, p 4.

37. Ibid, p 4.

38. ICM, op. cit., pp 1–3.

39. Ibid, p 4.

40. Chiarella M, 1995, op. cit.

41. NMBA Codes of Conduct for Nurses and Midwives, op. cit.

42. Australian Health Practitioner Regulation Agency (Ahpra) website, 'Registration standards', https://www.ahpra.gov.au/Registration/Registration-Standards.aspx.

43. Forster D, McKay H, Davey M-A, Small R, Cullinane F, Newton M, Powell R and McLachlan H, 'Women's views and experiences of publicly-funded homebirth programs in Victoria, Australia: a cross-sectional survey', (2019) *Women and Birth* 32(3):221–30.

44. Currie J, Chiarella M and Buckley T, 'Workforce characteristics of privately practicing nurse practitioners in Australia: results from a national survey', (2016) *Journal of the American Association of Nurse Practitioners* 28:546–53.

45. ICM, 2008, op. cit., p 2.

46. ICN, 2021, op. cit., p 18.

Section 2

COMMENCING AS A PROFESSIONAL

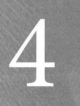

4

PROFESSIONAL REGULATION OF NURSES AND MIDWIVES

LEARNING OBJECTIVES

In this chapter, you will:

- examine the elements of professional regulation
- consider mechanisms for regulating those wishing to enter the professions of nursing and midwifery
- examine the standards required for registration and ongoing practice
- reflect on the specific requirements related to the regulation of midwifery
- explore mechanisms for making notifications and/or complaints about nurses and midwives.

INTRODUCTION

This chapter describes the Australian National Registration and Accreditation Scheme (the National Scheme), the first of its kind in a federated system in the world. The scheme has been in operation for 12 years at the time of writing and has had a number of reviews and legislative changes over that time.

On 1 July 2010 the National Scheme came into being as a result of legislation that passed in the Queensland Parliament. The scheme now entails fifteen health professional registration boards and one overarching management organisation — the Australian Health Practitioner Regulation Agency (Ahpra) — to support the boards and employ the staff members who work in the scheme. Ahpra is the organisation responsible for implementing the National Scheme across Australia.[1]

RELEVANT LEGISLATION AND STRUCTURE OF THE SCHEME

Legislation

Ahpra's operations are governed by the *Health Practitioner Regulation National Law Act 2009* (Qld) (hereafter the *National Law*), as in force in each state and territory, which came into effect on 1 July 2010. This law means that one Act of parliament governs the full operation and implementation of the National Scheme across the selected health professions, which, to date, are Aboriginal and Torres Strait Islander health practitioners, Chinese medical practitioners, chiropractors, dental practitioners (including dentists, dental hygienists, dental prosthetists and dental therapists), medical practitioners, medical radiation practitioners, nurses and midwives (including enrolled and registered nurses, endorsed midwives and rural and isolated practice nurses and nurse practitioners), occupational therapists, osteopathists, paramedics, pharmacists, physiotherapists, podiatrists and psychologists.

The object of the *National Law* is set out in Part 1, section 3(1) of the Schedule:

> … *to establish a national registration and accreditation scheme for —*
> a. *the regulation of health practitioners; and*
> b. *the registration of students undertaking —*
>   i. *programs of study that provide a qualification for registration in a health profession; or*
>   ii. *clinical training in a health profession.*

The objectives of the National Scheme are set out in section 3(2):

a. *to provide for the protection of the public by ensuring that only health practitioners who are suitably trained and qualified to practise in a competent and ethical manner are registered; and*

b. *to facilitate workforce mobility across Australia by reducing the administrative burden for health practitioners wishing to move between participating jurisdictions or to practise in more than one participating jurisdiction; and*

c. *to facilitate the provision of high quality education and training of health practitioners; and*

d. *to facilitate the rigorous and responsive assessment of overseas-trained health practitioners; and*

e. *to facilitate access to services provided by health practitioners in accordance with the public interest; and*

f. *to enable the continuous development of a flexible, responsive and sustainable Australian health workforce and to enable innovation in the education of, and service delivery by, health practitioners.*

The traditional purpose of a professional regulatory scheme is to protect the public; it has been said that those presiding over disciplinary tribunals and committees for the purpose of professional regulation exercise a 'protective jurisdiction'.[2] However, while the National Scheme upholds that tradition, it also has a number of other objectives relating to workforce mobility and flexibility. The system now works in the same way as the Australian drivers' licensing system — a person registers in one state, but their licence enables them to drive anywhere in Australia. Similarly, now, although a person might register, say, with the Northern Territory State Board of the Nursing and Midwifery Board of Australia, they will be able to practise nursing and/or midwifery in any jurisdiction in Australia. Thus, the National Scheme is intended to facilitate workforce mobility. This is clearly a desirable outcome. It was a new development to have this objective made explicit in a scheme that has traditionally been about protecting the public — a scheme which has on occasion been argued to limit access to certain professions and create monopolies.[3]

Structure

A Ministerial Council comprising Health Ministers from each state and territory and the Commonwealth has oversight of the National Scheme under the National Law. They currently meet as the Health Ministers Meeting (HMM).[4] The HMM may direct Ahpra and/or the Nursing and Midwifery Board of Australia (NMBA)[5] to implement policies and about matters regarding administrative processes, procedures or particular proposed accreditation standards or amendments. The matters cannot be about a particular person, qualification, application, notification or proceeding. In addition, the Health Ministers Meeting is required to approve registration standards recommended by the national board established for a particular health profession, but has the discretionary power to ask a national board to review an approved or proposed registration standard. The Health Ministers Meeting is comprised of the Health Ministers from each jurisdiction and the Federal Health Minister.[6]

The HMM has a number of specific roles and responsibilities, some of which have developed in direct response to the COVID-19 pandemic. It is supported by two main bodies, the Health National Cabinet Reform Committee (HNCRC) and the Health Chief Executives Forum (HCEF). The HNCRC is a National Cabinet committee that undertakes specific, time-limited tasks assigned directly by the National Cabinet. It manages matters of national significance that need all governments to work together. The HMM works with the HNCRC to align national priorities and achieve complementary work programs. The HCEF is an inter-governmental forum for joint decision-making and strategic policy discussions that helps to deliver health services efficiently in Australia. It is made up of the health department Chief Executive Officers from each state and territory and the Australian Government.[7] As previously stated, the National Scheme is administered by Ahpra, which is overseen by the Australian Health Practitioner Regulation Agency Board. This Board comprises at least five members — a Chairperson, two people with expertise in health and/or education and training, and two with business or administrative expertise. Current or recently registered health practitioners are not permitted to be the Board Chair or the two non-health Board members.[8] The functions of Ahpra (*inter alia*) are set out in **Box 4.1**.

BOX 4.1

FUNCTIONS OF THE AUSTRALIAN HEALTH PRACTITIONER REGULATION BOARD[9]

(a) to provide administrative assistance and support to the National Boards, and the Boards' committees, in exercising their functions;

(b) in consultation with the National Boards, to develop and administer procedures for the purpose of ensuring the efficient and effective operation of the National Boards;

(c) to establish procedures for the development of accreditation standards, registration standards and codes and guidelines approved by National Boards, for the purpose of ensuring the national registration and accreditation scheme operates in accordance with good regulatory practice;

(d) to negotiate in good faith with, and attempt to come to an agreement with, each National Board on the terms of a health profession agreement;

(e) to establish and administer an efficient procedure for receiving and dealing with applications for registration as a health practitioner and other matters relating to the registration of registered health practitioners;

(f) in conjunction with the National Boards, to keep up-to-date and publicly accessible national registers of registered health practitioners for each health profession;

(g) in conjunction with the National Boards, to keep up-to-date national registers of students for each health profession;

(h) to keep an up-to-date and publicly accessible list of approved programs of study for each health profession;

(i) to establish an efficient procedure for receiving and dealing with notifications against persons who are or were registered health practitioners and persons who are students, including by establishing a national process for receiving notifications about registered health practitioners in all professions;

(j) to give advice to the Ministerial Council on issues relating to the national registration and accreditation scheme;

(k) if asked by the Ministerial Council, to give to the Ministerial Council the assistance or information reasonably required by the Ministerial Council in connection with the administration of the national registration and accreditation scheme;

(ka) to do anything else necessary or convenient for the effective and efficient operation of the national registration and accreditation scheme;

(l) any other function given to the National Agency by or under this Law.

The National Boards

At the time of writing, there are 15 national boards. The one relevant to nurses and midwives is the Nursing and Midwifery Board of Australia.[10] Ahpra's national office provides support to the national boards, and the state, territory and regional offices provide support to the corresponding local boards of the national boards. Because of the sheer numbers of nurses and midwives in Australia, there is a committee of the NMBA in each jurisdiction. These committees are somewhat confusingly also called boards and they are tasked with administering the *National Law* by delegation from NMBA. The state and territory boards make all registration and notification decisions about individual nurses and midwives.[11]

The only exceptions are in New South Wales and Queensland, where co-regulatory models have been established to manage complaints, or notifications as they are called under the *National Law*. Notifications

in New South Wales and Queensland are managed by the Health Professional Councils Authority (HPCA) and the Office of the Health Ombudsman respectively.

Notifications about nurses and midwives in New South Wales are reviewed and determined by the Nursing and Midwifery Council of NSW. The HPCA provides administrative support to the 15 New South Wales Councils in their primary role to protect the public. The Councils, in cooperation with the Health Care Complaints Commission (HCCC), receive and process any notifications about registered health professionals.[12]

The Office of the Health Ombudsman is an independent statutory body and the agency that receives complaints by Queenslanders about a health service provider or health service provided to them, a family member or someone in their care.[13]

The powers of the national boards are governed by the *National Law* and their functions are set out in **Box 4.2**.

BOX 4.2
FUNCTIONS OF THE NATIONAL BOARDS[14]

35 (1) The functions of a National Board established for a health profession are as follows —

(a) to register suitably qualified and competent persons in the health profession and, if necessary, to impose conditions on the registration of persons in the profession;

(b) to decide the requirements for registration or endorsement of registration in the health profession, including the arrangements for supervised practice in the profession;

(c) to develop or approve standards, codes and guidelines for the health profession, including —

　(i) the approval of accreditation standards developed and submitted to it by an accreditation authority; and

　(ii) the development of registration standards for approval by the Ministerial Council; and

　(iii) the development and approval of codes and guidelines that provide guidance to health practitioners registered in the profession;

(d) to approve accredited programs of study as providing qualifications for registration or endorsement in the health profession;

(e) to oversee the assessment of the knowledge and clinical skills of overseas trained applicants for registration in the health profession whose qualifications are not approved qualifications for the profession, and to determine the suitability of the applicants for registration in Australia;

(f) to negotiate in good faith with, and attempt to come to an agreement with, the National Agency on the terms of a health profession agreement;

(g) to oversee the receipt, assessment and investigation of notifications about persons who —

　(i) are or were registered as health practitioners in the health profession under this Law or a corresponding prior Act; or

　(ii) are students in the health profession;

(h) to establish panels to conduct hearings about —

　(i) health and performance and professional standards matters in relation to persons who are or were registered in the health profession under this Law or a corresponding prior Act; and

　(ii) health matters in relation to students registered by the Board;

(i) to refer matters about health practitioners who are or were registered under this Law or a corresponding prior Act to responsible tribunals for participating jurisdictions;

(j) to oversee the management of health practitioners and students registered in the health profession, including monitoring conditions, undertakings and suspensions imposed on the registration of the practitioners or students;

(k) to make recommendations to the Ministerial Council about the operation of specialist recognition in the health profession and the approval of specialties for the profession;

(l) in conjunction with the National Agency, to keep up-to-date and publicly accessible national registers of registered health practitioners for the health profession;

(m) in conjunction with the National Agency, to keep an up-to-date national register of students for the health profession;

(n) at the Board's discretion, to provide financial or other support for health programs for registered health practitioners and students;

(o) to give advice to the Ministerial Council on issues relating to the national registration and accreditation scheme for the health profession;

(p) if asked by the Ministerial Council, to give to the Ministerial Council the assistance or information reasonably required by the Ministerial Council in connection with the national registration and accreditation scheme;

(q) to do anything else necessary or convenient for the effective and efficient operation of the national registration and accreditation scheme;

(r) any other function given to the Board by or under this Law.

PRINCIPLES OF THE NATIONAL SCHEME

The National Scheme has one main guiding principle and three other guiding principles, set out in the Schedule under the National Law, part one, s 3(a):

> (1) *The main guiding principle of the national registration and accreditation scheme is that the following are paramount—*
>   (a) *protection of the public;*
>   (b) *public confidence in the safety of services provided by registered health practitioners and students.*
> (2) *The other guiding principles of the national registration and accreditation scheme are as follows —*
>   (a) *the scheme is to operate in a transparent, accountable, efficient, effective and fair way;*
>   (aa) *the scheme is to ensure the development of a culturally safe and respectful health workforce that —*
>   (i) *is responsive to Aboriginal and Torres Strait Islander Peoples and their health; and*
>   (ii) *contributes to the elimination of racism in the provision of health services;*
>   (b) *fees required to be paid under the scheme are to be reasonable having regard to the efficient and effective operation of the scheme;*
>   (c) *restrictions on the practice of a health profession are to be imposed under the scheme only if it is necessary to ensure health services are provided safely and are of an appropriate quality.*[15]

The National Scheme is intended to provide uniformity through consistent national standards for registration and professional conduct and efficiency as a result of less 'red tape' and more streamlined processing. The scheme is also designed to increase collaboration through regular sharing and learning, thereby fostering more understanding between professions.

The concept of consistency is not intended to mean that 'one size fits all'. Despite a number of uniform requirements across the professions, such as professional indemnity insurance (PII) arrangements, continuing professional development (CPD), a minimum English Language Standard, criminal record and identity checks, and notifications, there is still a degree of difference in the way the professions impose their requirements. For example, nursing and midwifery have their own international respective codes of ethics (as was discussed in **Chapter 3**).

THE NATIONAL REGISTERS

Under the National Scheme there are national registers that the public can access online. Anyone can check a practitioner's registration status, simply by entering their name into a search engine and viewing the results.[16] The search will confirm that the person is registered and identify whether there are any *endorsements, notations, conditions, undertakings* or *reprimands* on their registration. If a health practitioner has the word 'registered' in the column 'registration status' they are registered and legally able to practise. This does not apply to practitioners on the non-practising register or those with a condition that stops them from practising, or where a registration has been suspended. However, health matters are not recorded there. The five terms written in italics are derived from the *National Law* and defined in a glossary on Ahpra's website.[17] The definitions are reproduced in **Table 4.1**.

There are now separate registers for nursing and midwifery. This means that a person can be registered as either a nurse or a midwife, or both. In addition, a person can opt to be practising or non-practising for the first time nationally. This means that people who wish to retain the title of registered nurse (RN) or registered midwife (RM) will be able to do so for a nominal fee even when they are not intending to practise.[18] However, if they wish to return to the practising register they would need to meet the requirements for re-entry to practice, which means that (*inter alia*) they must be able to demonstrate recency of practice.[19] In addition to being registered as an RN, it is also possible to be registered as an enrolled nurse (EN) (either solely or concurrently) and endorsed as a nurse practitioner (NP), which would primarily require registration as an RN. In addition to being registered as a midwife, it is also possible to be endorsed as a midwife practitioner and notated and endorsed to prescribe as a midwife.

TABLE 4.1
Definition of Key Terms that May Appear on a Health Practitioner's Registration

Key Term	Definition from Ahpra Glossary
Condition	A national board or an adjudication body can impose a condition on the registration of a practitioner or student, or on an endorsement of registration. A condition aims to restrict a practitioner's practice in some way, to protect the public.
	Conditions can be placed on a practitioner's registration for disciplinary reasons, such as because a national board has found that a practitioner has departed from accepted professional standards.
	Conditions can also be placed on a practitioner's registration for reasons that are not disciplinary, such as for a practitioner who is returning to practice after a break.
	Current conditions which restrict a practitioner's practice of the profession are published on the register of practitioners. When a national board or adjudication body decides they are no longer required to ensure safe practice, they are removed and no longer published.
	Examples of conditions include requiring the practitioner to: ■ complete specified further education or training within a specified period ■ undertake a specified period of supervised practice ■ do, or refrain from doing, something in connection with the practitioner's practice ■ manage their practice in a specified way ■ report to a specified person at specified times about the practitioner's practice, or ■ not employ, engage or recommend a specified person, or class of persons
	There may also be conditions related to a practitioner's health (such as psychiatric care or drug screening). The details of health conditions are not usually published on the register of practitioners.
	Also see the definition of Undertaking.
Endorsement	An endorsement of registration recognises that a person has an extended scope of practice in a particular area because they have an additional qualification that is approved by the national board ...
	There are a number of different types of endorsement available under the National Law, including: ■ scheduled medicines[1] ■ nurse practitioner ■ acupuncture, and ■ approved area of practice.
	In psychology, these are divided into 'subtypes' which describe additional qualifications and expertise ...
	An endorsement can include more than one 'subtype' ...
Notation	Is used by national boards to describe and explain the scope of a practitioner's practice by noting the limitations on that practice. The notation does not change the practitioner's scope of practice but may reflect the requirements of a registration standard.
Reprimand	A reprimand is a chastisement for conduct, a formal rebuke. Reprimands issued since the start of the National Scheme (1 July 2010 or 18 October 2010 in WA) are published on the Registers of Practitioners.
Undertaking	National boards can seek and accept an undertaking from a practitioner to limit the practitioner's practice in some way if this is necessary to protect the public. The undertaking means the practitioner agrees to do, or to not do something in relation to their practice of the profession. Current undertakings which restrict a practitioner's practice of the profession are published on the register of practitioners. When a national board or adjudication body decides they are no longer required to ensure safe practice, they are revoked and are no longer published. Current undertakings which relate to a practitioner's health are mentioned on the national register but details are not provided.
	An undertaking is voluntary, whereas a condition is imposed on a practitioner's registration.

[1]For registered nurses, there is an additional endorsement subtype to supply scheduled medicines (rural and isolated practice).

Both these qualifications require the applicant primarily to be registered as a midwife. Under section 15 of the *Health Practitioner Regulation National Law and Other Legislation Amendment Bill 2017*, section 113 of the *National Law* is amended to recognise the following protected titles: for midwifery the titles of midwife and midwife practitioner and for nursing the titles of nurse, registered nurse, nurse practitioner and enrolled nurse.

The Nursing and Midwifery Board of Australia

The NMBA was established on 1 July 2009 and commenced operation on 1 July 2010. It comprises one practitioner member from each jurisdiction (from among whom the Chair is appointed) and currently three community members. All members are permitted to hold office for three 3-year terms, although not all serve the three terms, as there is a need to ensure corporate memory among NMBA members through a staged renewal process.

Although the functions of all national boards as set out in the legislation (see **Box 4.2**) are the same, not all boards choose to exercise all functions. At the time of writing, NMBA has three sub-committees that provide the infrastructure for the determinations of the NMBA, and each of these sub-committees functions as a high-level policy and governance committee, using a 'hub and spoke' model for its day-to-day business. The NMBA provides the strong policy 'hub': oversight and endorsement of the registration and notification decisions of its state and territory boards. In turn, the state and territory boards provide the strong operational 'spokes' and implement the codes, policies and guidelines developed by the NMBA.

As was stated above, NMBA functions in a co-regulatory model, with a number of other organisations being involved in the regulatory process. For example, the element of professional regulation that comprises the accreditation of programs leading to registration, enrolment and endorsement is now undertaken by an independent authority, the Australian Nursing and Midwifery Accreditation Council (ANMAC).[20] This is discussed briefly at the end of this chapter, but it is important to differentiate between the role of ANMAC, which is to conduct the accreditation processes, and the role of the NMBA, which is only to endorse the recommendations of ANMAC in relation to the accreditation of programs.

The NMBA meets monthly and is supported in its work by a number of Ahpra staff, including an Executive Officer and designated policy support officers. In addition, the NMBA works closely with other senior executive staff of Ahpra and the other health professional regulatory bodies, at both national and jurisdictional levels.

Student Registration

Under the *National Law*, students undertaking courses leading to qualification as registered health practitioners have been registered from 2011. The only student group not to be registered is psychology students. (The Psychology Board of Australia has determined to register these students through provisional registration.) There are no fees for student registration.

Any student who is currently enrolled in an approved program of study is required to be registered. Students need not apply for registration personally, as Ahpra works directly with education providers to do this. The other group who must be registered as students comprises those who are not enrolled in an approved program of study, but are undertaking a clinical placement where they do not hold registration in that profession. It is the responsibility of the education provider (or the person or organisation providing the clinical placement) to advise Ahpra of students who need to be registered.

Ahpra advice is that the definition of an education provider in the *National Law* is broad. It includes education providers delivering board-approved programs of study leading to registration, and education providers, health services and other organisations, and in some cases individuals, who provide clinical experience placements for people who are undertaking 'clinical training', but are not enrolled in a board-approved program of study leading to registration and do not hold registration in Australia in that profession. The National Law has no definition of 'clinical training', but Ahpra has advised that section 91 has been taken to mean that it is:

> *any form of clinical experience (also known as clinical placements, rotations etc.) in a health profession AND where the person does not hold*

registration in the health profession in which the clinical training is being undertaken. This might apply, for example:

■ when an overseas student arranges a clinical placement as part of the course requirements set out by the education provider in their home country.[21]

THE ELEMENTS OF PROFESSIONAL REGULATION

Professional regulation is not solely the domain of those who usually claim to be professional regulators, such as health professions' boards and colleges. Governments already play a significant role in regulating health professionals through:

■ industrial and commercial remuneration systems;
■ legislation that grants access to therapeutic drugs and devices;
■ admission and visiting rights to hospitals and other healthcare facilities;
■ processes such as routine adverse event and clinical incident reporting; and
■ investigations and recommendations from commissions of inquiry.

Indeed, it has been argued that the serial killings committed by Dr Harold Shipman put an end to any possibility of medical self-regulation in the United Kingdom.[22] In the UK now, the ten statutory authorities that are required to regulate health and care professionals are overseen by the Professional Standards Authority for Health and Social Care whose role, it states, is to:

… set standards for regulators and carry out performance reviews each year to assess how well they meet them. Performance reviews tell everyone how well the regulators are doing and, through our recommendations, help the regulators to improve. We also conduct audits and investigations and can appeal fitness to practise cases to the courts if we consider that sanctions are insufficient to protect the public and it is in the public interest.[23]

Thus, the model in most countries is arguably not one of self-regulation, but rather of co-regulation, most usually with government, through a range of government agencies. This is the case in Australia.

Within the domain of professional self-regulation are four key elements:

■ who should enter the profession (registration);
■ how they might properly conduct themselves as members of that profession (codes and guidelines);
■ what criteria would need to be breached for them to be excluded from the profession (complaints and notifications);
■ what those who enter might look like (accreditation).[24]

These elements are set out in **Figure 4.1**.[25]

Standards for Initial Registration

The first element of professional regulation to be discussed is registration. Since its inception, the NMBA has been required to set and subsequently review a number of standards under the *National Law* in order to enable applicants to register. Nurses and midwives who have been off the register and wish to renew, and those who are applying for the first time, either because they have just completed an approved course of study in Australia or because they are applying from overseas, are required to meet the national registration eligibility criteria, including certain registration standards, some of which, as already stated, are mandatory across all health professions.

The *National Law* states that:

An individual is **qualified** for general registration in a health profession if —
(a) the individual holds an approved qualification for the health profession; or
(b) the individual holds a qualification the National Board established for the health profession considers to be substantially equivalent, or based on similar competencies, to an approved qualification; or
(c) the individual holds a qualification, not referred to in paragraph (a) or (b), relevant to the health profession and has successfully completed an examination or other assessment required by the National Board for the purpose of general registration in the health profession; or

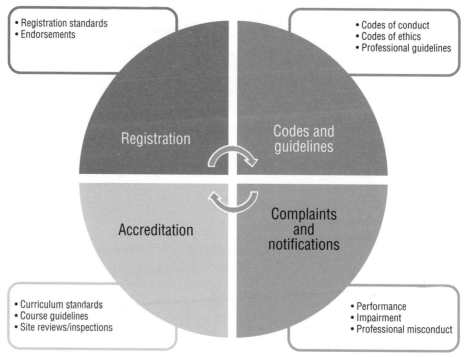

- Registration standards
- Endorsements

- Codes of conduct
- Codes of ethics
- Professional guidelines

Registration

Codes and guidelines

Accreditation

Complaints and notifications

- Curriculum standards
- Course guidelines
- Site reviews/inspections

- Performance
- Impairment
- Professional misconduct

Figure 4.1 ■ **Elements of professional regulation.**

(d) the individual —
(i) holds a qualification, not referred to in paragraph (a) or (b), that under this Law or a corresponding prior Act qualified the individual for general registration (however described) in the health profession; and
(ii) was previously registered under this Law or the corresponding prior Act on the basis of holding that qualification.[26]

In relation to internationally qualified nurses and midwives (IQNMs) wishing to apply for registration in Australia, a new system was introduced in 2020.[27] The new model of assessment includes an online self-check for all IQNMs, an orientation program for all IQNMs who are advised to continue with the assessment process, and an Outcomes Based Assessment (OBA) for some IQNMs. The OBA is a two-stage assessment process: a multiple-choice question exam (MCQ) and an objective structured clinical examination (OSCE). IQNMs must pass the first stage before moving to the

next stage. Stage one is a cognitive assessment, which is a computer-based MCQ exam. Stage two is a behavioural assessment in the form of an OSCE, which was developed to assess that an IQNM demonstrates the knowledge, skills and competence of a graduate-level Australian nurse or midwife.[28] In addition to the assessment, there is also a two-stage orientation program that IQNMs must undertake.[29] The first stage of the orientation process has to occur after the self-check and before the OBA, and the second stage within six months of becoming registered with the NMBA. The process has a range of fees attached to each stage of the assessment and these are set out on the NMBA website.[30]

In addition to being *qualified* for registration, section 52(1) of the *National Law* requires that a number of other requirements be met for a person to be *eligible* for registration:

1. An individual is eligible for general registration in a health profession if —
a. the individual is qualified for general registration in the health profession; and

b. *the individual has successfully completed —*
   i. *any period of supervised practice in the health profession required by an approved registration standard for the health profession; or*
   ii. *any examination or assessment required by an approved registration standard for the health profession to assess the individual's ability to competently and safely practise the profession; and*
c. *the individual is a suitable person to hold general registration in the health profession; and*
d. *the individual is not disqualified under this Law or a law of a co-regulatory jurisdiction from applying for registration, or being registered, in the health profession; and*
e. *the individual meets any other requirements for registration stated in an approved registration standard for the health profession.*[31]

CODES OF CONDUCT AND ETHICS AND COMPETENCY STANDARDS/ STANDARDS FOR PRACTICE

As seen in **Figure 4.1**, the second element of professional regulation is the setting of standards through the development of codes and guidelines. The NMBA sets standards for practice and provides codes, guidelines and advice.[32] In 2018 the NMBA published two new codes of conduct: one for nurses in Australia and one for midwives in Australia.[33] However, it has not updated its individual codes of ethics for nurses and midwives but has instead endorsed *The ICN code of ethics for nurses*[34] and the ICM's *International code of ethics for midwives*.[35] These international codes have been discussed and reviewed in **Chapter 3**.

The NMBA regularly reviews these key pieces of regulatory infrastructure and there is a strong commitment to redeveloping them and updating them, according to changes in the professions. To engage in comment on the NMBA's program of work and to see new documents when developed, check current consultations on the 'News' page of the NMBA website.[36]

As can be seen under section 52(1)(e), extracted above, there is an expectation that the profession will set one or more registration standards and that they will be approved by the HMM. The NMBA has developed five core registration standards, in addition to the obvious requirement for an approved qualification in nursing or midwifery. These are the:

- Continuing professional development (CPD) registration standard;
- Criminal history registration standard;
- English language skills (ELS) registration standard;
- Professional indemnity insurance (PII) arrangements registration standard;
- Recency of practice (RoP) registration standard.[37]

Each of these standards, apart from the CPD standard, needs to be met for a nurse or midwife to be eligible for registration. To be eligible for re-registration, the CPD standard is also required. While the Criminal history registration standard is identical across all professions, the CPD, ELS, PII and RoP standards may differ in their actual content.[38] The CPD, PII and RoP standards are discussed briefly here, but it is important for applicants to check the NMBA website as these registration standards are reviewed regularly and updated as new research and information becomes available. For example, a new ELS standard for nurses and midwives came into effect on 1 March 2019.[39]

It is important to note that these are standards for *registration* as a nurse or midwife and are not to be confused with standards for *endorsement* as an NP or as a prescribing midwife. These are both discussed separately; both take the requirements for eligibility for registration as the first step, after which the requirements for endorsement as an NP or prescribing midwife are cumulative.

Continuing Professional Development Registration Standard

The requirements for CPD are the same for ENs, RNs and RMs, although clearly the content will differ. This standard applies to all nurses and midwives who are on the register, but not to nurses and midwives applying to go onto the register. The requirements for the CPD standard are set out in **Box 4.3**.

Each registration standard is set out in a similar format, and each has an accompanying fact sheet. The fact sheets, published on the same page as the standard, are set out in a frequently asked questions (FAQ) format and contain definitions of key terms. An explanation of the 'context of practice', a term referred to in the

BOX 4.3
REQUIREMENTS OF THE CONTINUING PROFESSIONAL DEVELOPMENT REGISTRATION STANDARD[40]

All enrolled nurses, registered nurses and midwives must complete a minimum of 20 hours of CPD per registration period.

PRO RATA CPD REQUIREMENTS

If you have been registered for a period of less than 12 months prior to the renewal of registration, pro rata CPD requirements apply.

SPECIFIC REQUIREMENTS FOR NURSES WHO HOLD AN ENDORSEMENT

Registered nurses with an endorsement as a nurse practitioner or holding an endorsement for scheduled medicines must complete additional CPD requirements. These are described in the table below.

Nurses	CPD requirements	Total additional CPD hours	Total CPD hours
Nurse practitioner	Registered nurse — 20 hours Nurse practitioner endorsement — 10 additional hours relating to prescribing and administration of medicines, diagnostic investigations, consultation and referral	10 hours	30 hours
Registered nurse with scheduled medicines endorsement	Registered nurse — 20 hours Scheduled medicines endorsement — 10 additional hours relating to obtaining, supplying and administration of scheduled medicines	10 hours	30 hours

SPECIFIC REQUIREMENTS FOR MIDWIVES WHO HAVE A NOTATION OR HOLD AN ENDORSEMENT

If you have a notation as an eligible midwife or hold an endorsement as a midwife who holds an endorsement for scheduled medicines, you must complete additional CPD requirements. These are described in the table below.

Midwives	CPD requirements	Total additional CPD hours	Total CPD hours
Midwife with a notation and/or scheduled medicines endorsement	Midwife — 20 hours Endorsement and/or notation — 10 additional hours relating to context of practice, prescribing and administration of medicines, diagnostic investigations, consultation and referral	10 hours	30 hours

SPECIFIC REQUIREMENTS FOR PEOPLE REGISTERED AS BOTH A NURSE AND A MIDWIFE

If you are registered as either an enrolled nurse or a registered nurse and a midwife, you must complete the required amount of CPD for both nursing and midwifery.

If your CPD activities are relevant to both the nursing profession and the midwifery profession, you may count those activities as evidence for both nursing and midwifery CPD hours.

EVIDENCE OF CPD

Records of CPD activities must be kept for a period of 5 years from the date of the CPD completion. All CPD records must be available for audit or if needed by the NMBA as part of an investigation arising from a notification (complaint). All evidence of CPD should be verified, and must demonstrate that the nurse or midwife has:

- identified and prioritised their learning needs, based on their self-reflection and evaluation of their practice against the relevant competency or professional practice standards;
- developed a learning plan based on identified learning needs;
- participated in effective learning activities appropriate to their learning needs; and
- reflected on the value of the learning activities or the effect that participation will have on their practice.

The format of this evidence is not defined by the NMBA and may take many forms. Evidence of CPD activities should be kept, such as certificates of attainment and/or attendance and notes from self-directed CPD activity such as a literature review, case study or journal articles. Any notes submitted should provide a comprehensive summary of the key points of the review and reflect the learning from the activity.

CPD guideline, is included in the CPD fact sheet. It is defined as follows:

> Context of practice refers to the conditions that define an individual's nursing and/or midwifery practice. These include:
> - the type of practice setting (e.g. clinical care, management, administration, education, research)
> - the location of the practice setting (e.g. urban, rural, remote)
> - the characteristics of patients (e.g. health status, age, learning needs)
> - the focus of nursing and/or midwifery activities (e.g. health promotion, research, management)
> - the degree to which practice is autonomous, and
> - the resources that are available, including access to other healthcare professionals.[41]

Professional Indemnity Insurance (PII) Arrangements Registration Standard

Under the National Scheme, all health practitioners are required to state on their application and renewal forms that they will not practise their profession unless they have appropriate PII arrangements in place.

PII may be obtained in two main ways: an employer may agree to indemnify an employee as part of the employment contract, and also as a result of the doctrine of vicarious liability (see **Chapter 7**); or it may be purchased as a commercial product, in the same way as any other form of insurance, for nurses and midwives whose employment status indicates that they are not indemnified through the doctrine of vicarious liability. The requirements of the PII standard for nurses and midwives are set out in **Box 4.4**.

PII arrangements are defined in the PII standard as:

> … arrangements that secure for the practitioner's professional practice, insurance against civil liability incurred by, or loss arising from, a claim that is made as a result of a negligent act, error or omission in the conduct of the practitioner. This type of insurance is available to practitioners and organisations across a range of industries and covers the cost and expenses of defending a legal claim, as well as any damages payable. Some government organisations under policies of the owning

government are self-insured for the same range of matters.[42]

The PII standard applies to RNs and ENs, RNs endorsed as NPs, and RMs. It does not apply to students of nursing and midwifery, nurses and midwives who have non-practising registration, and RMs who are exempted under the *National Law*.[43] It is important that nurses and midwives check the NMBA website regularly for the most up-to-date advice, as it is a relatively recent development for nursing and midwifery regulatory authorities to become involved in advice about PII.

PII for privately practising midwives (PPMs) is particularly complex and is discussed later in this chapter.[44]

Recency of Practice Registration Standard

The RoP standard requires nurses and midwives to keep up to date with their practice for a minimum period of 450 hours within the past 5 years.[45] Alternatively they could demonstrate successful completion of a program or assessment approved by the NMBA or successful completion of a period of supervised practice approved by the NMBA.[46]

This seems to be a sensible means of ensuring that nurses and midwives stay in touch with professional practice.

The RoP standard applies to nurses and midwives seeking registration, endorsement of registration or renewal of registration.[47] It does not apply to recent graduates from nursing or midwifery programs in Australia applying for registration for the first time, persons holding student registration, nurses or midwives holding non-practising registration, or applicants for non-practising registration. 'Practice' is defined very broadly under the standard as:

> … any role, whether remunerated or not, in which the individual uses their skills and knowledge as a health practitioner in their profession. Practice in this context is not restricted to the provision of direct clinical care. It also includes using professional knowledge (working) in a direct non-clinical relationship with clients, working in management, administration, education, research, advisory, regulatory or policy development roles, and any other roles that impact on the safe, effective delivery of services in the profession.[48]

BOX 4.4

REQUIREMENTS OF PROFESSIONAL INDEMNITY INSURANCE ARRANGEMENTS REGISTRATION STANDARD[49]

1. When you practise as a nurse and/or a midwife, you must be covered by either your own or third party PII arrangements that meet this standard:
   a. for all aspects of your practice
   b. that cover for all locations where you practise
   c. that provide cover for you whether you are working in the private sector, non-government sector and/or public sector, and
   d. that provide cover for you whether you are practising full-time, part-time, self-employed, employed, or in an unpaid or volunteer capacity, or any combination of these factors.
2. Your PII cover must include:
   a. civil liability cover
   b. appropriate retroactive cover for otherwise uncovered matters arising from prior practice, and
   c. automatic reinstatement
   or
   d. the equivalent of 2a to 2c above under third party PII arrangements.

3. If you are covered by a third party PII arrangement, it must meet this standard. If you are in any doubt about whether the third party cover meets this standard, you should always ask what is covered by the third party PII arrangement.
   If the third party cover does not meet this standard you must take out additional cover to ensure this standard is met.
4. If any area of your practice is specifically excluded from your PII cover, you must not practise in that area.
5. If your PII arrangements are provided by your employer, and you intend to practise outside your stated employment, you must have individual PII arrangements in place to cover that practice. This may include cover for undertaking:
   ■ practical components of continuing professional development
   ■ study involving patient treatment, or
   ■ volunteer work (unless already separately covered in that capacity, for example, by the volunteering organisation).

The requirements for the RoP standard are set out in **Box 4.5**.[50]

The requirements for those in clinical practice are further explained in the fact sheet on the RoP standard.[51] A new re-entry to practice policy was released in February 2019 for those nurses who do not meet the RoP registration standard. The new policy lays out the paths to be taken by people in different 'assessment categories' returning to practice:

■ people who are no longer on the register and have not practised for a period of between 5 and 10 years;
■ persons holding general registration who have not practised for between 5 and 10 years;
■ nurses and midwives holding non-practising registration who have not practised for between 5 and 10 years seeking general registration as a registered nurse, enrolled nurse, or midwife; and
■ persons who have not practised for a period of 10 years or more.[52]

The policy sets out fairly unequivocal rules about the paths to be taken by each category.

ENDORSEMENTS UNDER SECTION 94 OF THE *NATIONAL LAW*

Along with the five registration standards that relate to nursing and midwifery entry requirements, there are also other registration standards that relate to specific categories of RNs and RMs that impose further requirements upon them. Under section 94, the NMBA has previously issued two endorsements: the rural and isolated practice nurses (RIPN) Registration standard for endorsement for scheduled medicines for registered nurses (rural and isolated practice)[53] and the Registration standard for endorsement for scheduled medicines for midwives,[54] which is discussed later in this chapter.

Section 94 of the *National Law* states that:

1. *A National Board may, in accordance with an approval given by the Ministerial Council under section 14, endorse the registration of a registered health practitioner registered [by the Board], as being qualified to administer, obtain,*

BOX 4.5

REQUIREMENTS OF RECENCY OF PRACTICE REGISTRATION STANDARD[55]

Practice hours are recognised as meeting this standard if:

- the nurse or midwife holds current and valid registration with a recognised nursing or midwifery regulatory authority (either in Australia or overseas), or
- the nurse or midwife's role involves the application of nursing and/or midwifery knowledge and skills, or
- the nurse or midwife has carried out postgraduate education leading to an award or qualification that is relevant to the practice of nursing and/or midwifery.

The NMBA acknowledges two main areas of practice in the profession for the purposes of this registration standard.

NURSES AND MIDWIVES IN CLINICAL PRACTICE

Enrolled nurses, registered nurses and midwives will fulfil the recency of practice requirements if they can demonstrate one or more of the following:

- completion of a minimum of 450 hours of practice within the past five years;

- successful completion of a program or assessment approved by the NMBA;
- successful completion of a period of supervised practice approved by the NMBA.

NURSES AND MIDWIVES IN NON-CLINICAL PRACTICE

Nurses and midwives working in non-clinical practice are required to meet the recency of practice standard. If they have recent clinical practice they are deemed to be recent in non-clinical practice.

During the yearly registration renewal process all nurses and midwives must declare whether they continue to meet this registration standard.

Nurses and midwives should retain records as evidence that the requirements of this standard are met for five years in case an audit occurs.

---

possess, prescribe, sell, supply or use a scheduled medicine or class of scheduled medicines if the practitioner —

a. holds either of the following qualifications relevant to the endorsement —
    i.   an approved qualification;
    ii. another qualification that, in the Board's opinion, is substantially equivalent to, or based on similar competencies to, an approved qualification; and
b. complies with any approved registration standard relevant to the endorsement.

Note. The endorsement of a health practitioner's registration under this section indicates the practitioner is qualified to administer, obtain, possess, prescribe, sell, supply or use the scheduled medicine or class of medicines specified in the endorsement but does not authorise the practitioner to do so. The authorisation of a health practitioner to administer, obtain, possess, prescribe, sell, supply or use scheduled medicines in a participating jurisdiction will be provided for by or under another Act of that jurisdiction.

Health practitioners registered in certain health professions will be authorised to administer,

obtain, possess, prescribe, sell, supply or use scheduled medicines by or under an Act of a participating jurisdiction without the need for the health practitioners to hold an endorsement under this Law.

2. An endorsement under subsection (1) must state —
    a. the scheduled medicine or class of scheduled medicines to which the endorsement relates; and
    b. whether the registered health practitioner is qualified to administer, obtain, possess, prescribe, sell, supply or use the scheduled medicine or class of scheduled medicines; and
    c. if the endorsement is for a limited period, the date the endorsement expires.

In 2022 the NMBA made the announcement that (finally) it would retire the endorsement for scheduled medicines for registered nurses in rural and isolated practice. RNs who currently held the RIP endorsement were able to renew for the 2022 renewal period if they wished to do so. Victoria and Queensland, the two states that had still required RNs to hold the RIP endorsement, developed alternative contemporary regulatory mechanisms for RNs to obtain, supply and administer certain scheduled medicines in rural and isolated practice settings without the RIP endorsement. Such changes enabled the model of care in remote and isolated practice to continue without the need for regulation by the NMBA. Thus, the day-to-day practice of previously RIP endorsed RNs did not change.

However, RNs who did not renew their RIP endorsement during the registration renewal period were still able to continue their medicines practice in rural and isolated practice settings and their day-to-day practice did not change. NMBA made the following announcement on its website in 2021.

> All Australian states and territories can now regulate the safe use of medicines by rural and isolated practice registered nurses (RNs) through local medicines and poisons legislation, policies and protocols. Therefore, there is no longer a need for additional regulation by the NMBA, and the Registration standard …
>
> Queensland changes
>
> In September 2021, Queensland established a new medicines and poisons regulatory framework that enables rural and isolated practice RNs to continue to obtain, supply and administer certain medicines via an extended practice authority. Under the new framework, the day-to-day practice of Queensland RNs who hold the RIP endorsement remains unchanged. For further information, please see Queensland Health's website.
>
> Victorian changes
>
> In February 2022, Victoria finalised changes to its drugs and poisons regulatory scheme. A new legal mechanism called a secretary approval, now enables scheduled medicines practice including conditions of practice such as experience, qualifications, location, type of medicines and clinical circumstances.
>
> Under Victoria's new drugs and poisons regulatory scheme, the current practice of rural and isolated practice RNs remains unchanged. For further information, please see the Victorian Department of Health's website.[56]

As can be seen from the note in section 94 above, even where an RN is endorsed as qualified under this standard, the relevant legislation to authorise the endorsed RN to undertake those activities still resides with the employing jurisdiction, usually under relevant drugs and poisons legislation.

ENDORSEMENT AS A NURSE PRACTITIONER UNDER SECTION 95 OF THE *NATIONAL LAW*

Under section 95 of the *National Law* there is a nationally consistent standard for endorsement as an NP. (There is also provision for endorsement as a midwife practitioner under section 96 of the *National Law*. However, as is explained later in this chapter, this provision has not been used as there is only one midwife practitioner currently endorsed in Australia, and this person transitioned across from a jurisdictional registration.)

Section 95 of the *National Law* states that:

1. *The Nursing and Midwifery Board of Australia may endorse the registration of a registered health practitioner whose name is included in the Register of Nurses as being qualified to practise as a nurse practitioner if the practitioner —*
   a. *holds either of the following qualifications relevant to the endorsement —*
      i. *an approved qualification;*
      ii. *another qualification that, in the Board's opinion, is substantially equivalent to, or based on similar competencies to, an approved qualification; and*
   b. *complies with any approved registration standard relevant to the endorsement.*
2. *An endorsement under subsection (1) must state —*
   a. *that the registered health practitioner is entitled to use the title 'nurse practitioner'; and*
   b. *any conditions applicable to the practice by the registered health practitioner as a nurse practitioner.*

Under section 95(1)(b), the NMBA has developed the *Endorsement as a nurse practitioner registration standard*[57] that applies to all applicants seeking endorsement

BOX 4.6
REQUIREMENTS FOR ENDORSEMENT AS A NURSE PRACTITIONER[58]

When applying for endorsement as a nurse practitioner, a nurse must be able to demonstrate all of the following.

1. Current general registration as an RN in Australia with no conditions or undertakings on their registration relating to unsatisfactory professional performance or unprofessional conduct.
2. The equivalent of three years' (5,000 hours) full-time experience at an advanced practice level, within the past six years, from the date when the application seeking endorsement as an NP is received by the NMBA.

Note: Advanced practice hours that are part of an NMBA-approved program of study cannot be included as evidence towards the 5000 hours of advanced practice.

3. Successful completion of:
   - Pathway 1: an NMBA-approved program of study leading to endorsement as an NP, or
   - Pathway 2: a program that is substantially equivalent to an NMBA-approved program of study leading to endorsement as an NP, as determined by the NMBA.
4. Compliance with the NMBA Nurse practitioner standards for practice.

ONGOING REQUIREMENTS FOR ENDORSEMENT

Ongoing endorsement by the NMBA is conditional on the nurse practitioner complying with the current:

1. NMBA-approved Continuing professional development registration standard, Recency of practice registration standard, Criminal history registration standard and Professional indemnity insurance arrangements registration standard, and
2. Safety and quality guidelines for nurse practitioners and any other applicable codes and guidelines approved by the NMBA.

---

as an NP. The requirements for endorsement are set out in **Box 4.6**.

The *Nurse practitioner standards for practice* were most recently revised in 2021[59] and the definition of advanced practice was also updated.[60] The new definition of advanced practice reads as follows:

> *Advanced practice is where nurses incorporate professional leadership, education, research and support of systems into their practice. Their practice includes relevant expertise, critical thinking, complex decision-making, autonomous practice and is effective and safe. They work within a generalist or specialist context and they are responsible and accountable in managing people who have complex healthcare requirements. Advanced practice in nursing is demonstrated by a level of practice and not by a job title or level of remuneration. Advanced practice for the purpose of the nurse practitioner endorsement requires 5000 hours clinically-based advanced practice in the past six years.*[61]

In 2016, the NMBA revised the safety and quality guidelines (SQG) for NPs.[62] The guidelines comprise the following elements:

- scope of practice;
- context of practice;
- codes of professional conduct and ethics;
- standards for practice;
- annual declaration;
- NMBA audit process;
- mandatory reporting;
- notification and management of performance, conduct or health matters;
- professional indemnity insurance;
- recency of practice;
- continuing professional development;
- Medicare Australia and Pharmaceutical Benefits Scheme arrangements;
- collaborative arrangements; and
- prescribing authority and compliance with state and territory legislation.[63]

There is also a definition section that makes specific reference to scope of practice. Scope of practice is defined as follows:

> **Scope of practice** *is the full spectrum of roles, functions, responsibilities, activities and decision-making capacity that individuals within that profession are educated, competent and authorised to perform. Some functions within the scope of practice of any profession may be shared with other professions or other individuals or groups. The scope of practice of all health professions is influenced*

by the wider environment, the specific setting, legislation, policy, education, standards and the health needs of the population. The scope of practice of an individual is that which the individual is educated, authorised and competent to perform. The scope of practice of an individual nurse or midwife may be more specifically defined than the scope of practice of their profession. To practise within the full contemporary scope of practice of the profession may require individuals to update or increase their knowledge, skills or competence. Decisions about both the individual's and the profession's practice can be guided using the Decision-making framework (DMF). When making these decisions, nurses and midwives need to consider their individual and their respective profession's scope of practice.[64]

As with the provisions under section 94, authority to prescribe medicines is conferred under the relevant drugs and poisons legislation of the Australian state or territory in which the NP practises. The conditions under which each authority is granted and the scope of that authority will depend on the requirements of the specific piece of legislation. These may range from a blanket authority limited by the NP's scope of practice to a prescribing authority based on a formulary or protocol, or related to a specific context of practice (such as being applicable only in a certain practice setting). To specify a distinct formulary of medicines for each area of specialty of NPs is outside the provisions of the *National Law*. However, nurse practitioners are clearly expected to function within the requirements of the legislation in their jurisdiction.[65]

The NMBA's *Guidelines: For nurses applying for endorsement as a nurse practitioner* explain (*inter alia*) the processes and evidence required both for initial and ongoing endorsement as an NP.[66]

The NMBA recognises that nurses obtain and develop specialist qualifications and expertise throughout the course of their careers and expects NPs to be competent in their specific area of practice to meet the needs of their client group. Nurses seeking endorsement as NPs must have completed 3 years advanced practice in their specific area of practice (within the preceding 6 years) before applying for endorsement.[67] The NMBA states that advanced practice requires the following evidence to be provided:

You are required to provide evidence of practising at the advanced practice level in accordance with the NMBA definition.

This means you must clearly document examples of the following in your application:
- *Leadership*
- *Education activities*
- *Research*
- *Support of systems*
- *Autonomous practice*
- *Complex decision-making*
- *Management of, and direct clinical care of people with complex health conditions*

You can provide this evidence in your CV or through case studies. If you choose to provide case studies these cannot be the same as case studies used for your Master of Nursing (NP) program.

Statement/s of service

The Statement of service is provided as part of your application to support your 5000 hours of advanced practice. The Statement of service should clearly reflect the evidence you have provided in your CV and:
- *be on the employer's letterhead*
- *be dated and signed by the Director of Nursing or equivalent*
- *detail the title of your advanced practice, dates of employment and hours*
- *detail any periods of extended leave (e.g. long service leave, maternity/paternity or extended sick leave)*
- *provide a breakdown/percentage of hours of any position that includes indirect or non-clinical components, such as management or education*
- *be correctly certified — refer to Ahpra's guidance on certification of documents.*

Note: Self-employed nurses may provide a statutory declaration as their proof of service.[68]

Given the dynamic nature of healthcare and the evolving role of NPs, a scope of practice notation is not included on the endorsement. Nevertheless, there is an expectation that the NP will practise only in that specific area and in accordance with the NP SQG. The SQG makes it clear that, should an NP decide to expand or change their scope of practice to meet the needs of their client group, they must make sure they have the appropriate skills, knowledge and education to ensure they remain safe and competent to practise at the advanced practice level, which may include the NP undertaking further postgraduate education and skill development. If the NP is employed, their employer is also obligated to ensure that the NP is educated, authorised and competent to perform any change to their scope of practice if this is required to meet the needs of their client group.[69] NPs planning to change scope must use the NMBA-approved *National framework for the development of decision-making tools for nursing and midwifery practice* to ensure they are competent in their proposed expanded or new scope of practice.[70]

NPs must also meet the NMBA's requirements for annual renewal of registration and endorsement. Failure to comply with the NP SQGs will incur disciplinary action by the NMBA that, if proven, carries considerable consequences for NPs.[71]

NURSE PRACTITIONERS' ACCESS TO THE AUSTRALIAN GOVERNMENT MEDICARE BENEFITS SCHEME (MBS) AND PHARMACEUTICAL BENEFITS SCHEME (PBS)

Endorsement as an NP with the NMBA confers eligibility to apply for approval by the Health Minister as a 'participating nurse practitioner' under the *Health Legislation Amendment (Midwives and Nurse Practitioners) Act 2010* (Cth). This is a significant development in terms of equity of access to patients cared for by NPs, as it means that they are able to obtain Medicare rebates for the services of an NP as well as subsidised medicines via the PBS through prescriptions written by an NP. At the time of writing, this applies only to NPs who are in private practice, but it is hoped that this will extend to NPs who are employees working in community settings, particularly in relation to prescribing.

What this participation means is that a participating NP has access to the MBS and, where the NP has an authority to prescribe, the PBS. These arrangements will enable patients of NPs who are approved MBS and/or PBS participants to access certain MBS rebates and PBS prescriptions.

To bill under Medicare, nurse practitioners must:

- complete approved education
- be recognised as a nurse practitioner by Services Australia
- be registered with the Nursing and Midwifery Board of Australia
- have a Medicare provider number to bill for services listed on the Medicare Benefits Schedule (MBS)
- enter into a collaborative arrangement with a medical practitioner.

Services Australia has Medicare information for nurse practitioners, including eligibility requirements and guides on bulk billing. Its Health Professional Education Resources Gateway also has guides on MBS items for nurse practitioners.[72]

Currently the access to MBS item numbers and PBS prescriptions is very limited. Services Australia acknowledges this on its website where it states that 'if you're an eligible nurse practitioner or midwife you can access some items under the Medicare Benefits Schedule and limited items under the Pharmaceutical Benefits Scheme on the PBS website'.[73]

Each NP must apply to Medicare Australia for a provider and/or prescriber number. The discretion to authorise access to the MBS and PBS remains with Medicare. This process of authorisation is additional to the NMBA's endorsement process. Medicare monitors and reviews the system to ensure that services and medicines provided by any health professional with access to the MBS and PBS are effective, efficient, appropriate and within benchmarking limits.

As part of the co-regulatory requirements of the NMBA and Medicare, any issues related to conduct, performance or health that may impact on the performance of an individual NP, as a prescriber or provider of Medicare services or medicines, is notified by either body to the other. For example, if Medicare has cause to investigate a particular provider, NMBA will be notified of that investigation, and vice versa. However, should there be an issue related to the performance, health or conduct of an NP, the notification will be referred to the NMBA, who will oversee the assessment of the notification and any subsequent investigation or disciplinary action.[74] It is sincerely hoped that the new government will make concerted efforts to enable NPs to practise to full scope of practice to facilitate equity and access for the client groups they serve.[75]

THE REGULATION OF MIDWIFERY

Midwifery has been recognised nationally as a profession distinct from, but aligned with, nursing. This has now been enacted into the *National Law*. Under section 15 of the *Health Practitioner Regulation National Law and Other Legislation Amendment Bill 2017*, both midwife and midwifery are recognised as protected titles and the Act also formalises the recognition of midwifery as a separate profession by inserting the term 'National Board for the midwifery profession' when midwives are mentioned separately. This is congruent with many other developed countries that recognise both direct entry and postgraduate pathways into nursing and midwifery.[76] The major difference in Australia's National Scheme is that there are now separate registers for nursing and midwifery, which means that people who have a sole qualification in midwifery are able to register solely as a midwife. Formerly in some jurisdictions, this was not possible and created difficulties for overseas-qualified midwives who did not have a nursing qualification but who may otherwise have wished to practise midwifery in Australia.

In addition, the option to be on the non-practising register will mean that, from a workforce perspective, there is a better understanding of the size of the practising midwifery workforce, rather than simply having a sense of how many people hold a midwifery qualification.

The requirements to be eligible to register as a midwife are similar to those to be eligible to register as a nurse — namely, the applicant must meet the eligibility requirements set out under section 52 of the *National Law*. The difference is that the approved program of study referred to in section 53 is in midwifery, rather than in nursing, and that recency of practice relates to midwifery practice. Upon renewal, the requirements for CPD also need to relate to a midwifery context of practice, although if a midwife is also registered as a nurse and any CPD undertaken for nursing also relates to midwifery practice it can be claimed for both contexts.[77]

Where the major differences occur are in relation to the *Registration standard for endorsement for scheduled medicines for midwives* under section 94[76] and the PII requirements for PPMs, particularly those who wish to provide homebirth services.[78] In 2017 the NMBA released *Registration standard: endorsement for scheduled medicines.*[79]

Registration Standard for Endorsement for Scheduled Medicines for Midwives Under Section 94

This registration standard, under section 94 of the *National Law*, is the means by which midwives are able to be endorsed to prescribe selected medications. The wording to appear on the register is:

> *An endorsed midwife qualified to prescribe schedule 2, 3, 4 and 8 medicines and to provide associated services required for midwifery practice in accordance with relevant state and territory legislation.*[80]

The requirements of this endorsement are set out in **Box 4.7**.[81] Two key issues in relation to this endorsement are worthy of note. First, a newly graduated midwife cannot be endorsed. A minimum equivalent of 3 years full-time midwifery experience after the initial registration as a midwife is required. Second, midwives need to complete an NMBA-approved program of study leading to endorsement (or substantially equivalent program of study).

Professional Indemnity Insurance Requirements for Privately Practising Midwives

To practise, a registered health practitioner is required under the *National Law* to have appropriate PII arrangements in place.[82] This is not usually a problem for midwives who are employees of large organisations, because the doctrine of vicarious liability likely applies (see Chapter 7).

From 1 July 2010, privately practising midwives have had access to Australian Government-supported PII and can purchase insurance from Medical Insurance Group Australia (MIGA). However, the Government-supported insurance does not cover the planned delivery of babies in the home.

BOX 4.7
ENDORSEMENT FOR SCHEDULED MEDICINES FOR MIDWIVES

1. Current general registration as a midwife in Australia with no conditions or undertakings relating to unsatisfactory professional performance or unprofessional conduct
2. Registration as a midwife that is the equivalent of three years' full-time clinical practice (5,000 hours) in the past six years that is either:
   ■ across the continuum of care, or
   ■ in a specified context of practice from the date when the complete application seeking endorsement for scheduled medicines is received by the NMBA.
3. Successful completion of:
   ■ an NMBA-approved program of study leading to endorsement for scheduled medicines, or

■ a program that is substantially equivalent to an NMBA-approved program of study leading to endorsement for scheduled medicines as determined by the NMBA.

Ongoing endorsement by the NMBA is conditional on the midwife complying with the current:

1. NMBA-approved Continuing professional development registration standard, Recency of practice registration standard, Criminal history registration standard and Professional indemnity insurance arrangements registration standard
2. any other applicable codes and guidelines approved by the NMBA, and
3. for midwives who are privately practising midwives the Safety and quality guidelines for privately practising midwives.

There are a number of specific requirements that midwives must meet to qualify for this insurance cover. Section 284 of the *National Law* outlines a number of requirements making it possible for midwives in private practice to be able to provide intrapartum care at a homebirth for women and their infants, without having the PII cover required for all other aspects of midwifery care across antenatal care and postnatal care.

As previously stated, under section 284 of the *National Law,* there are a set of requirements that provide for exemption from PII arrangements for midwives practising private midwifery, but they are strictly limited to those who provide intrapartum services for women planning to have homebirths. Midwives working in private practice will still require appropriate insurance to provide antenatal and postnatal care to women in their care, regardless of the planned location of the birth.[83]

Section 284 of the *National Law* is a transitional provision and this exemption will be available only from 1 July 2010 to 30 June 2025.[84]

As stated above, to be granted an exemption from holding PII for homebirths, PPMs are required to meet a set of specified requirements under section 284(1)(b) and (c) of the *National Law*. Section 284(1)(b) states that 'the woman in relation to whom the midwife is practising private midwifery' must have given

'informed consent'. The *National Law* defines 'informed consent' in section 284(5) as:

… written consent given by a woman after she has been given a written statement by a midwife that includes:

■ *a statement that appropriate professional indemnity insurance arrangements will not be in force in relation to the midwife's practise of private midwifery; and*

■ *any other information required by the National Board.*

Section 284(1)(c)(i) requires the midwife to comply with 'any requirement in a code or guideline about reports to be provided by midwives practising private midwifery'. The Board has a number of codes and guidelines specifically for midwives, some of which have been discussed earlier, such as the *Code of conduct for midwives* and the *ICM Code of ethics for midwives*.

For the PII exemption to apply under the National Scheme and satisfy NMBA requirements, midwives in private practice will be required to demonstrate they meet all obligations in another set of guidelines, the NMBA's *Safety and quality guidelines for privately practising midwives*.[85]

Despite the specific differences, there are also many similarities in the law regulating nurses and midwives, and indeed other health professionals. The NMBA has adopted and/or developed a number of other guidelines for nurses and midwives, some of which make separate reference to the two professions and others which are generic.

OTHER NMBA GUIDELINES FOR NURSES AND MIDWIVES

The NMBA has a significant number of helpful documents on its website under the tab of professional codes and guidelines, ranging from policies about mothercraft nurses to a joint statement with CATSINAM on culturally safe care.[86]

All of these documents together form the professional practice framework for nurses and midwives, who should be familiar with those pertaining to their practice area. Although all of these documents are developed to protect the public, it is fair to say that using them and abiding by them will also protect the nurse or midwife.

COMPLAINTS AND NOTIFICATIONS ABOUT NURSES AND MIDWIVES

The third element of professional regulation (see **Figure 4.1**) is the management of complaints and notifications, which includes expressions of concern about the health, performance or conduct of a registered health professional.[86] The general public, including other health professionals, has a right (and in some instances a duty) to notify the relevant registration authority of a concern about a health practitioner's:

- conduct, if it appears in some way to be putting the public at risk;
- health, insomuch as it affects their ability to practise safely;
- clinical competence or performance.

Case example 4.1 summarises a 2013 case involving unsatisfactory professional conduct and professional misconduct.

Ahpra explains in simple terms what a notification can be about. These are set out in **Box 4.8**.

Health Care Complaints Commission (HCCC) V Shah [2013] NSWNMT 1 (12 March 2013)[87]

In the first of four complaints against him, Mr Shah was accused of unsatisfactory professional conduct in providing dishwashing liquid to Patient A after failing to check whether it was Patient A's prescribed medication, or checking that the dose administered was correct, and subsequently failing to notify a senior nurse when Patient A complained of nausea and feeling unwell.

The second complaint asserted a failure by Mr Shah to satisfactorily complete the IELTS (international English language testing system) examination to the standard required. This failure is asserted to constitute unsatisfactory professional conduct.

The third complaint asserts that, due to Mr Shah's actions, and lack of appropriate action after Patient A consumed the dishwashing liquid, and his failure to complete the IELTS examination to the required standard, he is not competent to practise nursing.

Complaint four asserts that Mr Shah is guilty of professional misconduct based on the particulars in the first two complaints, or that he had engaged in more than one instance of unsatisfactory professional conduct which, considered together, amounted to conduct of a sufficiently serious nature to justify suspension or cancellation of his registration.

Mr Shah was found guilty of professional misconduct and his name was ordered to be removed from the register for a period of at least 12 months prior to re-application.

> **BOX 4.8**
> **WHAT CAN A NOTIFICATION BE ABOUT?[88]**
>
> - A practitioner's behaviour is placing the public at risk
> - A practitioner is practising their profession in an unsafe way, or
> - A practitioner's ability to make safe judgements about their patients might be impaired because of their health.

The notification process is quite complex and also differs between certain states, such as New South Wales and Queensland, which have co-regulatory processes with the National Scheme.[89] A notification can be made electronically, by mail, by telephone or in person. There are forms that need to be completed but Ahpra staff can assist the public where necessary.

When a notification is received, Ahpra will assess it to determine whether a Board must consider taking immediate action to protect public health or safety. This may result in suspending or imposing conditions on the registration status of a student or practitioner. If immediate action is not required, Ahpra will assess the notification thoroughly to enable the relevant Board to make an informed decision about it. Each investigation is tailored to the notification received, and complex matters take more time. Notwithstanding the differences mentioned in New South Wales and Queensland, there is a nationally consistent process across the National Scheme for managing notifications, which can include the following stages:

- lodgement;
- assessment;
- health complaints entity (HCE) consultation;
- investigation;
- health or performance assessment;
- immediate action;
- panel hearings; and
- tribunal hearings.[90]

There is also a requirement under the *National Law* for mandatory notifications in some situations. Practitioners and employers must report a registrant whom they reasonably believe has engaged in notifiable conduct. Under section 140, notifiable conduct in relation to a registered health practitioner means that the practitioner has been:

(a) *practising the practitioner's profession while intoxicated by alcohol or drugs; or*

(b) *engaging in sexual misconduct in connection with the practice of the practitioner's profession; or*

(c) *placing the public at risk of substantial harm in the practitioner's practice of the profession because the practitioner has an impairment; or*

(d) *placing the public at risk of harm by practising the profession in a way that constitutes a significant departure from accepted professional standards.*

The Ahpra website provides useful information in relation to notifications, but it is important to remember that the advice on the NMBA website in relation to professional standards is there specifically to protect the public. Practitioners who practise within their professional practice framework, while not being immune from public dissatisfaction or concern, would be less likely to attract disapprobation.

THE ACCREDITATION OF NURSING AND MIDWIFERY COURSES

Prior to the National Scheme coming into operation, each jurisdiction used to accredit its own courses leading to registration or enrolment as a nurse or registration as a midwife. Under the National Scheme, ANMAC has been established as a new independent accreditation authority for nursing and midwifery. Although it is beyond the scope of this chapter to describe this work in detail, nurses and midwives should understand that the approval of programs leading to qualifications that go onto the registers is rigorous, systematic and now nationally consistent. Information about ANMAC is available on its website.[91]

CONCLUSION

It is evident that there have been substantial and exciting changes to the regulation of nurses and midwives in Australia. The National Scheme is well established but undergoes regular review, so it is important that nurses and midwives check the relevant websites on a regular basis to keep abreast of updates.

CHAPTER 4 REVIEW QUESTIONS

Following your reading of **Chapter 4**, consider these questions in reaching the objectives of this chapter. Guidance on which part of the chapter will assist you in answering the questions can be found at http://evolve.elsevier.com/AU/Staunton/law/. You may, of course, consider other sources as part of your considerations.

1. What are the elements of professional regulation? (See **Figure 4.1**.)

2. Do you find the standards required for registration and ongoing practice helpful or onerous?

3. To what extent can you understand the specific requirements related to the regulation of midwifery?

4. When would you be required to make a mandatory notification about a fellow health professional? (See section 140, *Health Practitioner Regulation National Law.*)

5. Do you consider the mechanisms used to control entry to the professions of nursing and midwifery to be adequate or too stringent?

ENDNOTES

Note: all links were last accessed on 26 March 2023.

1. Australian Health Practitioner Regulation Authority (Ahpra), click on 'About' Tab, then 'What we do', https://www.ahpra.gov.au/About-Ahpra/What-We-Do.aspx. For an extensive description of the history and development of the scheme, particularly in relation to complaints and notifications, see Satchell C, Walton M, Kelly P, Chiarella M, Pierce S, Nagy M, Bennett B and Carney T, 'Approaches to management of complaints and notifications about health practitioners in Australia', (2016) *Australian Health Review* 40(3):311–18, doi: 10.1071/AH15050.

2. Nursing and Midwifery Council of NSW, 2018, *Hearing members professional development: acting fairly*, 2018, https://hpca-useruploads.s3-ap-southeast-2.amazonaws.com/s3fs-public/qrg_-_module_3_-_acting_fairly_-_nmc.pdf.

3. Joselin D, *Breaking down monopolies in the medical profession*, Institute of Economic Affairs, 2014, https://iea.org.uk/blog/breaking-down-monopolies-in-the-medical-profession.

4. Australian Government Department of Health and Aged Care, *Health Ministers Meeting: ministerial authorities and national bodies who report to the HMM*, 2022, https://www.health.gov.au/committees-and-groups/health-ministers-meeting-hmm#ministerial-authorities-and-national-bodies-who-report-to-the-hmm.

5. *Health Practitioner Regulation National Law Act 2009* (Qld), Schedule, Part 2, s 11.

6. Australian Government Department of Health and Aged Care, *Health Ministers Meeting: members*, 2022, https://www.health.gov.au/committees-and-groups/health-ministers-meeting-hmm#members

7. Australian Government Department of Health and Aged Care, *Health Ministers Meeting: related-committees-or-groups*, 2022, https://www.health.gov.au/committees-and-groups/health-ministers-meeting-hmm#related-committees-or-groups

8. *Health Practitioner Regulation National Law Act 2009* (Qld), op. cit., Part 4, s 29.

9. *Health Practitioner Regulation National Law Act 2009* (Qld), op. cit., Part 4, s 25.

10. Nursing and Midwifery Board of Australia (NMBA) website, home page, 2021 https://www.nursingmidwiferyboard.gov.au/.

11. NMBA website, 'About' tab, State and Territory Nursing and Midwifery Board members, 2021, https://www.nursingmidwiferyboard.gov.au/About/State-and-Territory-Nursing-and-Midwifery-Board-Members.aspx.

12. HPCA website, *How councils manage complaints*, https://www.hpca.nsw.gov.au/how-councils-manage-complaints-hpca.

13. Office of the Health Ombudsman website, 'About us' tab, Office of the Health Ombudsman, https://www.oho.qld.gov.au/about-us.

14. *Health Practitioner Regulation National Law Act 2009* (Qld), op. cit., Part 5, s 35 (1).

15. *Health Practitioner Regulation National Law Act 2009* (Qld), op. cit., Part 1, s 3 (a).

16. Ahpra website, home page, 2022, https://www.ahpra.gov.au/.

17. Ahpra website, Glossary, http://www.ahpra.gov.au/Support/Glossary.aspx.

18. NMBA website, 'Registration & endorsement' tab, https://www.nursingmidwiferyboard.gov.au/Codes-Guidelines-Statements/FAQ/Non-practising-registration-for-nurses-and-midwives.aspx.

19. NMBA website, Re-entry to practice Fact Sheet, https://www.nursingmidwiferyboard.gov.au/Codes-Guidelines-Statements/FAQ/fact-sheet-reentry-to-practice.aspx.

20. Australian Nursing and Midwifery Accreditation Council (ANMAC) website, 'About us' tab, https://www.anmac.org.au/about-anmac/about-us.

21. Ahpra website, 'Registration' tab, Student registration, https://www.ahpra.gov.au/Registration/Student-Registrations.aspx.

22. Chamberlain J, *Medical regulation, fitness to practice and revalidation: a critical introduction*, Policy Press, Bristol, 2015.

23. Professional Standards Authority for Health and Social Care website, What we do, https://www.professionalstandards.org.uk/what-we-do.

24. Chiarella M and White J, 'Which tail wags which dog? Exploring the interface between professional regulation and professional education', (2013) *Nurse Education Today*, 33(11):1274–8.

25. Ibid, p 1275.

26. *Health Practitioner Regulation National Law Act 2009* (Qld), op. cit., Part 7, s 53.

27. NMBA website, 2020, Transition to a new assessment model for internationally qualified nurses and midwives, https://www.nursingmidwiferyboard.gov.au/Codes-Guidelines-Statements/FAQ/Transition-to-a-new-assessment-model-for-internationally-qualified-nurses-and-midwives.aspx.

28 Ibid.

29 NMBA website, Orientation to health care in Australia, https://www.nursingmidwiferyboard.gov.au/Accreditation/IQNM/Orientation-Part-1-and-Part-2.aspx.

30. NMBA website, Internationally qualified nurses and midwives, https://www.nursingmidwiferyboard.gov.au/Accreditation/IQNM.aspx

31. *Health Practitioner Regulation National Law Act 2009* (Qld), op. cit., Part 7, s 52 (1).

32. NMBA website, 'Professional codes & guidelines' tab, Safety and quality standards https://www.nursingmidwiferyboard.gov.au/

33. NMBA website, Professional standards, https://www.nursingmidwiferyboard.gov.au/Codes-Guidelines-Statements/Professional-standards.aspx.

34. International Council of Nurses, *The ICN code of ethics for nurses*, 2021, https://www.icn.ch/system/files/2021-10/ICN_Code-of-Ethics_EN_Web_0.pdf

35. International Confederation of Midwives, International code of ethics for midwives, 2008, https://www.internationalmidwives.org/assets/files/general-files/2019/10/eng-international-code-of-ethics-for-midwives.pdf.

36. NMBA website, 'News' tab, https://www.nursingmidwiferyboard.gov.au/News/Current-Consultations.aspx. The 'Current consultations' section lists those consultations open for comment.

37. NMBA website, 'Registration standards' tab, https://www.nursingmidwiferyboard.gov.au/

38. Ahpra website, 'Registration tab', Registration standards, https://www.ahpra.gov.au/Registration/Registration-Standards.aspx. Ahpra provides advice about the revision of registration standards and publishes the relevant standard for each profession.

39. NMBA website, 'Registration standards' tab, English language skills, https://www.nursingmidwiferyboard.gov.au/Registration-Standards/English-language-skills.aspx.

40. NMBA website, 'Registration standards' tab, Registration standard: continuing professional development, 2016, https://www.nursingmidwiferyboard.gov.au/Registration-Standards/Continuing-professional-development.aspx.

41. NMBA website, 'Professional codes and guidelines' tab, https://www.nursingmidwiferyboard.gov.au/Codes-Guidelines-Statements/FAQ/CPD-FAQ-for-nurses-and-midwives.aspx.

42. NMBA website, 'Registration standards' tab, Registration standard: professional indemnity insurance arrangements, 2016, https://www.nursingmidwiferyboard.gov.au/Registration-Standards/Professional-indemnity-insurance-arrangements.aspx, p 4.

43. Ibid, p 1.

44. An exemption exists under section 284 of the National Law for midwives providing private intrapartum services for women planning homebirths. For more information see: NMBA website, 'Professional codes and guidelines' Additional documents Fact sheet: Professional indemnity insurance arrangements (updated 2022), https://www.nursingmidwiferyboard.gov.au/Registration-Standards/Professional-indemnity-insurance-arrangements.aspx.

45. NMBA website, 'Registration standards' tab, Registration standard: recency of practice, 2016, https://www.nursingmidwiferyboard.gov.au/Registration-Standards/Recency-of-practice.aspx, p 1.

46. Ibid.

47. NMBA website, 'Registration standards' tab, Registration standard: recency of practice, 2016, op. cit., p 1.

48. Ibid, p 3.

49. Ibid.

50. NMBA website, 'Professional codes and guidelines' tab, Additional documents Fact sheet: recency of practice, 2016, https://www.nursingmidwiferyboard.gov.au/Registration-Standards/Recency-of-practice.aspx.

51. NMBA website, 'Professional codes and guidelines', *Re-entry to practice for nurses and midwives*, 2019, https://www.nursingmidwiferyboard.gov.au/Codes-Guidelines-Statements/Policies/reentry-to-practice-policy.aspx.

52. NMBA website, 'Registration standards' tab, *Registration standard: endorsement for scheduled medicines for registered nurses (rural and isolated practice)*, 2011, https://www.nursingmidwiferyboard.gov.au/Registration-Standards/Endorsement-for-scheduled-medicines.aspx

53. NMBA website, 'Registration standards' tab, *Registration standard: endorsement for scheduled medicines for midwives*, 2017, https://www.nursingmidwiferyboard.gov.au/Registration-Standards/Endorsement-for-scheduled-medicines-for-midwives.aspx

54. NMBA website, *Endorsement for scheduled medicines for registered nurses (rural and isolated practice)*, https://www.nursingmidwiferyboard.gov.au/Registration-Standards/Endorsement-for-scheduled-medicines.aspx.

55. NMBA website, 'Registration standards' tab, *Registration standard: endorsement as a nurse practitioner*, 2016 https://www.nursingmidwiferyboard.gov.au/Registration-Standards/Endorsement-as-a-nurse-practitioner.aspx.

56. NMBA website, *Codes, guidelines, statements and professional standards*, https://www.nursingmidwiferyboard.gov.au/Codes-Guidelines-Statements/Professional-standards/nurse-practitioner-standards-of-practice.aspx

57. Ibid.

58. Ibid.

59. Ibid.

60. NMBA website, Safety and quality guidelines for nurse practitioners, https://www.nursingmidwiferyboard.gov.au/Codes-Guidelines-Statements/Codes-Guidelines/Safety-and-quality-guidelines-for-nurse-practitioners.aspx.

61. Ibid.

62. NMBA website, Safety and quality guidelines for nurse practitioners, https://www.nursingmidwiferyboard.gov.au/

Codes-Guidelines-Statements/Codes-Guidelines/Safety-and-quality-guidelines-for-nurse-practitioners.aspx. See Definitions.

63. NMBA website, Safety and quality guidelines for nurse practitioners, https://www.nursingmidwiferyboard.gov.au/Codes-Guidelines-Statements/Codes-Guidelines/Safety-and-quality-guidelines-for-nurse-practitioners.aspx.

64. NMBA website, 'Professional codes and guidelines' tab, Guidelines, Guidelines: For nurses applying for endorsement as a nurse practitioner, 2016, https://www.nursingmidwifery-board.gov.au/Codes-Guidelines-Statements/Codes-Guidelines/Guidelines-on-endorsement-as-a-nurse-practitioner.aspx

65. NMBA website, 'Professional codes and guidelines' tab, Guidelines, Guidelines: For nurses applying for endorsement as a nurse practitioner, 2016, op. cit., p 1.

66. Ibid.

67. NMBA website, Safety and quality guidelines for nurse practitioners, https://www.nursingmidwiferyboard.gov.au/Codes-Guidelines-Statements/Codes-Guidelines/Safety-and-quality-guidelines-for-nurse-practitioners.aspx.

68. NMBA website, 'Professional codes and guidelines' tab, Frameworks, National framework for the development of decision-making tools for nursing and midwifery practice, 2013.

69. NMBA website, 'Professional codes and guidelines' tab, Guidelines, Safety and quality guidelines for nurse practitioners, 2016, https://www.nursingmidwiferyboard.gov.au/Codes-Guidelines-Statements/Codes-Guidelines/Safety-and-quality-guidelines-for-nurse-practitioners.aspx.

70. Australian Department of Health and Aged Care website, Medicare access for nurse practitioners, https://www.health.gov.au/topics/medicare/access-practitioners-industry/nurse-practitioners.

71. Services Australia website, Bulk billing for nurse practitioners and midwives, https://www.servicesaustralia.gov.au/bulk-billing-for-nurse-practitioners-and-midwives.

72. NMBA website, 'Professional codes and guidelines' tab, Guidelines, Safety and quality guidelines for nurse practitioners, 2016, https://www.nursingmidwiferyboard.gov.au/Codes-Guidelines-Statements/Codes-Guidelines/Safety-and-quality-guidelines-for-nurse-practitioners.aspx.

73. Chiarella M and Griffin K, 'The strengthening Medicare Task-force: Making everyone equal at the front door of the health system', (2022) Pearls and Irritations, https://johnmenadue.com/the-strengthening-medicare-taskforce-making-everyone-equal-at-the-front-door-of-the-health-system/.

74. UNFPA, State of the world's midwifery, 'Global health systems must invest in midwives', 2022, unfpa.org.

75. NMBA website, 'Professional codes and guidelines' tab, Fact sheets, https://www.nursingmidwiferyboard.gov.au/Codes-Guidelines-Statements/FAQ/CPD-FAQ-for-nurses-and-midwives.aspx

76. NMBA website, 'Registration standards' tab, Registration standard: endorsement for scheduled medicines for midwives, https://www.nursingmidwiferyboard.gov.au/Registration-Standards/Endorsement-for-scheduled-medicines-for-midwives.aspx.

77. NMBA website, 'Professional codes and guidelines' tab, Fact sheets, Fact sheet: Professional indemnity insurance arrangements, 2019, op. cit.

78. NMBA website, 'Registration standards' tab, Registration standard: endorsement for scheduled medicines for midwives, https://www.nursingmidwiferyboard.gov.au/Registration-Standards/Endorsement-for-scheduled-medicines-for-midwives.aspx.

79. NMBA website, 'Professional codes and guidelines' tab, Fact sheets, https://www.nursingmidwiferyboard.gov.au/Codes-Guidelines-Statements/FAQ/Fact-sheet-Endorsement-for-scheduled-medicines-for-midwives.aspx.

80. NMBA website, 'Registration standards' tab, Registration standard: endorsement for scheduled medicines for midwives, 2017 https://www.nursingmidwiferyboard.gov.au/Registration-Standards/Endorsement-for-scheduled-medicines-for-midwives.aspx.

81. NMBA website, 'Registration standards' tab, Registration standard: professional indemnity insurance arrangements, 2016, https://www.nursingmidwiferyboard.gov.au/Registration-Standards/Professional-indemnity-insurance-arrangements.aspx, p 4.

82. NMBA website, Guidelines: For Midwives applying for endorsement for scheduled medicines, https://www.nursingmidwiferyboard.gov.au/Codes-Guidelines-Statements/Codes-Guidelines/Guidelines-for-Midwives-applying-for-endorsement-for-scheduled-medicines.aspx.

83. NMBA website, Safety and quality guidelines for privately practising midwives, https://www.nursingmidwiferyboard.gov.au/Codes-Guidelines-Statements/Codes-Guidelines.aspx.

84. Department of Health and Aged Care, Supporting privately practising midwives to work to their full scope, 2023, https://www.health.gov.au/ministers/the-hon-ged-kearney-mp/media/supporting-privately-practising-midwives-to-work-to-their-full-scope.

85. NMBA website, home page, https://www.nursingmidwiferyboard.gov.au/.

86. Health Practitioner Regulation National Law Act 2009 (Qld), op. cit., Schedule, Part 8.

87. Health Care Complaints Commission (HCCC) v Shah [2013] NSWNMT 1 (12 March 2013), https://www.austlii.edu.au/cgi-bin/viewdoc/au/cases/nsw/NSWNMT/2013/1.html.

88. Ahpra website, 'Concerns about practitioners' tab, How we manage a concern, 2021, https://www.ahpra.gov.au/Notifications/Concerned-about-a-health-practitioner.aspx.

89. Ahpra website, 'Concerns about practitioners: are you in New South Wales or Queensland and have a complaint about a practitioner?' https://www.ahpra.gov.au/Notifications/Further-information/NSW-and-Qld.aspx. See also Satchell CS, Walton M, Kelly P, Chiarella M, Pierce S, Bennett B & Carney T, 'Approaches to management of complaints about health practitioners in Australia', (2015) Australian Health Review, http://dx.doi.org/10.1071/AH15050.

90. Ahpra website, 'How we manage concerns', 2021, https://www.ahpra.gov.au/Notifications/How-we-manage-concerns.aspx. See also Nagy M, Chiarella M, Bennett B, Walton M & Carney T, 'Health care complaint journeys for system comparison', (2018) International Journal of Health Care Quality Assurance 31(8).

91. ANMAC website, About ANMAC, 2016, https://www.anmac.org.au/about-anmac.

5

THE CONTRACT OF EMPLOYMENT INCLUDING WORKPLACE HEALTH AND SAFETY AND WORKERS COMPENSATION

LEARNING OBJECTIVES

In this chapter, you will:

- gain an understanding of the legal principles that must exist to create a binding contract
- learn about the legal obligations of an employer and employee that arise in the contract of employment
- gain an awareness of the legal structure and process that create employment contracts for the majority of employees in Australia
- examine how an employment contract is terminated including the relevant principles of unfair dismissal
- gain an awareness of the employer's obligations in relation to workplace health and safety
- consider the legal basis of an employee's right to workers compensation.

INTRODUCTION

Essentially, a contract is an agreement that gives rise to rights and obligations between the parties to the agreement. Such rights and obligations will be protected and enforced by the law. Most people enter into a wide variety of contracts every day of the week, ranging from simple contracts when purchasing goods from the local supermarket to a more complex contract when purchasing a new home.

The principles of the law of contract apply to you as a nurse or midwife in relation to the contract of employment between you and your employer.

The issues addressed in this chapter are related to the working conditions as well as the working environment of nurses and midwives.

THE CONTRACT OF EMPLOYMENT

The employer–employee relationship is based on the agreement that is created between the two parties when the employer engages an employee to perform work under the employer's direction and control. Such a relatively simple statement is influenced and constrained by legislation and a range of legal principles as well as the administrative machinery that deals with issues that arise as a result of contractual relationships.

The contract of employment is generally found within the context of industrial relations. Industrial relations has implications in every facet of an organisation's activities because it is concerned not only with demands made in relation to wages and conditions of employment but also with the ability of an organisation to create a working environment which is safe, harmonious and constructive for the employer and employee.

In any general consideration of the employer–employee relationship it is essential to keep in mind the distinction between an employee and an independent contractor. That distinction has been clearly spelled out in relation to the doctrine of vicarious liability in **Chapter 7**.

The great majority of registered and enrolled nurses as well as midwives working in Australia are employees, but those nurses or midwives working as private duty nurses, homebirth midwives or, in some circumstances, agency nurses are more often than not independent contractors. Any dispute on that threshold issue would have to be determined having regard to the facts and circumstances of the particular situation.

Quite apart from the doctrine of vicarious liability, the major reason it is necessary to make the distinction between the two is that an independent contractor is unable to claim the benefits and conditions of an industrial award or workplace agreement and, in most cases, the statutory entitlements of long service leave, sick leave, annual leave, parental leave and so on.

The legal principles relating to the formation of a contract of employment apply in exactly the same way as they do to the formation of any other contract. These five conditions must exist:

1. There must be an offer and an acceptance. In the contract of employment, it is the employee who makes the employer an offer to work, which the employer can accept or reject.
2. There must be valuable consideration, that is, money or money's worth. In the contract of employment, the consideration is the exchange of services for money; that is, salary or wages, together with any other conditions that are agreed to apply.
3. There must be an intention to create a legal relationship. In the contract of employment, a person who volunteers to 'help out' in emergencies or other situations would not normally be deemed to be intending to create a legal relationship and therefore would not be an employee. Some exceptions arise to that statement for occupational health and safety and workers compensation purposes, but not otherwise.
4. The parties must have the legal capacity to enter into the contract. In the contract of employment relating to nurses and midwives, there is generally no difficulty on this issue. The issues that affect a person's legal capacity to enter into a contract may be briefly and primarily categorised as:
    a. persons who are children;
    b. persons who are deemed to be mentally ill or suffer from a developmental disability; or
    c. drunkards or persons so affected by any other drug or substance as to be incapable of understanding the nature of the agreement.
5. There must be no illegality. In the contract of employment, the work to be performed must not be an unlawful act.

Terms and Conditions of the Contract of Employment

An important part of establishing the contractual relationship is determining the terms and conditions of the contract that create obligations on the parties to the contract. Some obligations in any contract of employment arise impliedly (or automatically) by the operation of long-established common law principles — for example, an employee's obligation to obey all lawful and reasonable directions of an employer. Such obligations do not necessarily have to be written down in a contract for them to apply. In many instances, however, such common law obligations are found embodied within contracts of employment.

For most employees, including nurses and midwives, the contract of employment is within the industrial award or workplace agreement covering their place of work. The document may be referred to as an industrial award, enterprise agreement or workplace agreement.

There are also statutory provisions that complement the terms and conditions found in industrial awards or agreements. For example, an employer's obligation to provide a safe place of work is reaffirmed in occupational health and safety legislation in all states and territories as well as Commonwealth workplaces.

Although most contracts of employment are in writing in one form or another, it is possible, though unusual, to create a legally binding contract of employment simply by verbal agreement between the employer and the employee.

Employees' Obligations Under the Contract of Employment

In many instances, the employee's obligations may or may not be expressly spelled out in any contract of employment, be it an industrial award, workplace agreement or otherwise. Nevertheless, if not expressly spelled out, they apply as implied conditions or obligations imposed on the employee in the contractual relationship with the employer. The employee's obligations may be expressed as:

■ the duty to obey all lawful and reasonable directions of the employer. The significant words are 'lawful' and 'reasonable'. In most workplaces, many of the employer's lawful and reasonable commands are conveyed to the employee via written policies, procedures and protocols, and the employee is required to comply with them. What would be reasonable would depend on the facts and circumstances of the situation under consideration;

- the duty to display due care and diligence in the performance of his or her work and to perform it competently;
- the duty to account to the employer for all monies and property received in the course of employment;
- the duty to make available to the employer any process or product invented by the employee in the course of employment;
- the duty to disclose to the employer information received by the employee relevant to the employer's business;
- the duty to be faithful and loyal to the employer's interests.

Employers' Obligations Under the Contract of Employment

Generally speaking, an employer's obligations have been almost totally reinforced by the creation of industrial awards or workplace agreements and by legislation. The employer's obligations may be generally expressed as:

- the duty to pay salary or wages and provide any other conditions of employment agreed on or expressly provided for by statute or otherwise;
- the duty to provide a safe system of work; and
- the duty not to discriminate against people in employment on various grounds such as gender, sexuality, religion, race or disability.

Discrimination in Employment

Each of the states and territories as well as the Commonwealth has legislation that imposes a duty on employers not to discriminate against people in employment on various grounds such as gender, sex, religion, race or disability. The legislation generally covers the same areas but some offer more extensive protection than others (see Box 5.1).

How Discrimination Complaints Are Dealt With

Complaints made in relation to issues of discrimination are dealt with by the commission or board established under the legislation of each of the states and territories, and the Commonwealth.

In the Australian Capital Territory, there is a Discrimination Commissioner and New South Wales has the Anti-Discrimination Board. Queensland has an Anti-Discrimination Commission as does the Northern Territory. South Australia, Victoria and Western Australia have an Equal Opportunity Commissioner.

If a complaint is unable to be successfully conciliated, it is generally referred to a tribunal for hearing and determination. If a complaint is made under the Commonwealth legislation, it is dealt with in the first instance by the Australian Human Rights Commission. If it is unable to be conciliated, the complaint may then be taken to the Federal Court or to a judge of Division 2 of the Federal Circuit and Family Court of Australia.

THE CREATION OF AN INDUSTRIAL AWARD OR WORKPLACE AGREEMENT

Employment contracts known as industrial awards, enterprise agreements or workplace agreements apply to almost 80% of employees in Australia. People who are self-employed and professionals whose associations set their scale of fees do not belong in this category.

An employer's obligation to pay wages and provide any other conditions agreed upon between employer and employee has, in most cases, long been embodied in industrial awards or workplace agreements. In some circumstances it may be an individual contract between the employer and the employee concerned.

Generally, an industrial award or workplace agreement is a document setting out the wages and conditions of employees of a particular industry or workplace.

In Australia, the creation of industrial awards and workplace agreements has been overseen by industrial tribunals of the states, territories and the Commonwealth within the constraints of their respective constitutional powers and supported by an associated legislative framework.

In 2010 the industrial regulation of the majority of employees in Australia was transferred to Commonwealth legislative control under the *Fair Work Act 2009*. Most of the states, with the exception of Victoria,

BOX 5.1
STATE, TERRITORY AND COMMONWEALTH DISCRIMINATION LEGISLATION

- **Australian Capital Territory** *Discrimination Act 1991:* The employer is not to discriminate on the grounds of sex, sexuality, gender identity, relationship status, status as a parent or carer, pregnancy, breastfeeding, race, religious or political conviction, disability, industrial activity, age, profession, trade, occupation or calling, spent convictions, and religious practice in employment.
- **New South Wales** *Anti-Discrimination Act 1977:* The employer is not to discriminate on the grounds of race (including colour, nationality, descent and ethnic, ethno-religious or national origin), gender, marital or domestic status, disability, homosexuality, carer's responsibility and compulsory retirement on the ground of age. Also, conduct deemed unlawful includes sexual harassment and vilification of homosexuality, race and transgender or HIV/AIDS status.
- **Northern Territory** *Anti-Discrimination Act:* The employer is not to discriminate on the grounds of race, sex, sexuality, age, marital status, pregnancy, parenthood, breastfeeding, impairment, trade union or employer association, religious belief or activity, political opinion, affiliation or activity and irrelevant medical or criminal history.
- **Queensland** *Anti-Discrimination Act 1991:* The employer is not to discriminate on the grounds of sex, relationship status, pregnancy, parental status, breastfeeding, race, age, impairment, religious belief or activity, political belief or activity, trade union activity, lawful sexual activity, gender identity, sexuality and family responsibilities. Sexual harassment is deemed unlawful conduct under the Act.
- **South Australia** *Equal Opportunity Act 1984:* The employer is not to discriminate on the grounds of sex, chosen gender, sexuality, marital or domestic status, pregnancy, race, age and disability. Sexual harassment is deemed unlawful conduct under the Act.

- **Tasmania** *Anti-Discrimination Act 1998*: The employer is not to discriminate on the grounds of race, age, sexual orientation, lawful sexual activity, gender and gender identity, intersex, marital, relationship and parental status, pregnancy, breastfeeding, family responsibilities, disability, industrial activity, irrelevant criminal or medical record, political activity, belief or affiliation and religious activity, belief or affiliation. Sexual harassment or inciting hatred on the basis of race, disability, sexual orientation or religion is deemed unlawful conduct under the Act.
- **Victoria** *Equal Opportunity Act 2010*: The employer is not to discriminate on the grounds of sex, sexual orientation, gender identity, pregnancy, breastfeeding, marital status, status as a carer, age, race, parental status, physical features, expunged homosexual conviction, religious belief or activity, political belief or activity, disability, employment activity, industrial activity and lawful sexual activity. Sexual harassment is deemed unlawful conduct under the Act.
- **Western Australia** *Equal Opportunity Act 1984*: The employer is not to discriminate on the grounds of sex, sexual orientation, marital status, pregnancy, race, religious or political conviction, age, racial harassment, impairment, family responsibility or family status and gender history. Sexual harassment is deemed unlawful conduct under the Act.
- **Commonwealth** legislation dealing with discrimination is overseen by the Australian Human Rights Commission:
  - *Age Discrimination Act 2004*
  - *Australian Human Rights Commission Act 1986*
  - *Disability Discrimination Act 1992*
  - *Racial Discrimination Act 1975*
  - *Sex Discrimination Act 1984.*

have retained a state-based Industrial Relations Commission or Employment Tribunal structure to provide industrial regulation for state public servants and some public sector employees, including local government employees not already employed under a federal industrial award or workplace agreement. Western Australia's Industrial Relations Commission also provides industrial regulation for small businesses that are not incorporated.

In Victoria, the Northern Territory and the Australian Capital Territory, the Commonwealth *Fair Work Act* applies to public servants and public as well as private sector employees.

Industrial Regulation of Nurses and Midwives in Australia

In relation to nurses and midwives, the situation varies as between the states and territories and as between nurses and midwives employed in the public and private sectors.

In New South Wales, Queensland, South Australia, Tasmania and Western Australia, nurses and midwives employed in the public sector continue to be covered by state industrial awards determined by their state-based industrial relations tribunal (or commission). In Victoria and the two territories, federal awards or agreements apply.

In relation to the private sector, in all states (including New South Wales) and the territories, where the employer is a 'constitutional corporation' (i.e. an incorporated business) the Commonwealth's *Fair Work Act* applies. Healthcare industry employers in the private sector, be they private hospitals, nursing homes, medical centres or community-based care centres, are all invariably operating as corporations, which is the catalyst for invoking the Commonwealth *Fair Work Act* provisions. Accordingly, nurses or midwives employed in any of those workplaces would be covered by the terms and conditions of a federal industrial award or workplace agreement.

There would also be a number of nurses or midwives in the private sector, particularly in relatively small medical centres and/or general practice areas, who would be employed pursuant to a federally registered employment agreement.

Whatever the circumstances of employment are, a nurse or midwife should, at the commencement of employment, take steps to ascertain the nature of the employment contract and its terms and conditions. In most circumstances, particularly in the public sector, it will be an industry-wide award or enterprise agreement. In the private sector, it may be an agreement relating just to the individual hospital, nursing home or healthcare centre, or the agreement may relate to all staff employed in private hospitals or nursing homes owned and/or operated by an industry-wide corporation — for example, Ramsay Health Care in relation to private hospitals owned by that group, or the Uniting Church of Australia in the aged care industry.

In all states and territories, advice about employment wage rates together with terms and conditions of employment for nurses and midwives working in either the public or private sector can be obtained from the state or territory branch of the Australian Nursing and Midwifery Federation.[1]

National Employment Standards and Employment Provisions Established by the *Fair Work Act*

One of the major changes established by the *Fair Work Act* was to identify National Employment Standards and other provisions that must be included in industrial awards or enterprise agreements or work-related contracts. Relevantly, the Fair Work Act was amended in 2022 by the provisions of the *Fair Work Legislation (Secure Jobs, Better Pay) Act 2022*. When taken together, the standards required to be incorporated in all industrial awards, enterprise agreements or work-related contracts include:

- maximum weekly hours of work;
- the right to request flexible working arrangements as well as offers and requests for casual conversion;
- parental leave and related entitlements;
- annual leave;
- personal carer's leave, unpaid family and domestic violence leave and compassionate leave;
- community service leave;
- long service leave;
- public holidays;
- notice of termination and redundancy pay;
- provision of a Fair Work information statement, which details the rights and entitlements of employees under the new system and how to seek advice and assistance.

Additionally, the 2022 amendments to the *Fair Work Act* significantly curtail the ability of employers to engage employees on fixed-term contracts. As well, from March 2023, sexual harassment in connection with work will be expressly prohibited and employers will be held vicariously liable for it unless they can prove they have taken all reasonable steps to prevent the conduct. Additionally, breastfeeding, gender identity and intersex status are now protected attributes under the anti-discrimination provisions of the *Fair Work Act*.

The *Fair Work Act* also permits an employee to file a claim for unfair dismissal if the employee has completed a minimum employment period of 12 months with a small business and 6 months in all other cases. A small business is defined as a business with fewer than 15 employees.

The Dispute Resolution Role of Industrial Tribunals

In addition to any role it may have in determining industrial awards or workplace agreements, an industrial tribunal may be called upon to deal with other issues that arise out of the contract of employment. In general terms, such issues result from a disagreement or dispute that arises between the employer and a union on behalf of an individual employee or on behalf of all employees covered by a particular award or workplace agreement. Such disputation can arise for a variety of reasons, for example:

- disagreement over the proper interpretation of a provision in an award or workplace agreement;
- measures implemented by the employer against an individual employee or employees generally that are believed to be harsh and unreasonable — for example, forced redundancy, termination of employment, demotion; or
- disagreement between the employer and employee about increases or changes in wages or conditions of employment.

When industrial disputes arise and are unable to be resolved by negotiation between the employer and employee(s), the employer will often seek the intervention of the appropriate industrial tribunal requesting that the employees concerned be ordered to return to work or lift work bans. In such a situation, the industrial tribunal will endeavour to resolve the conflict by calling the parties together in proceedings known as a **compulsory conference**. At a compulsory conference the parties are encouraged to discuss the issues openly and frankly in an attempt to reach agreement. If that should fail, then a recommendation or order as to what should be done by one or both parties may be made by the industrial tribunal. If such a recommendation or order is ignored by one or both of the parties to the dispute, then the industrial tribunal may proceed to arbitrate the issue. That is, it hears evidence from both sides to the dispute and then makes a decision that is binding on both parties.

HOW THE CONTRACT OF EMPLOYMENT IS TERMINATED

All contracts that are entered into, whether they be contracts of employment or otherwise, ultimately come to an end either by the operation of law or by the actions of either party to the contract.

The ways that a contract of employment may be terminated are as follows.

(i) A Contract for a Fixed Period or a Specific Undertaking

A good example of a contract for a fixed period as far as a nurse or midwife is concerned would be where she or he was employed for the period of maternity leave of another nurse or midwife. Once the contract period has expired, it comes to an end.

An example of employment for a specific undertaking might be where a nurse or midwife is employed for the duration of a research program. When the program is completed, the contract of employment is terminated.

(ii) Death

It is obvious that the employment contract is terminated on the death of an employee. Equally, if the employer is an individual, the employer's death will put an end to the contract. Where the employer is a company or government department or quasi-government authority, the death of a company director or department secretary does not affect the contract.

(iii) Transfer of Business

At common law, a termination of employment is deemed to occur when one company transfers its business to another. However, legislation and award provisions have intervened in relation to this issue, particularly where leave entitlements are concerned. In most circumstances, the industrial award or workplace agreement will provide that service with the prior employer shall, on change of ownership of the business, transfer to the new owner for the calculation of leave entitlements.

(iv) Frustration or Impossibility of Performance

The usual situation that constitutes frustration or impossibility of performance is that an illness or incapacity of the employee is of such a nature and of such duration as to render that employee unable to work. As a consequence, the obligation of the employee to perform under the contract is frustrated by his or her prolonged ill-health. Obviously, normal sick leave provisions are not contemplated here but rather an extended and seemingly continuing incapacity of the employee to carry out the work for which he or she was engaged.

(v) Consent

A contract of employment may be terminated by the mutual consent of both parties.

(vi) Redundancy

A contract of employment may be terminated because the position occupied by the employee is made redundant — generally because the employer is restructuring its business or where the business is being wound down. In such circumstances, an employee may be entitled to a redundancy payment that is generally based on 1 or 2 weeks' pay for every full year of service with a maximum entitlement capped at a set number of weeks or months.

Very often, where an employer wishes to downsize its workforce, it will call for expressions of interest from its employees, who can then register their interest in being made redundant. When that occurs, the employer may then choose to offer a redundancy payment to an employee once the employee registers such an interest. As a general rule, the employer cannot be compelled to offer a redundancy payment unless provision is made for it in the industrial award or workplace agreement; however, under the *Fair Work Act* National Employment Standards, redundancy pay is one of the mandatory conditions of employment that must be provided for in awards and workplace agreements.

It is important to remember that, in a redundancy, the position is deemed to be redundant, not the person who fills it.

Before offering a redundancy, an employer may offer alternative and financially comparable employment to ensure continuing employment and negate the need for a redundancy payment.

(vii) Termination by Notice

If a period of notice is not expressly stated, the presumption is that a contract of employment may be terminated by reasonable notice of either party. Once again, statute and particular awards have modified this presumption so that all awards now state a specific period of notice that either party must give to terminate the contract of employment.

The period of notice required to be given can vary, but for most employers and employees the requisite period is 1 or 2 weeks.

The obvious exception to the necessity to give notice is where the employer has the right to summarily dismiss an employee on the grounds of misconduct. There is no general legal definition of misconduct as each case would have to be looked at in the light of its own particular facts and circumstances. The type of conduct that has justified summary dismissal has ranged between:

- a wilful refusal by an employee to obey a lawful and reasonable direction from the employer;
- insubordination;
- breach of confidence in disclosing an employer's trade or other secrets;
- drunkenness affecting the employee's ability to work;
- fraud or dishonesty by the employee in his or her employment; and/or
- conviction of a crime, but only if the conduct constituting the crime is inconsistent with the proper performance of his or her duties as an employee.

Apart from circumstances that would warrant summary dismissal, there is still the right of the employer or employee to terminate the contract between them. As far as the employer is concerned, that right has been constrained to some extent by the statutory power given to industrial tribunals to reinstate employees. The major factor that has to be established in asking an industrial tribunal to reinstate an employee is that the employee's dismissal is harsh and unfair. In other words, whatever the employee did or failed to do did not warrant the ultimate penalty of dismissal.

In certain circumstances a tribunal may order compensation to the employee in lieu of reinstatement.

What Constitutes an 'Unfair' Dismissal Warranting Reinstatement

As always in such matters, there are no hard-and-fast principles that determine whether an employee has been treated fairly. Each case has to be judged on its own facts and circumstances, and very rarely are two situations exactly the same. However, in arriving at a decision as to whether or not an employee has been treated fairly, these factors would warrant consideration:

- The employee's length of service and previous conduct; obviously an employee with many years of loyal and good service to the employer would warrant more favourable consideration than an employee with a short period of service and previous disciplinary problems.

■ Has the employer clearly spelled out the duties and responsibilities expected of the employee? It may be that an employee's failure to perform a particular duty is due to the failure of the employer to inform the employee that the particular duty is expected of him or her, rather than the employee's refusal or inability to perform it.

■ Has the employer drawn the alleged breach of duty to the employee's attention? If an employer condones a course of conduct by an employee over a long period and then attempts to use this conduct to justify dismissal, it would not, in most situations, be sufficient to warrant dismissal.

■ Once the alleged breach of duty has been drawn to the employee's attention, has he or she been given the opportunity to rectify the problem?

■ Is there anything the employer could or should have done to rectify the problem? For example, it may be that an employee's excessive absences from work are due to domestic problems which may be eased or resolved with advice from the personnel department or staff counselling.

■ If the employee's alleged breach of duty continues without good reason, the employer should firmly warn the employee in writing that his or her continued employment is in jeopardy and request an improvement.

■ A further continuation of the alleged breach of duty on the part of the employee, without good reason, would normally be sufficient grounds to justify dismissal.

As long as the employer can show that the steps taken leading up to the employee's dismissal were fair and reasonable considering the employee's conduct, an industrial tribunal will not interfere with an employer's right to dismiss an employee.

As well as determining whether or not an employee has been treated fairly, an industrial tribunal is also concerned to ensure, should an employee be reinstated, that harmonious working relationships will prevail. Industrial tribunals are concerned with solving industrial disputes, not creating them. If it was thought that the reinstatement of a dismissed employee would create further industrial disruption at the workplace, an industrial tribunal may be reluctant to reinstate the employee even if it was established that the employee had been unfairly treated. In such circumstances, monetary compensation may be awarded.

THE LEGAL PERSPECTIVES OF WORKPLACE HEALTH AND SAFETY

In addition to the relevant legislation in place in all of the states and territories as well as for Commonwealth workplaces, workplace health and safety should be understood from three legal perspectives:

1. An employer is obligated to provide a safe place of work pursuant to the relevant workplace health and safety legislative provisions. A breach of these obligations will render the employer liable to criminal prosecution and a significant financial penalty if the offence is found to be established.

2. An employee has the right to claim compensation for work-related injuries. That right and subsequent entitlement arises under the relevant workers compensation legislation of each state and territory or, where applicable, the Commonwealth.

3. An employee has the right to claim monetary damages from an employer for personal injury arising from an employer's failure to provide a safe place of work.

WORKPLACE HEALTH AND SAFETY LEGISLATION

Each of the states, territories and the Commonwealth has enshrined in legislation employer and employee obligations for the health and safety of people in a workplace.

In 2008, the Commonwealth and the states and territories agreed to harmonise their workplace health and safety laws to overcome confusion and compliance issues that had arisen for employers who had a business that operated across state and territory borders as well as Commonwealth instrumentalities.

Following a comprehensive review of workplace health and safety laws across Australia, a model *Work Health and Safety Act* was developed and unanimously endorsed by the Commonwealth together with all the states and territories. The intention was for the nationally harmonised laws to take effect in all jurisdictions from 1 January 2012.

That process took some time but, as of March 2022, all of the states (except Victoria) and territories, together with the Commonwealth have enacted a new *Work Health and Safety Act* that replicates the agreed model legislation.

Victoria does not propose to adopt the model Act but supports much of what is contained within it. It has instead incorporated relevant changes into its existing occupational health and safety legislation rather than adopt the model Act in its entirety. The relevant legislation in Victoria is the *Occupational Health and Safety Act 2004.*

In this text, we refer to the model *Work Health and Safety Act.* A reference to a section of the *Work Health and Safety Act* has the same title, section number and content in the work health and safety legislation of all of the states and territories and the Commonwealth except for Victoria.

While Victoria has retained its *Occupational Health and Safety Act*, the duties and obligations imposed on employers and employees are in relatively similar terms although the section numbers will differ.

The Need for a Comprehensive Workplace Health and Safety System

Overall, to be effective, a proper approach to workplace health and safety should incorporate these elements:

- clear and comprehensive occupational health and safety policies and protocols that are regularly reviewed;
- effective workplace communication and consultation;
- adequate training and dissemination of information to ensure workers know how to adequately protect themselves at work;
- proper and adequate hazard identification and risk assessment;
- risk control and management flowing from the risk assessment process; and

- continuous reinforcement of the importance of workplace safety.

Duty of Care Owed by an Employer Under the *Work Health and Safety Act*

The Act refers to the 'duty of care' owed by a 'person conducting a business or undertaking' (PCBU). In section 5 of the Act, a person conducting a business or undertaking includes an employer, a corporation, an association, partners in a partnership, a sole trader and certain volunteer organisations. A volunteer organisation that employs a person or people to carry out work is a PCBU, but a volunteer organisation that operates with volunteers and does not employ anyone is not.

For the purposes of this text, we refer to a PCBU as an employer.

The employer has the 'primary duty of care' under the Act (s 19) and must ensure 'so far as is reasonably practicable' the health and safety of workers and 'other persons' (for example, customers or visitors) by removing or reducing risks from work being carried out as part of the person's business or undertaking. Such a duty encompasses, but is not limited to:

- a work environment without risks to health and safety which would include psychosocial hazards, for example, bullying, aggression, violence or sexual harassment;
- safe plant and structures;
- safe systems of work;
- safe use, handling and storage of plant, structures and substances;
- the provision of adequate facilities for the welfare at work of workers;
- information, training, instruction or supervision necessary to protect all persons at the workplace; and
- the monitoring of workplace health to prevent illness or injury (s 19(3)).

There are also duties imposed on an employer who:

- manages or controls a workplace (s 20);
- manages or controls fixtures, fittings or plant at a workplace (s 21);
- designs, manufactures, imports or supplies plant, substances or structures (ss 22–25);
- installs, constructs or commissions plant or structures for a workplace (s 26).

The duty imposed on the above categories of people is to ensure 'so far as is reasonably practicable' that a workplace is safe and without risks to the health and safety of any person.

Central to the wide and general obligation placed on an employer to ensure a safe and healthy workplace 'so far as is reasonably practicable' is the obligation to identify and control risks to safety in the workplace.

Risks to safety can occur at many levels in a workplace. For example, a piece of plant or equipment may be inherently unsafe because of inadequate guarding of dangerous parts, or the system of work adopted for a particular task may be unsafe because employees have not been given sufficient information, instruction, training or supervision to ensure the task is done safely and without risk to their health.

To address its workplace health and safety obligations proactively, an employer is required to approach the workplace from the perspective of identifying hazards and then undertake risk analysis to determine how the hazards can be eliminated or controlled.

Workplace hazards are many and varied and include:

- mechanical hazards relating to plant and equipment;
- chemical hazards such as toxic substances, flammable and explosive materials;
- environmental hazards such as dust and fibres from mining and agricultural activities;
- hazards associated with manual handling, weight lifting and occupational overuse syndrome;
- biological hazards including infectious diseases from animals or non-infectious allergic reactions from coming into contact with substances;
- illness arising from exposure to transmissible viral infections, specifically, in more recent times, COVID-19.

COVID-19 Precautions Relating To an Employer's Obligation To Provide a Safe System of Work and Safe Place of Work

The emergence of COVID-19 in late 2019 created a serious public health risk to the wider community and particularly to staff employed in the health and aged care system (among other areas). It was declared a pandemic and a public health emergency. All of the states and territories have a Public Health Act (or equivalent) which gave power to governments to issue orders to limit public gatherings, certain operations and movements as well as directions for certain workers in a number of industries to be vaccinated against COVID-19. The health and aged care industry was one industry identified.

In the health and aged care industry, the risk to safety posed by COVID-19 was twofold. In the first instance, COVID-19 posed a risk to the health and safety of the general public who, in turn, required access to healthcare and treatment, thereby introducing the virus to the healthcare system and all who worked in it. Secondly, exposing healthcare workers (as well as other categories of workers) to the virus required government and employers to take drastic measures to address the risk to the safety and wellbeing of staff and other persons or patients who accessed healthcare facilities. Such measures included the implementation of risk management strategies designed to protect staff and patients such as personal protective equipment (PPE), infection control measures, isolation and compulsory vaccination. The last issue was contentious for those employees and workers who opposed compulsory vaccination. In some instances, a refusal to be vaccinated against the COVID-19 virus resulted in the loss of employment for those workers. A number of legal arguments were raised challenging the employer's right to mandate COVID-19 vaccination. In weighing the competing rights of the individual to refuse a vaccination against the employer's obligation to provide a safe system and safe place of work, the courts acknowledged the working environment of the healthcare system where staff are directly exposed to the virus and ruled in favour of the employer requirement of compulsory vaccination. In doing so, it acknowledged that the outcome could be different where, for example, the employee worked from home and did not have direct and close contact with members of the public.

What is Meant by 'Reasonably Practicable'?

Section 18 of the Act defines 'reasonably practicable' as 'that which is, or was at a particular time, reasonably able to be done' taking into account and weighing up all relevant matters including:

a. the likelihood of the hazard or risk concerned occurring;

b. the degree of harm that might result from the hazard or risk;

c. what the person concerned knows, or ought reasonably to know, about the hazard or risk, and ways of eliminating or minimising the risk;

d. the availability and suitability of ways to eliminate the risk; and

e. after assessing the extent of the risk and the available ways of eliminating or minimising it, the cost associated with doing so, including whether the cost is grossly disproportionate to the risk.

Definition and Duties of 'Worker' Under the Act

Under the Act an employee is included in the definition of 'worker'.

Section 7 of the Act defines a 'worker' as someone who carries out work for a 'person conducting a business or undertaking'. A 'worker' includes an employee, labour hire staff, volunteer, apprentice, work experience student, subcontractor, contractor and outworker.

The duties of a 'worker' (s 28) include that he or she must:

- take reasonable care for their own health and safety;
- ensure that they do not adversely affect the health and safety of others;
- comply with any reasonable instruction and cooperate with the employer's work health and safety policies and procedures.

Under the Act, 'other persons' at a workplace include clients, customers and visitors. Their workplace responsibilities (s 29) are similar to those of a 'worker'. That is, they must:

- take reasonable care for their own and others' health and safety;
- take reasonable care not to adversely affect the health and safety of others;
- comply with any reasonable instruction given by the employer, as far as they are reasonably able.

The Employer's Obligation To Consult with Workers

A duty is placed on an employer to consult with workers in relation to workplace health and safety 'so far as is reasonably practicable' (s 47). If there is a health and safety representative (HSR) at the workplace, he or she must be involved in the consultation (s 48(2)). Section 48 provides for the nature of the consultation that must occur; that is:

- relevant information must be shared with workers;
- workers must be given a reasonable opportunity to express their views in relation to health and safety matters and be able to contribute to decision-making;
- the views of workers are to be taken into account in relation to health and safety;
- the workers are to be advised of the outcome of consultation in a timely manner.

Consultation with workers is required in any of the following matters (s 49). When:

- identifying hazards and assessing risks to health and safety arising from the work carried out or to be carried out;
- making decisions about ways to eliminate or minimise those risks;
- making decisions about the adequacy of facilities for the welfare of workers;
- proposing changes that may affect the health or safety of workers;
- making decisions about the procedures for consulting with workers, resolving health and safety issues, monitoring the health of workers, monitoring the conditions at any workplace under the management or control of the employer, and/or providing information and training for workers.

Requirement for Health and Safety Representative(s) in a Workplace

A worker or workers may request that one or more HSRs be elected for the workplace (s 50). The number to be elected would depend on the size and layout of the workplace, and all workers are eligible to stand for election and vote.

Requirement for Work Groups To Be Established

Workers may request the establishment of work groups. The purpose of a work group (s 51) is to facilitate the representation of the workers by one or more HSRs. If workers request the establishment of one or more work groups, the employer is required to do this (s 51).

Work groups are to be established by negotiation and agreement between the employer and the workers or their representatives. Although the Act itself does not specify the circumstances that might give rise to the establishment of one or more work groups, s 56(4) does state that the Regulations accompanying the Act 'may prescribe matters that must be taken into account' in negotiations for and determinations of work groups.

Reference to regulation 16 provides that negotiations for and determination of work groups must be directed at ensuring the workers are grouped to most effectively and conveniently enable their health and safety concerns to be represented, and that an HSR for a work group be 'readily accessible' to workers in that work group.

Regulation 17 states that matters to be taken into account when establishing work groups include the size and nature of the workplace, the diverse skill sets of the workers and work arrangements such as shift work.

The Powers and Functions of Health and Safety Representatives

The powers and functions of HSRs are considerable. They:

- are required to undergo training to undertake the full range of their functions and powers;
- represent workers in a work group in relation to workplace health and safety;
- monitor safety measures, investigate complaints from workers in the work group relating to health and safety and inquire into risks to safety in the workplace.

In undertaking those functions, HSRs may:

- inspect a workplace;
- accompany an appointed Workplace Inspector in his or her investigations in a workplace;
- be present at interviews with a worker relating to health and safety;
- receive information relating to the health and safety of workers in a relevant work group (s 68(2));

- where there is a serious risk to health and safety, direct a cessation of work (s 85); and
- may, in some circumstances, issue a Provisional Improvement Notice (PIN) (s 90). Such a notice requires an employer to remedy a health and safety contravention, prevent a likely contravention, or take steps to remedy those matters causing the contravention.

Requirement for a Workplace Health and Safety Committee

A workplace health and safety committee must be established if requested by an HSR or five or more workers (s 75). The constitution of such a committee may be agreed by negotiation between the employer and the workers or their representatives (s 76). If there is an HSR in place, he or she must be on the committee. If there are two or more HSRs, they may choose one or more of them to be on the committee. Subsection (4) states that at least half the committee must be made up of workers who are not nominated by the employer.

The role and functions of a workplace health and safety committee are:

- to facilitate cooperation between the employer and the workers in relation to health and safety issues at the workplace;
- to assist in the development of standards, rules and procedures for the workplace relating to health and safety (s 77); and
- to act as an advisory body, to make recommendations and to maintain a watching brief over workplace health and safety programs and their effectiveness.

Overall, the objective is to provide the workplace with an effective occupational health and safety management system that is acceptable to management and workers because it has had input from both. The committee itself is not responsible for workplace health and safety — the employer remains responsible for the health and safety of workers and others at all times.

Compliance Provisions under Workplace Health and Safety Legislation

To ensure employers comply with their legal obligations in relation to workplace safety, the legislation provides (s 156) for Workplace Inspectors to be appointed by the relevant state, territory or Commonwealth authority. Workplace Inspectors have a general and specific authority to enter a workplace and, where necessary, enforce the relevant health and safety laws.

The overall functions and powers of Workplace Inspectors are:

- to provide information and advice in relation to workplace health and safety;
- to assist in the resolution of health and safety issues at a workplace;
- to assist in the access of workplaces by HSRs and to deal with disputed right of entry issues in relation to authorised union officers;
- to review disputed PINs;
- to require compliance with the Act by the employer by the issuing of notices;
- to investigate contraventions of workplace safety; and
- to monitor compliance with the Act (s 160).

Workplace Inspectors are also authorised under the Act (s 163) to enter workplaces without notice and to request help from individuals and take photographs and copies of business records (s 165). They may even remove equipment. Also, they have the power to give legally binding directions by the issuing of notices as follows:

- prohibition notices mean that work must stop until the problem has been fixed (s 195);
- improvement notices mean that work can continue while the problem is being fixed (s 191);
- non-disturbance notices mean a workplace situation must not be disturbed while a matter is being investigated (s 198).

The Act also requires an employer to notify the relevant authority in each state or territory of any workplace accidents resulting in death or serious injury or a serious incident defined as a 'notifiable incident' (s 35). The notification must be done 'immediately' after the incident by 'the fastest possible means' (s 38).

Entry by an Authorised Union Officer

Authorised union representatives are able to enter workplaces where they have members and investigate occupational health and safety matters.

To do so, however, the union official must first possess a work health and safety (WHS) entry permit (s 117). To obtain such a permit, the union may apply to the authorising authority and the nominated union official must have completed prescribed health and safety training (s 131).

Holding a WHS entry permit allows the union official to enter a workplace where a contravention of workplace health and safety laws is suspected. When exercising a right of entry, the WHS permit holder may inspect the workplace, consult with workers and the employer, copy relevant documents and warn any person at the workplace of exposure to the risk to his or her health or safety (s 118).

An employer cannot obstruct a union official with a WHS entry permit in undertaking investigatory tasks in relation to occupational health and safety.

Penalties for Non-Compliance

If an employer or an individual is charged with an offence for breaching their respective obligations under the workplace health and safety legislation, and the offence is proved according to the criminal standard, significant monetary penalties apply to the corporate body.

For an individual found guilty of an offence under the Act, a period of imprisonment is provided for.

The maximum penalty for the most serious offence by a corporation where death or serious injury has occurred, a Category 1 offence, is \$3 million. If an individual who is an employer is found guilty of a Category 1 offence, the maximum penalty is a fine of \$600 000 or 5 years imprisonment, or both (s 31).

WORKERS COMPENSATION

Workers compensation is a form of statutory compensation that, subject to certain conditions, is available to an employee who is injured at work.

The first workers compensation legislation emerged in Germany in the nineteenth century under Bismarck's administration. In Australia, all of the states, territories and the Commonwealth (with respect to Commonwealth employees) now have workers compensation legislation in place, incorporating changes over recent years.

Workers Compensation Versus Other Types of Compensation for Injury at Work

Workers compensation is but one of four entitlements an employee may be able to claim when he or she suffers an injury at work and is unable to work. The other three entitlements are:

1. sick leave in accordance with the conditions set out in the relevant industrial award or workplace agreement;
2. social security payments — for example, disability pension, unemployment benefits; and
3. compensation in the form of damages arising from a civil negligence claim against the employer and/or a third party alleging that the employee suffered harm caused by an unsafe system of work.

How Does a Person Qualify for Workers Compensation Payments?

The three essential criteria that must be established to entitle a person to receive workers compensation are that:

1. the person must be an employee;
2. the person must suffer an injury or disease; and
3. the injury or disease must arise out of or in the course of employment, or the disease must occur in the course of employment and the employment must be a contributing factor or it must have contributed to a substantial degree.

Each of those criteria is further considered.

The Person Must Be an Employee

For the purposes of entitlement to workers compensation, the employer–employee relationship must exist. Once again the major distinction must be made between an employee and an independent contractor. (See **Chapter 7**.) Each of the relevant *Workers Compensation Acts* of the states, territories and Commonwealth defines those persons who are eligible for workers compensation under the synonymous title of 'workers' or 'employees'.

The Employee Must Suffer an Injury or Disease

To be entitled to receive workers compensation payments, the worker must suffer an injury which, as generally prescribed in the relevant legislation, arises out of or in the course of employment, *or* a disease that occurs in the course of employment and to which the employment was a contributing factor. Additionally, the legislation generally provides for workers compensation to be paid to cover the aggravation, exacerbation, deterioration or general worsening of a disease process if the employment was a contributing factor or the employment contributed to a substantial degree.

Meaning of Injury. The term 'injury' is generally interpreted in accordance with its ordinary everyday meaning — that is, it includes all physical or psychological damage sustained to the body arising out of or in the course of employment. There is a definition of injury in the relevant workers compensation legislation.

Apart from the 'physical blow' situation often associated with the concept of injury, conditions such as dermatitis, hepatitis and viral infections have been deemed to be injuries in that they all involve trauma to the body.

A good example of the broad view taken by the courts in relation to the meaning of 'injury' for workers compensation purposes was a case decided by the High Court of Australia in 1976.[2] The court determined that viral meningeal-encephalitis contracted by an employee arising from his employment was an injury within the ordinary meaning of the word. In coming to that decision, the court said:

> *The meningeal-encephalitis is neither idiopathic nor autogenous. It was the result of the introduction into the employee's body of a foreign body, the virus … This attack by, or reception of, the virus was the injury.*[3]

Meaning of Disease. For the purposes of workers compensation, 'disease' has been widely interpreted to cover a range of illnesses, such as heart disease, viral infections, cancer and epilepsy. The list is not exhaustive. A definition of disease is generally included in each piece of workers compensation legislation. For example, the *Workers' Compensation and Injury Management Act 1981* of Western Australia defines disease as including 'any physical or mental ailment, disorder, defect, or morbid condition whether of sudden or gradual development' (s 5).

A good example of how the meaning of disease is considered by the courts is the decision of the Compensation Court of New South Wales in 1992 where the judge found, on the balance of probabilities, the applicant had demonstrated that he had acquired the HIV virus in the course of his employment as a first-aid officer.[4]

Briefly, the facts of that case were that the applicant was diagnosed as being a sufferer of the disease AIDS. He claimed that he acquired it by blood-to-blood infection in the course of conducting his duties as a first-aid officer. He said that, from time to time, he was required to treat open wounds which were bleeding and that, at such times, he was open to infection by reason of the fact that he was an inveterate nail biter who bit his nails down so far as to cause injury to his nail bed and surrounding parts of his fingers, causing frequent bleeding from those areas.

Depending on the definitions in the relevant workers compensation legislation, there are conditions that can be both an injury and a disease.

Where a disease is claimed, it is necessary to establish not only that the disease was contracted in the course of employment, but also that the employment was a contributing factor in contracting the disease.

With an injury, it is only necessary to establish that it arose out of the employment or occurred in the course of employment.

The Injury Must Arise out of or Occur in the Course of Employment

The courts' interpretation in recent years of what constitutes 'arising out of or occurring in the course of employment' has widened considerably in that more and more activities are accepted as being work related. As a general rule, 'arising out of employment' will be established where a worker can show 'that the fact of his being employed in the particular job caused, or to some material extent contributed to, the injury'.[5] Equally, 'in the course of employment' has been stated as meaning:

> ... where a worker, while not performing the actual duties of his employment, was caused

> injury at a time and a place doing something which might be regarded as reasonably incidental to, consequential upon or ancillary to, his employment.[6]

In most situations when a worker suffers an injury at work, there is no dispute that he or she is engaged in the course of employment. Other situations are not so clear and need to be examined individually, particularly considering the wide and variable interpretation given by the courts in such matters. The more obvious examples are injuries sustained while travelling to and from work, during lunch or recognised rest periods, while attending work-related training or seminars, or as a result of being assaulted at work, or while participating in sporting activities related to employment.

Travelling to and From Work. This is generally referred to as a journey claim.

The long-standing provision that a worker who suffers an injury travelling to and from work is still within the course of employment and entitled to claim workers compensation for injuries occurred during that journey has been generally abolished in some states over recent years.

In Tasmania, Victoria, Western Australia, Northern Territory and the Commonwealth, an employee who incurs an injury while travelling to and from work is not covered for workers compensation purposes. In the Northern Territory, injuries from motor vehicle accidents while on a normal journey to or from work may be claimed under the *Motor Accidents (Compensation) Act* that provides for a no-fault scheme of compensation regardless of who caused the accident.

In New South Wales and South Australia, the legislation provides that there is no compensation payable on a journey to or from work where the injury is attributable 'to the serious and wilful misconduct of the worker'. Further, there has to be 'a real and substantial connection between the employment and the accident or incident out of which the personal injury arose'. Examples of how this provision has been interpreted can be found in **Case examples 5.1** and **5.2**.

CASE EXAMPLE 5.1

Dewan Singh and Kim Singh t/as Krambach Service Station v Wickenden[7]

In 2014, the NSW Workers Compensation Commission considered the issue of journeying to and from work in this case involving an employee who worked at a service station. She usually finished at 2.30 pm and travelled home in daylight hours. For a period of time, she was required to work outside her 'normal' hours resulting in her finishing work at a later time and having to travel home in darkness. While driving home from work in the dark one evening, she was injured when a car swerved onto her side of the road. She made a claim for workers compensation and her employer rejected the claim on the basis she was travelling home from work.

The employee appealed and was successful. The Commission found there was a connection between the injury and her employment, which, at that time, required her to drive home in darkness thereby exposing her to a danger which contributed to the accident.

A later case involving a claim for workers compensation relied on both the journey to work provisions and claiming the injury arose out of the course of employment.[8] In this matter, a worker driving to perform overtime was involved in a head-on collision where he sustained injuries and two passengers in the oncoming vehicle died as a result of their injuries. The worker had been speeding at the time of the accident as well as being on his mobile phone to his supervisor either at the time or shortly before the accident. Apart from the criminal proceedings that followed, the worker claimed workers compensation asserting that his injuries arose out of the course of employment or, in the alternative, that his injuries had occurred on a journey to work and he was entitled to be compensated. His employer claimed the worker was not entitled to claim workers compensation under the journey to work provisions as his injuries were due to his 'serious and wilful misconduct' evidenced by his speeding and talking on his mobile phone. On appeal, the court agreed but did find the worker was entitled to be compensated as

CASE EXAMPLE 5.2

Smith v Woolworths Ltd[9]

In May 2017, Ms Smith was employed by Woolworths at the Kiama Village Shopping Centre. She drove her car to the centre and parked in the staff car park. She then walked along a walkway outside the shopping mall on her way to entering the mall and to her place of work. Prior to entering the shopping mall, she was attacked by a bird and sustained a severe injury to her right eye. When Mrs Smith claimed workers compensation for her injury, two issues arose for determination:

1. Was Ms Smith still on a journey to work at the time of her injury?
2. Was Ms Smith's employment a substantial contributing factor to her injuries and did her injury arise out of the course of employment?

In the first instance, it was determined that Ms Smith had completed her journey to work once she had parked her car and exited her vehicle. Once she had completed her journey to work, Ms Smith was deemed to be in the course of her employment. Accordingly, Ms Smith's claim for compensation was not considered to be a journey claim as she had already arrived at her place of work.

In relation to the second issue raised, it was determined that Ms Smith's employment had brought her to the place where the injury occurred. That is, Ms Smith's injuries inflicted by the bird would not have occurred had she not been in the course of employment at the time of the injury. Accordingly Ms Smith was entitled to claim workers compensation payments.

---

his injuries were causally related to his employment. That is, he was calling his employer for a work-related purpose on a work issued mobile phone at the time of the accident. Given those facts, the court found the worker's injuries 'arose out of his employment' and whether the worker's conduct took him out of the course of employment was irrelevant.

In the Australian Capital Territory and Queensland, a worker who incurs an injury travelling to and from work is entitled to claim workers compensation.

Travelling to and from work is generally confined to travelling between the worker's home and place of employment. Problems can arise in establishing entitlement where a worker deviates during his or her usual journey to and from work or instances where the employee broke the law while in control of the vehicle and contributed to the accident.

Circumstances where a worker may be entitled to claim workers compensation for a work-related injury include the following.

Injuries Incurred During Lunch Periods or Recognised Rest Periods. As a general rule, if a worker suffers an injury during a recognised lunch or recreation period which occurs on the employer's premises, or in a situation which may be said to be incidental to the worker's employment, then the worker would be entitled to claim workers compensation. In a decision given in 1962, the High Court upheld a claim for workers compensation made by a worker who had been injured playing cricket during the lunch break, even though the employer had prohibited the playing of such games.

In that matter, the employer had erected a sign prohibiting the playing of games in the lunch hour, but had never bothered to enforce the rule. For some 2 years, during the lunch break, workers had engaged in a variety of sports of which the employer was aware. When a worker was injured, the employer denied workers compensation payments on the basis that playing sport in the lunch period was not in the course of employment. In its decision in favour of the worker, the High Court said:

> ... a worker who is having lunch on his employer's premises with his employer's sanction is, save in exceptional cases, 'doing something which he was reasonably required, expected or authorised to do in order to carry out his duties' ... if this is to be said about taking lunch, why should not it also be said about taking a walk, dozing in the sun, or playing a game of tennis or cricket ...[10]

As always, where a dispute arises, the court will consider the matter on the basis of the particular facts and circumstances of that situation.

Injuries Incurred While Attending Work-Related Training or Seminars or Where Travel to a Destination Where Attendance is Required by the Employer. Workers who are required to attend a trade or training school as part of their contract of employment and who are injured while attending or travelling to or from the school would generally always be considered to be in the course of employment (except in Victoria, where an injury incurred while travelling to or from an educational institution that the worker is attending for an employment-related purpose is not covered for workers compensation purposes).

Equally, workers sent away on seminars, conventions, conferences and so on would normally be said to be acting within the course of employment.

Obviously a worker who is required to travel as part of his or her employment and suffers an injury during that journey would be covered for workers compensation purposes.

Injuries Incurred as a Result of Being Assaulted at Work. If a worker is carrying out duties or activities related to his or her employment and is assaulted, the worker is clearly acting in the course of employment and is entitled to workers compensation payments. Accordingly, a nurse or midwife who is attacked and injured by a patient or third party while carrying out his or her duties is clearly in the course of employment.

Aggression and assault in the healthcare environment is an issue of increasing concern to employers as part of providing a safe place of work in the health system. Healthcare staff, particularly nursing staff, can be, and occasionally are, subject to verbal and physical assault by patients as well as relatives and friends of patients.

This issue is a particular problem in accident and emergency units, psychiatric care areas and nursing homes with a high proportion of residents with dementia. It is an issue that cannot be ignored by employers, who should put in place effective policies and risk-prevention strategies for dealing with the problem.

However, a worker who is injured on the employer's premises as a result of an assault by another person would not necessarily be entitled to claim workers compensation unless that worker was carrying out duties or activities related to his or her employment. An example is the case of *Bill Williams Pty Ltd v Williams*.[11] The relevant facts are set out in **Case example 5.3**.

Injuries Incurred While Participating in Sporting Activities Related to Employment. There can be no hard-and-fast rule in relation to this area. Many employers actively encourage their employees to participate in competitive sport or in sporting teams associated with the employer.

As a general rule, it could be said that an employee who is participating in a sporting activity is not acting within the course of his or her employment, even where the employer actively encourages such participation. However, where an employee, as part of his or her contract of employment, is expected to participate in sporting activities or does so with the express approval of the employer and is paid while doing so, then the employee could be said to be acting in the course of his or her employment and be entitled to claim workers compensation. Similarly, participation in social activities, work picnics and the like must be considered on the facts of each case.

Defences to a Claim for Workers Compensation Payments

It is no defence to a claim for compensation for an employer to say that the worker was the author of his or her own misfortune. It does not matter in workers compensation claims that the worker may have been negligent. It is, however, a defence if the employer can show that the injury was caused by the worker's own serious and wilful misconduct.

Making a Workers Compensation Claim

If in doubt, always seek legal advice as to your entitlement to workers compensation. If you are a member of the relevant union in your state or territory, it will always provide you with advice and assist you with making a claim. Also bear these points in mind:

- Time limits for making a claim — different provisions apply in respect to the giving of notice of injury or disease and, in some cases, the making of a claim for compensation.
- Incapacity and the payment of benefits — workers compensation benefits will be paid when the injury or disease sustained by a worker in relation to his or her employment results in the worker's incapacity for work. Incapacity for work can be either total or partial and is deemed to arise when the injury or disease prevents an employee from:
  - performing the full range of his or her employment duties; or
  - obtaining other employment.
- **Total incapacity** is where the injury or disease prevents the employee from performing all of his or her pre-injury duties.
- **Partial incapacity** is where the injury or disease prevents the employee from performing some, but not all, of his or her pre-injury duties. For example, when a nurse suffers a work-related back injury, the nurse is often told he or she can return to work as long as he or she performs only 'light duties', which usually means no heavy lifting or excessive bending. Whether or not the employer can provide such work and the rate of pay the nurse may be able to earn as a result of the partial incapacity is significant for the purposes of determining the nurse's workers compensation entitlements.
- Workers compensation payments can be made on a weekly or lump sum basis and may be made to either the worker or the dependants of a deceased worker.

CASE EXAMPLE 5.3

Bill Williams Pty Ltd v Williams

Williams was the managing director of a company and on one occasion, when he was at work on the company's premises, he was approached by a man named O'Neill who made allegations that Williams was having an affair with O'Neill's wife. An argument ensued between them and Williams assaulted O'Neill. O'Neill had a rifle and threatened to shoot Williams. Williams ran out of the premises. O'Neill followed and shot him in the back. Williams later claimed workers compensation payments for the injuries received.

The court rejected his claim on the basis that while Williams was clearly within the course of employment during the time he was on the employer's premises, the argument with O'Neill was unrelated to his employment and had interrupted the course of employment.

■ Additional payments that may be made to cover costs arising from a workers compensation injury will include such matters as:
  ■ medical expenses, including artificial aids such as limb prosthesis, false teeth, etc.;
  ■ alterations to the injured worker's home necessitated by the long-term effects of the injury, such as ramps or handrails;
  ■ the cost of rehabilitation and/or the need to provide domestic assistance; and
  ■ funeral expenses.

PRACTICAL CONSIDERATIONS AND ADVICE CONCERNING WORKERS COMPENSATION

■ Any injury suffered at work, no matter how slight it may appear, should be recorded and reported. Even apparently minor injuries can lead to unforeseen consequences. The procedure for recording incidents is a matter for individual hospital policy. It may be an accident report book at local level or an accident report form sent to central administration.

■ Statistical reports of injuries received at the workplace should be used by the employer as a guide when implementing occupational health and safety measures.

■ Some work-related injuries, particularly back injuries, occur gradually over a long period of time. Nurses and midwives are often inclined to treat mild back pain themselves by staying home from work for 1 or 2 days. As most employers generally do not require a medical certificate for up to 2 days' sick leave, no medical attention is sought. As a result, the leave taken is recorded as sick leave and the nurse's sick leave record is reduced. More importantly, no report is given to the employer of the work-related back pain and no record is made of that fact on the nurse's file. In due course the injury is diagnosed and long periods off work and/or surgery may be required. The question then arises as to how the injury occurred and when it was reported. In summary:
  ■ do not treat a work-related injury by yourself;
  ■ report and record all instances of work-related pain — particularly back pain;

■ ensure that all time taken off with work-related injuries is claimed as workers compensation leave and not sick leave. If sick leave is initially debited for a workers compensation injury, it should be re-credited by the employer when the workers compensation is paid.

■ On occasion, a worker may be off work for many months with a workers compensation injury. If there is no likelihood of the worker's return to work after a reasonable period of time, the employer may decide to terminate the worker's employment. Most employers wait until the expiration of the period of full pay before making any decision in that regard. In some of the recent legislative changes in this area, restrictions have been placed on the right of the employer to terminate the employment of a worker following a workers compensation injury.

■ On occasion, an employer will ask a worker to resign if it appears that the worker is unlikely to return to work in the foreseeable future. As a rule, a worker should not resign but wait for the employer to terminate the employment.

■ When recovering from a work-related injury, a worker is often advised by his or her medical practitioner that he or she is fit for 'light duties' which means the worker is partially, but not totally, incapacitated. The worker knows that the employer has no work that can be considered light duties. Nevertheless, the worker should present such a certificate to the employer. In some instances the employer's inability to provide light duties may mean that the worker is deemed to be totally incapacitated.

■ Termination of employment because of a workers compensation injury will not terminate the worker's entitlement to continue to receive workers compensation payments. Such payments will continue as long as the incapacity to work continues and as determined by the medical evidence.

If in any doubt concerning a workers compensation entitlement, always seek advice from the appropriate organisation in your state or territory.

THE EMPLOYER'S OBLIGATION TO PROVIDE A SAFE SYSTEM OF WORK

In addition to an employer's obligations under workplace health and safety legislation, with its potential for criminal penalties, an employer may be found liable to an employee for monetary damages where an employee establishes that he or she suffered a work-related personal injury as a result of the employer failing to provide a safe system of work.

An entitlement to bring such a claim is in addition to any workers compensation claim an employee may have for a work-related injury.

There is nothing to preclude an employee bringing both a workers compensation claim and a claim for damages based on an allegation of an unsafe system of work. However, if both proceed and monies are paid under both claims, the money paid in workers compensation is offset against any monies paid for personal injury damages.

Any claim for personal injury damages based on an unsafe system of work would need to be pursued as a claim in civil negligence by establishing the legal principles discussed in **Chapter 7**. Also, such a claim would be subject to the threshold requirement of having to show, as a result of the work-related injury arising from the employer's negligence, that the worker suffered the percentage of whole person impairment as required by the civil liability legislation.

An unsafe system of work can take many forms. First, one must understand the nature of the duty of care owed by an employer to the employees. This principle is precisely stated in the decision of the High Court in *Rae v Broken Hill Proprietary Co Ltd*.[12] The facts of the appeal do not need to be stated. The relevant passage of the decision is as follows:

> *The question always is whether an employee's injury has resulted from some failure on the part of the employer to take reasonable care for the safety of the former. Such a failure may be shown by establishing, in appropriate cases, a failure to observe commonly recognised precautions or safeguards or, in others, by showing that the performance of his work by an employee has exposed him to risk of injury which might reasonably have been foreseen and avoided.*[13]

What Constitutes an Unsafe System of Work for Nurses and Midwives?

Situations that pose a risk to safety and give rise to an allegation of an unsafe system of work can vary from workplace to workplace. Some examples are the failure to:

1. provide for the proper 'trapping' and control of anaesthetic gases in operating theatres;
2. properly earth and maintain all electrical equipment used by staff;
3. provide proper instruction, lifting equipment or appropriate staff in the lifting or care of patients;
4. reasonably and adequately protect staff against the transmission of infectious diseases such as hepatitis and, since 2019, COVID-19 or other transmissible viruses;
5. provide adequate safety and security to protect staff from aggressive work-related incidents from either fellow employees or patients or members of the public; and
6. ensure safe-handling protocols are in place and provide suitable protective clothing and monitoring where nurses or midwives are required to handle cytotoxic drugs or work in diagnostic radiology.

The example given in point 3 is probably the most contentious area as far as injuries to nursing and midwifery staff are concerned. There is no doubt that back injuries constitute a large percentage of injuries suffered by nurses and midwives in the course of employment. In most situations the person concerned will claim and be paid workers compensation. It is arguable, in some instances, and depending on the facts and circumstances, that the nurse or midwife may also have the right to bring an action in civil negligence alleging an unsafe system of work.

In determining what is a reasonable standard of a safe system of work, these factors should be borne in mind:

- the degree of likelihood of harm occurring in relation to a particular procedure or incident;
- the steps taken to reduce the likelihood of harm in relation to a particular procedure or incident; for example, in the lifting of patients, it is worth considering whether the employer provides:
  - adequate and proper instructions for lifting patients;

■ adequate lifting devices as circumstances warrant;

■ working facilities built to accommodate difficulties in lifting; for example, bathrooms may need structural alterations to allow patients to be lifted in and out of the bath without undue difficulty;

■ adequate instructions to staff about procedures to be followed if difficulties arise; and

■ adequate additional staff, such as wards people, available as circumstances require;

■ any failure on the employer's part to take all reasonable steps to eliminate the likelihood of the harm occurring;

■ any failure on the employee's part to take all reasonable steps to prevent injury occurring.

CONCLUSION

The importance for nurses and midwives to understand their rights and obligations under their contract of employment cannot be overstated. A knowledge of workplace health and safety legislation, particularly the duty of the employer to provide a safe place of work, can provide a nurse or midwife with the necessary information to communicate, and if need be negotiate, with an employer about safety matters of concern in the workplace. Also, work-related injuries, particularly back injuries, can seriously impair the ongoing employment of a nurse or midwife. Understanding the basis of workers compensation entitlements is an important consideration if a work-related injury should eventuate.

CHAPTER 5 REVIEW QUESTIONS

Following your reading of **Chapter 5**, consider these questions in reaching the objectives of this chapter. Guidance on which part of the chapter will assist you in answering the questions can be found at http://evolve.elsevier.com/AU/Staunton/law/. You may, of course, consider other sources as part of your considerations.

1. If an employer has a 'primary duty of care' to provide a safe place of work under the Work Health and Safety Act, what types of matters would have to be addressed by an employer to identify risks to safety in the workplace?

2. An employer's obligation is to identify and reduce risks to the health and safety of persons in the workplace. In considering the diverse range of workplaces nurses and midwives may

work in, identify five potential 'risks to safety' that may arise and how that risk might be safely managed.

3. As a nurse or midwife, if you encountered a situation in your workplace that you believed constituted a risk to your safety and the safety of others, what steps would you take to draw the matter to your employer's attention for appropriate action to be taken?

4. What criteria must be present to entitle a person to claim workers compensation benefits?

5. In your state or territory, are employees entitled to claim workers compensation benefits for injuries received when travelling to and from work — otherwise known as journey claims?

ENDNOTES

1. See the Australian Nursing and Midwifery Federation website for a list of the state and territory branches, https://www.anmf.org.au/about.
2. *Favelle Mort v Murray* (1976) 8 ALR 649, at 652.
3. Ibid, at 652.
4. *A v R* (Compensation Court of New South Wales, McGrath J, 15 May 1992, unreported).
5. *Nunan v Cockatoo Docks* (1941) 41 SR (NSW) 119, at 124.
6. *Hickox v Education Department* [1974] VR 426, at 430.
7. *Dewan Singh and Kim Singh t/as Krambach Service Station v Wickenden* [2014] NSWWCCPD 13.
8. *Ballina Shire Council v Knapp* [2018] NSWWCC F 35.
9. *Smith v Woolworths Ltd* [2017] NSWWCC 290.
10. *Commonwealth v Oliver* (1962) 107 CLR 353, at 363.
11. *Bill Williams Pty Ltd v Williams* (1972) 126 CLR 146.
12. *Rae v Broken Hill Proprietary Co Ltd* (1957) 97 CLR 419.
13. Ibid, at 430.

Section 3   PROFESSIONAL PRACTICE

SECTION OUTLINE

6

CONSENT TO TREATMENT (INCLUDING THE RIGHT TO WITHHOLD CONSENT, END-OF-LIFE PLANNING, NOT-FOR-RESUSCITATION ORDERS, AND THE RIGHT TO DETAIN AND RESTRAIN PATIENTS WITHOUT THEIR CONSENT)

LEARNING OBJECTIVES

In this chapter, you will:

- gain an understanding of the purpose of the tort of trespass to the person
- explore the relevance of consent to the clinical practice of health professionals
- identify and examine the elements required for valid consent
- study the right to refuse consent, including the right to use advance directives
- examine the introduction of voluntary assisted dying into Australia, with particular reference to the requirements for consent
- consider how the tort of false imprisonment impacts on the use of restraint in clinical practice.

INTRODUCTION

This chapter provides a comprehensive overview of the medico-legal concept of consent. Consent is, in the reality of our healthcare world particularly, a defence to actions in trespass to the person. The chapter explores the importance of consent; the elements of consent, including mental capacity and consent in relation to children; and the right to refuse consent, including the use of advance directives and the introduction of voluntary assisted dying into Australian jurisdictions.

Finally, it briefly discusses the tort of false imprisonment, with particular emphasis on the use of restraint.

WHY IS CONSENT IMPORTANT?

The area of law studied in this chapter is an area of civil law relating to a trio of civil wrongs or torts, which fall under the collective heading of trespass to the person. These torts, which are divided into assault, battery and false imprisonment, exist to protect people's 'personal space'. However, for nurses and midwives, this topic is often referred to as 'consent' because the consensual aspect of the law is more readily identified as relevant to people working in healthcare. From a legal perspective, the consent to treatment is a defence to actions in assault, battery or false imprisonment, which explains why it becomes so important to health professionals in their daily work. This area of the law is based on common law principles which have been either enforced or extended by individual state or territory legislation in some areas, particularly in relation to children.

Assault and Battery

Assault is most often contemplated as a criminal offence. However, as far as healthcare staff members are concerned, assault as a crime fortunately does not have general application. The criminal offence of assault would not only consist of the application of force to another person without their consent, but would include the actual intent to cause harm to the person assaulted, or a very high degree of reckless indifference to the probability of harm occurring to the person assaulted. It is fortunately rare for such an intention or attitude to prevail among health professionals. Where it does, it would undoubtedly become a professional disciplinary matter as well as a criminal matter.

As far as the civil law is concerned, there is a technical distinction to be made between assault and battery, although in common parlance no such distinction is made, and the word 'assault' is often (inaccurately) used to embrace both actions. To explain the technical distinction, an **assault** can be committed merely by intentionally putting a person in fear for their physical wellbeing — for example, shaking a fist in front of a person's face and threatening to punch the person could well constitute an assault. If such a threat were to be carried out, the actual application of the blow to the person's body would constitute the technical offence of **battery**. The offence of battery, it was famously said, 'exists to keep people free from "unconsented-to touchings".[1] However, more recently it has been argued that the requirement for consent performs three separate functions in healthcare — legal, ethical and administrative.[2] The legal aspects are as discussed, but the authors also add an ethical dimension — of protecting autonomous decision-making and ensuring patient-defined goals, and also an administrative dimension of 'a systems-level check to ensure that a consent process has occurred'.[3]

Regardless of its limited or wider application, it becomes clear from the above why the defence of consent is so important to health professionals, who are often required to 'touch' people in what would normally be extremely private and personal ways in the course of examination, care and treatment. Often the circumstances in which they are required to perform these 'touchings' can also be quite unusual, such as in emergency departments or operating theatres, where the patient's mental state may be altered, intentionally or otherwise.

Any intentional treatment given to a patient without the patient's consent, or the consent of a person entitled to give such consent on behalf of the patient, constitutes a battery for which the patient is entitled to be compensated by an award of damages.

It is a well-established legal principle, which the courts will uphold, that 'every human being of adult years and sound mind has a right to determine what shall be done with his own body'.[4] There are some exceptions to that statement, which have largely been created by statute. Some of these are dealt with in this chapter and others in **Chapter 10**.

Relevance of Consent Generally

Consent as a defence in law has relevance far beyond the area of treatment to patients in hospitals or healthcare settings. For example, in the criminal law, the charge of aggravated sexual assault essentially comprises three elements:

1. that sexual intercourse took place;
2. that intercourse was without the complainant's consent; and
3. that the person committing the sexual assault either knew or was reckless to the fact that the person did not consent.[5]

It is the absence of consent which renders an otherwise legitimate act a crime or a tort (a civil wrong). Consent to the disclosure of specified private information negates the possibility of an action for breach of confidentiality in relation to that information. Consent as a defence also arises for consideration in relation to civil negligence, where it is otherwise known as the *defence of volenti*, explained in **Chapter 7**. Although such a defence has limited application in hospitals and healthcare settings, it is raised because it provides another example of the application of consent as a defence in a variety of legal situations, both criminal and civil.

NEGLIGENCE MUST BE DISTINGUISHED

Any consideration of the absence or otherwise of consent to treatment must not be confused with negligence. Negligence and assault and battery are two distinct and separate civil wrongs, and a negligent act does not have to precede a battery for a civil action alleging battery to succeed. As far as any treatment given to a patient is concerned, it is quite possible that such treatment was competently given, that the patient suffered no harm and recovered completely, yet the patient can still succeed in an action in battery if he or she has not consented to the treatment given. The fact that the specific type of touching occurred *without the patient's consent* means that a battery has occurred.

The main reason why patients undergo any form of medical treatment is their belief that their condition will be improved or at least palliated by that treatment. Often, if their condition is improved, most patients are happy to let the situation rest, even if they did not know the precise details of what had happened to them or even if their treatment was slightly different to that which they had anticipated. An exception to this is where treatment may be given in disregard of a person's moral or religious convictions and, even if the outcome were successful, the patient may still feel deeply aggrieved. In the Canadian case of *Malette v Shulman*, the facts of which are set out in **Case example 6.1**, a Jehovah's Witness was given a life-saving blood transfusion against her express wishes. She successfully sued in battery, with Robins JA making the observation that:

> *The patient manifestly made the decision on the basis of her religious convictions. It is not for the doctor to second-guess the reasonableness of the decision or to pass judgement on the religious principles which motivated it.*[6]

CASE EXAMPLE 6.1

Malette v Shulman[7]

Mrs Malette was seriously injured in a motor vehicle accident in which her husband was killed. She was taken by ambulance to hospital. She had severe head and facial injuries and was bleeding profusely. She was initially transfused with intravenous glucose and Ringers Lactate. On admission a nurse discovered a card in Mrs Malette's purse, which identified her as a Jehovah's Witness, and in which she requested, on the basis of her religious convictions, that she be given no blood transfusions under any circumstances. The nurse advised Dr Shulman, the doctor on duty, of the existence of the card and its contents.

Shortly after admission Mrs Malette's condition deteriorated sharply, and she became critically ill. Dr Shulman decided that a blood transfusion was necessary to replace Mrs Malette's lost blood and preserve her life and health. He personally administered blood transfusions to her despite the directions on the card found in her purse and a request by Mrs Malette's daughter, who had subsequently arrived

CASE EXAMPLE 6.1

Malette v Shulman (Continued)

at the hospital, that the transfusions be discontinued. When Mrs Malette recovered from her injuries, she successfully sued Dr Shulman in battery on the basis that she had specifically withheld her consent to blood transfusions as evidenced by the card in her purse and, in treating her contrary to that express request, Dr Shulman had committed a battery. Mrs Malette's action against Dr Shulman was not compromised by the fact that Dr Shulman had not been negligent in any way.

The judgment from *Malette v Shulman* states:

> *It is important to note here that Dr Shulman was not found liable for any negligence in his treatment of Mrs Malette: he had acted promptly and professionally and was well motivated throughout and his management of the case had been carried out in a competent, careful and conscientious manner in accordance with the requisite standard of care. His decision to administer blood in the circumstances confronting him was found to be an honest exercise of his professional judgment which did not delay Mrs Malette's recovery, endanger her life or cause her any bodily harm. Indeed, the doctor's treatment of Mrs Malette may well have been responsible for saving her life.*[8]

Notwithstanding this somewhat unusual situation, as a general rule, it is when something goes wrong, and patients suffer damage as a result of their treatment (now often referred to as an adverse event) that they start to seek further explanations and information. On some occasions, the care or treatment may have gone wrong because a practitioner had not exercised adequate care, and an action in negligence may be a possible outcome. On other occasions all the most prudent precautions and competence will still not prevent unforeseen problems arising. Nevertheless, when something does go wrong, invariably the patient will want to know what happened, why, who did what and when, or perhaps whether anyone failed to do something.

The process for managing adverse events and disclosing their occurrence to patients is discussed in

Chapter 9, specifically in relation to the practice of 'open disclosure'. Depending on the facts and circumstances and, more often than not, influenced by the degree of damage that has occurred and the way in which the adverse event was managed, the patient may seek legal advice about the appropriateness of making a complaint and/or suing the doctor, hospital and any other parties the patient feels may have been responsible for the damage that has occurred. However, the Australian Commission on Safety and Quality in Health Care, in its guide for health service managers, points out that:

There is no conclusive evidence that open disclosure either increases or decreases litigation. Current literature states that if a patient is told about an adverse event and they are treated quickly and harm prevented or minimised, the patient may be less inclined to pursue legal action.

In taking an active approach, you or your clinical staff may be able to talk to the patient in a way that defuses anger and restores trust. In some cases, it may be appropriate, after consultation with the clinical team, management and insurers, to recommend a prompt and fair out of court settlement. When you offer support for follow up or additional treatment, it doesn't necessarily mean your organisation is accepting liability … Litigation may be reduced if patients appreciate the fallibility and honesty of the clinician. If you or your clinical team do not disclose and serious mistakes come to light later on, the patient may think it is an attempt to cover up and become angry and litigious.[9]

If the patient chooses to make a complaint, this may be done locally to the hospital or through the relevant healthcare complaints body or registration authority. In such situations the patient is usually concerned that the same mistake does not happen again, and the purpose is often to improve patient safety, rather than to seek financial redress. Complaints of this nature are discussed in detail in **Chapter 4**.

If, on the other hand, the patient decides to take legal action, the legal action that may be contemplated will generally revolve around three potential considerations:

1. professional negligence, either by act or by omission;

2. assault and battery in the absence of a valid consent; and/or

3. breach of contract (where a contractual relationship exists between the patient and the provider of treatment).

Two potential causes of action, negligence and battery, often overlap, and this can confuse the layperson. This overlap is often described (erroneously in Australia) as **informed consent**. For legal purposes, as is demonstrated above, there are two distinct areas of law in play here.

The question of adequately informing a patient in 'broad terms of the nature of the procedure which is intended' is critical to the issue of obtaining a valid consent as a defence to an action in battery.[10] However, the failure of a medical practitioner to inform a patient adequately about the treatment he or she is to undergo, particularly the material risks involved and likely outcome of any proposed treatment, can and has been determined by the courts to be negligence.[11]

Such a failure will, more often than not, be deemed to be a breach of the doctor's duty of disclosure, as part of their duty of care to the patient. That important distinction, together with the relevant cases and the views expressed by the courts, is set out in **Chapter 7**.

Remember that, in any allegation of negligence, the patient must prove all the necessary elements, including the fact that he or she has suffered some form of recognisable damage. As far as any action in battery is concerned, the patient does not have to prove damage, but rather an intentional touching and the absence of consent to the treatment given. The amount of compensation awarded by a court in such a situation may be nominal when compared with the compensation awarded if the patient were damaged and could prove negligence. Nevertheless, it is possible for a patient to bring an action seeking compensation for battery in the absence of any negligence on the part of the person concerned and in the absence of any physical harm to the person bringing the action and solely on the basis that consent was not given to the type of touching which occurred. The case of *Malette v Shulman* (**Case example 6.1**) made precisely this point.[12] Although the decisions of Canadian courts are not binding on Australian courts, they would be considered to be persuasive precedent. This case is particularly interesting because it demonstrates the distinction between an action in negligence and battery and at the same time it reinforces the right of a person to withhold consent to treatment — in this case, a blood transfusion.

The court upheld Mrs Malette's claim against Dr Shulman on the basis that he had violated Mrs Malette's 'rights over her own body by acting contrary to the Jehovah's Witness card and administering blood transfusions that were not authorised'.[13] The court awarded Mrs Malette $20 000 in damages but declined to make any award of costs; that is, Mrs Malette would have had to pay her own legal costs out of the damages awarded. Compared with amounts awarded by courts today for negligence actions, damages of $20 000 for battery would certainly be considered nominal, particularly as Mrs Malette had to pay her own legal costs. In a number of more recent cases involving blood transfusions and Jehovah's Witnesses, not all the decisions are as clear-cut as this one.[14] Justice Basten pointed out in *X v The Sydney Children's Hospitals Network*:[15]

The interest of the state in preserving life is at its highest with respect to children and young persons who are inherently vulnerable, in varying degrees.[16]

Douglas J, in the Queensland Supreme Court in 2015,[17] cited the judgment of Basten J in determining these cases. He observed that Basten J:

... usefully then went on to consider the balancing considerations there between concepts of sanctity of life and the best interests of a young person, including balancing the issues raised by the religious beliefs of the child and the parents as matters which are clearly significant and should be taken into account. But here, in effect, it seems to me appropriate to conclude that the sanctity of J's life, in the end, is a more powerful reason for me to make the orders than is respect for the dignity of the beliefs so sincerely held by his parents and him.[18]

Notwithstanding these recent children's cases, *Malette v Shulman* does provide a clear example of what the tort of battery is intended to do, which is to uphold the right of individuals to control what happens to their own body.

WHAT INFORMATION IS AVAILABLE TO HELP PROFESSIONALS AND PATIENTS?

These matters are extremely complex, and there are many useful documents available to assist health professionals and consumers alike both to understand the law and to provide the best available information and practices.

For health professionals, there is a range of useful information — for example, the National Health and Medical Research Council (NHMRC), in its *National Statement on Ethical Conduct in Human Research*,[19] has a helpful section on General requirements for consent in Chapter 2.2.[20] Links to two further state policies are provided in the footnotes, and similar documents would be available in every jurisdiction.[21] These documents are extremely comprehensive and valuable resources for any health professional who wishes to understand not only the law but also how the law operates in practice. In addition, there are many useful consumer information documents — some developed by government and others by consumer organisations, such as Canberra Health Literacy, which provide accessible information about the law and what people are entitled to expect.[22] The Federal Government also publishes information for consumers on informed consent, including a list of questions to ask, via its *healthdirect* Australia website.[23]

HOW MAY CONSENT BE GIVEN?

It is helpful to remember that the word 'consent' comes from the Latin *consensere*, meaning 'to agree'. Thus, consent is an agreement between two parties, and requires a level of common understanding. It is generally stated that a patient must give **valid consent**. The term 'valid consent' simply denotes the necessity to ensure that any consent given comprises certain elements; otherwise, the consent will be invalid. The elements that comprise valid consent apply regardless of the way in which consent is given (see **Box 6.1**).

Implied consent to treatment can be given in a variety of ways and is most often used as the method of consenting to a simple procedure of common knowledge. For example, a nurse might request a patient to hold out their arm to have their blood pressure taken, or to roll over onto their back before being lifted out of bed, and the patient's compliance with such a request would normally imply consent to that process or intervention.

Even though a patient may appear to be implying consent for the intended procedure by their actions, it is good practice to explain fully what you are going to do, regardless of behaviour that you may take to imply consent. For example, if you asked to take someone's pulse, they would normally assume you meant a radial pulse and may not have imagined (for example) that you wished to check their femoral pulse, which would clearly involve a more personal procedure.

In addition, the element of common knowledge means that it is not enough to claim that a person has given consent to treatment 'simply by turning up at the hospital'. In the 1984 deep sleep therapy (DST) case of *Hart v Herron*, the Supreme Court held that turning up at the hospital was not sufficient to imply consent for treatment, and the defendant was found to be liable in battery for administering the DST.[24] DST does not constitute a simple procedure of common knowledge. Quite clearly it is not possible to consent to a procedure about which you have neither knowledge nor understanding, as a person cannot agree to that which they have not contemplated.

Verbal consent is probably the most common form of consent that occurs in relation to simple procedures in healthcare settings. Both verbal and written consents are often described as express consent — that is, the person has expressly indicated that they consent to the procedure or intervention, rather than the healthcare practitioner having to make assumptions by implication. See **Boxes 6.2** and **6.3** for differing examples of verbal consent.

A **consent in writing**, in the form of either a standard or specialised written consent form, is generally nothing more than documentary evidence of what has already been consented to verbally by the patient. In many ways the function served by a written consent form parallels the function of a contract made in writing. It is quite possible to create a legally binding contract between two parties by verbal agreement without recourse to a document, as long as the elements of a simple contract exist. There is no general legal principle that states that consent forms must exist and be signed before a patient can be treated, although there are now a number of situations where either law or policy requires consent in writing. For example, the Western Australian Department of Health's *WA Health consent to treatment policy* (s. 2.2.1)[25] requires explicit

---

BOX 6.4
DOES THE CONSENT NEED TO BE IN WRITING?[26]

The example below is taken from the NSW Health *Consent to medical and healthcare treatment manual.*

The general law on consent does not require consent or the provision of information, including warnings about risks, to be in writing. Consent to the treatment or procedure must still be sought notwithstanding it is not always required in writing. Patient consent can be express, either orally or in writing, or it can be implied from a person's conduct. For example, a patient may freely hold out their arm to receive an injection and this action could imply their consent. However, a written consent, using the consent forms attached to this Consent Manual (Attachments A-F) (or an electronic equivalent as discussed in section 4.11.1) will assist Health Practitioners in providing appropriate and adequate information to patients in line with community expectations and legal requirements. Written consent must be obtained for significant treatment and procedures as set out at section 4.5. Written consent should also be sought where a Person Responsible is consenting to treatment on behalf of a patient. There are some exceptions to this set out at section 7.5. Written consent may also assist if there are subsequent legal proceedings questioning the validity of consent. In such cases, written consent will provide strong contemporaneous evidence of what was discussed and the patient's consent and views. While a written consent is not a legal document, it can be used in legal proceedings as evidence. The absence of a written record of consent could give rise to the inference that the procedure has not been discussed or that consent has not been obtained.

---

consent to be sought and specifically recorded in certain situations. **Box 6.4** summarises situations where written consent is recommended.

The critical element that a completed written consent form provides is documentary evidence that consent was given, should a dispute arise over that point. Having said that, a written consent in no way guarantees that the consent given is a valid one — that is another issue completely.

It is true to say that a consent form is only as good or as valid as the quality of the consent or agreement that has been made and that it represents. It is the validity of the consent that goes to the heart of the procedural requirements, and not the signing of a piece of paper.

WHAT ARE THE ELEMENTS OF A VALID CONSENT?

The validity of any consent, however given, will be satisfied only if the three elements that constitute a valid consent are present. These elements are set out in **Box 6.5**. Each of these is now examined in turn.

Any Consent Given is Freely and Voluntarily Given

This means that any consent given by a patient must be given without any fraud, duress or coercion being

---

BOX 6.5
ELEMENTS OF A VALID CONSENT

1. That any consent given is freely and voluntarily given;
2. That any consent given is properly informed; and
3. That the person giving consent has the legal capacity to give it.

---

applied by the medical practitioner or any other member of staff to obtain the patient's consent. As a general rule, medical and nursing staff members do not deliberately seek to apply fraudulent or coercive measures on patients to obtain their consent but can do so unwittingly in a variety of ways. For example:

- if a healthcare practitioner advises a patient that he or she must have a particular form of treatment, or else they will be discharged;
- the authoritative role of a healthcare practitioner may introduce an element of coercion into the consent procedure on the basis of 'I know what's best for you'.

However, despite what might be the best intentions of the clinician, if it can be established that any coercion or duress was brought to bear on a patient to obtain their consent, that consent will be invalid.

Sadly, on occasions nurses have been involved in deceptions to obtain consent, as shown in the Royal Commission into Deep Sleep Therapy, which investigated the practices of a psychiatrist and his colleagues who admitted mentally ill patients to a private hospital (Chelmsford) and gave them the 'special treatment' of barbiturate-induced coma and sometimes adjuvant electroconvulsive therapy. Over the ensuing 16 years until 1979, at least 24 people died as a direct result of the DST. This excerpt from the testimony of one nurse gives an example of how deception was used to implement the DST.

> Some who did know, if they refused to sign the consent form, then the instruction was that you gave them some medication to quieten them down; that's what you would say, 'I'll give you this little injection now, it will calm you down. You will feel a lot better after it'. But of course, that little injection was sodium amytal and I think some Valium as well and then of course they were off on the sedation.[27]

While no action was taken against any nurses as a result of the events at Chelmsford, this excerpt provides a clear example of how deception might be employed to obtain consent to treatment. Such behaviour is clearly not acceptable and would invalidate any consent.

The Patient is Informed 'In Broad Terms of the Nature of the Procedure Which is Intended'[28]

This element probably gives the greatest concern to nursing staff, largely because of the problems that arise in relation to written consent forms. From a strictly legal perspective the term 'informed consent', which can be traced to early American decisions,[29] is no longer considered to be appropriate, confusing as it does the requirement for consent in defence to actions in battery and the requirement to give information about material risks, the absence of which forms one of the elements of an action in negligence. However, in the practicality of explaining a procedure to a patient there is an alignment of the two processes, as people need not only to be informed in broad terms (thus providing a defence against an action in battery), but also to be informed about the material risks (thus providing a defence against a potential action in negligence). Both

levels of information are in fact necessary before any therapeutic intervention can be undertaken.

Perhaps a helpful way to think about the issue is to consider the concept of giving information (and informed consent) in general, everyday terms. On a day-to-day basis, people make decisions on a whole variety of issues which affect their lives, whether it be to buy a house or a new car, take an overseas holiday, take out insurance or change jobs. In making decisions on such major issues, people obtain relevant information that will help them decide whether to go ahead with a particular proposal — for example, cost, finance available, repayments, access to public transport and schools, career opportunities and so on. A person will then assess the various alternatives available before coming to a final decision on the matter.

Gathering together the information needed to arrive at the most appropriate decision constitutes the informed element of the decision-making process. It is much the same situation when considering whether or not to consent to a particular medical treatment.

Obviously, the consequences of making a decision about healthcare are often more serious than deciding whether to buy a new car, thereby only increasing the need for information and care. Nevertheless, the principle is the same.

In Australia two questions arise from the fact that information must be given to a patient when he or she is being asked to give consent to a treatment:

1. How much information does the patient require to make a decision to consent to treatment?
2. Who is responsible for giving sufficient information to a patient?

Let us consider each in some detail.

How Much Information Does the Patient Need to Make a Decision to Consent to Treatment?

At this point, it is necessary to restate that, invariably, when this issue is considered, it is done within the context of **negligence**, having regard to the perceived duty of the doctor to inform the patient adequately about the material risks inherent in any proposed treatment, and readers should refer to the cases on this issue in **Chapter 7**. That is not to suggest that an action in **battery** cannot or should not be pursued. It simply reflects the views expressed by the courts in Australia and elsewhere, particularly in England, on this issue.

Indeed, the decision of the High Court of Australia in *Rogers v Whitaker* makes it quite clear that actions against medical practitioners alleging inadequacy of information about a proposed treatment should properly be considered as part of the medical practitioner's duty of care within the context of an action in negligence.[30] The facts of *Rogers v Whitaker* are set out in **Chapter 7** and should be referred to. The facts reveal that Mrs Whitaker received precisely the treatment to which she had consented, thus there could be no successful action in battery. In unanimously dismissing Dr Rogers' appeal, the High Court made the following comment on the issue of the term 'informed consent':

In this context nothing is to be gained by reiterating the expressions used in American authorities such as 'the patient's right of self-determination' or even the oft-used and somewhat amorphous phrase 'informed consent'. The right of self-determination is an expression which is, perhaps, suitable to cases where the issue is whether a person has agreed to the general surgical procedure or treatment but is of little assistance in the balancing process that is involved in the determination of whether there has been a breach of the duty of disclosure. Likewise, the phrase 'informed consent' is apt to mislead as it suggests a test of the validity of the patient's consent. Moreover, consent is relevant to actions framed in trespass, not in negligence. Anglo-Australian law has rightly taken the view that an allegation that the risks inherent in a medical procedure have not been disclosed to the patient can only be found an action of negligence and not in trespass; the consent necessary to negative the offence of battery is satisfied by the patient being advised in broad terms of the nature of the procedure to be performed.[31]

As a result of the clear direction of the law in relation to information giving and consent, there is a great deal of detail provided to clinicians by all of the jurisdictions. The NSW Health advice on the content of the information to be presented when obtaining consent to treatment is set out in **Box 6.6**. In addition, the document also provides valuable advice on presenting information in **Box 6.7** and withholding information, which is set out in **Box 6.8**.

BOX 6.6

CONTENT OF INFORMATION TO BE GIVEN WHEN OBTAINING CONSENT TO TREATMENT (NSW HEALTH)[32]

As a guide, health practitioners advising patients about proposed treatment should consider discussing:
- the possible or likely nature of the illness
- the proposed approach to investigation and treatment including – what the proposed approach entails – the expected benefits – common side effects and material risks – whether the procedure is conventional or experimental and, if novel or experimental, that some of the risks may be unknown – who will undertake the intervention
- alternative options for diagnosis and treatment
- the benefits and risks of different options, including options to defer the decision
- the degree of uncertainty of the diagnosis and any therapeutic outcome
- the likely outcome of not having the diagnostic procedure or treatment, or of not having any procedure or treatment at all
- the likelihood of complete resolution of the clinical problem and symptoms, or chance of improvement and chance of recurrence
- level of evidence for proposed intervention

- location of procedure and length of stay
- expected timeframe for recovery
- option of seeking a second opinion
- any significant long-term physical, emotional, mental, social, sexual, or other outcome which may be associated with the proposed intervention
- where the treatment involves an 'implantable device' (such as vaginal mesh, breast implants) the manufacturer's provided consumer information
- the time and cost involved, including any out-of-pocket expenses.

Clinical judgment about how to convey risks will be influenced by several factors. These include:
- the seriousness of the patient's condition
- the nature of the intervention (complex interventions require more information)
- the likelihood of harm and the degree of possible harm
- the questions asked by the patient
- the patient's Health Literacy level and the patient's cognitive capacity
- accepted medical practice.

BOX 6.7
ADVICE ON PRESENTING INFORMATION[33]

The Health Practitioner should:

- communicate information and clinical opinions in a form the patient should be able to understand, using plain language, without any medical or technical jargon
- allow the patient enough time to decide. The patient should be encouraged to reflect on opinions, ask more questions, and consult with their family, a friend or an adviser. The patient should be assisted in seeking another medical opinion where this is requested
- repeat key information to help the patient understand and remember it
- give written information or use diagrams/pictures/photos, where appropriate, in addition to talking to the patient
- pay careful attention to the patient's responses to help identify what has or has not been understood
- use a competent, registered interpreter when the patient is not fluent in English or use AUSLAN sign interpreter if required.

Prepared material about a procedure or treatment can be useful as a means of stimulating discussion and for guiding the Health Practitioner when informing the patient. Prepared material should:

- be up to date, accurate and appropriate for the patient

- be in plain language (Easy English) that is easy to understand or translate
- contain all inherent risks of the procedure.

If a risk is more likely and/or has significant consequences, additional detail should be included

- ideally be provided before meeting with the patient to give the patient time to consider the information and prepare questions for the Health Practitioner
- be available in a variety of languages and formats (for example, large print).

Providing prepared material, without discussion, will not be enough to discharge the Health Practitioner's duty to fully inform the patient about the proposed treatment. The Health Practitioner should assist the patient to understand the material and provide further explanation if required. Health Practitioners should also check that information is up to date and accurate. An inadequate, inaccurate or out-dated information sheet may undermine the assertion that a patient has been properly informed. If a patient is provided with a copy of prepared material as part of obtaining consent, this should be recorded in the Health Record and, ideally, a copy of the prepared material attached to the consent form.

BOX 6.8
WHEN IS IT ACCEPTABLE TO WITHHOLD INFORMATION FROM A PATIENT?[34]

There are two (2) situations where a Medical Practitioner may be justified in withholding information from a patient.

1. Where a patient does not want the information and expressly directs the treating Medical Practitioner to make decisions on their behalf. Even in this case, the Medical Practitioner should give the patient basic information about the diagnosis and treatment. Any direction or views expressed by the patient must be documented in the patient's Health Record.

2. Therapeutic privilege. Information could be withheld in rare circumstances where the Medical Practitioner holds a reasonable belief that providing information would be damaging to the patient's health. This will only arise in very limited circumstances and requires the Medical Practitioner to make a judgment, based on reasonable grounds, that the patient's physical or mental health might be seriously harmed by the information. The types of factors governing therapeutic privilege include the patient's personality, temperament or attitude;

their level of understanding; the nature of the treatment and the likelihood of adverse effects resulting from the treatment.

In these circumstances, the Medical Practitioner should clearly record the reasons for exercising therapeutic privilege in the patient's Health Record. Health Practitioners should consider seeking assistance in communicating with patients and families about difficult matters and consult with colleagues before making a decision on withholding information.

Information cannot be withheld from a guardian or Person Responsible making decisions on behalf of a patient under the *Guardianship Act 1987*. Where it is considered that the Person Responsible is not capable of performing their functions the Medical Practitioner should certify this in writing and the next person in the Person Responsible hierarchy should be consulted. Further advice should be sought from Ministry of Health Legal Branch or the local Director of Medical Services if there is any uncertainty about whether information can be withheld from a patient.

The issue of how much information a person needs to make a decision about consenting to treatment can be summarised as follows:

- the information element of a valid consent is the gathering together of the information needed to allow a patient to arrive at a decision they believe is in their own best interests;
- if there were to be any statement of general legal propositions applicable in Australia, it would be that, in obtaining a valid consent, a patient must be given sufficient information to be able to understand the nature and consequences of the proposed treatment; and
- failure to advise and inform a patient properly about the nature and consequences of the proposed treatment as well as its material risks would, in most instances, amount to a breach of the doctor's duty of care, which could, should damage ensue, make the doctor liable in negligence, quite apart from any action in battery.

Who is Responsible for Giving Sufficient Information to a Patient?

There is no doubt that the responsibility for giving the patient sufficient information to enable him or her to make an informed decision rests with the primary treating healthcare practitioner.

In some situations, where no doctor is involved, the responsibility would rest with the person in charge of the case. For example, in the case of a homebirth conducted by a homebirth midwife with no obstetrician involved, the responsibility for giving the patient sufficient and relevant information rests with the midwife. Likewise, where the treating healthcare practitioner was a nurse practitioner, the primary responsibility would rest with the nurse practitioner.

This situation has been recognised in policy. For example, the New South Wales Ministry of Health policy *Consent to medical and healthcare treatment manual*, states:

In most cases, the Health Practitioner who will perform the procedure, or provide the treatment should obtain or confirm the patient's consent for that procedure or treatment. Health Practitioners such as Nurse Practitioners and Midwives, and

allied health professionals perform procedures and some examinations as part of their usual scope of practice, such as central line insertion, lumbar puncture, and abdominal paracentesis. Any Health Practitioner who is appropriately experienced and trained to perform procedures within their scope of practice must obtain valid consent prior to performing those procedures. Consent may be implied from the patient acquiescing to the procedure. However, the criteria for obtaining a valid consent must still be met, the procedure must still be explained to the patient, and it is advisable for a written note to be made in the patient's Health Record documenting this.[35]

Until recently, the usual situation encountered in hospitals and healthcare settings would be that the treating doctor would be responsible for informing the patient about the treatment he or she has consented to undergo. Three questions set out in **Box 6.9** are regularly raised by nursing (and sometimes midwifery) staff in relation to this. The first question simply relates to the practicalities of signing the consent form. The second to the new concepts of electronic signatures, faxed signatures and other forms of communication.

The dilemma presented in the third question in **Box 6.9** often arises in relation to treatments which patients undergo on the advice of their treating doctor in

---

BOX 6.9

QUESTIONS RELATING TO INFORMATION GIVEN TO PATIENTS BY HEALTH PROFESSIONALS WHO ARE NOT THE TREATING PRACTITIONER

1. What is the scope of responsibility for a nurse (or other healthcare employee) who is asked to obtain a patient's signature for a consent form?
2. Can consent be captured electronically, and can a consent form be faxed or emailed?
3. What are the professional responsibilities of nurses and midwives to inform patients of aspects of their treatment if they believe they have not been fully explained by the treating healthcare practitioner? Alternatively, what are the nurses' and midwives' professional responsibilities when a patient asks them for advice about the appropriateness of the treatment he or she is having?

terminal illnesses — for example, chemotherapy, radiotherapy and radical surgery.

We examine each of these issues.

Written Consent Forms. For many years, hospitals insisted that nurses (or other administrative personnel) were responsible for obtaining a patient's signature on consent forms. It is pleasing to note that key policy documents have now placed the responsibility primarily where it rightfully belongs — with the medical officer or other treating practitioner concerned. The policy allows for delegation, but not abrogation, of responsibility. The New South Wales Ministry of Health policy, *Consent to medical and healthcare treatment manual*, has this to say:

> *Both the Admitting Medical Officer and the Medical Practitioner or Health Practitioner who ultimately performs the procedure have legal and professional responsibilities to the patient to obtain a valid consent. The extent of the legal responsibility of each practitioner will vary according to the facts and circumstances of each situation considering the complexity and seriousness of the procedure or treatment.*[36]

Legally, any person over the age of 18 years and of sound mind may witness a patient's signature on a consent form. This argument is the one most often raised by medical practitioners, who state that they should not be required to witness a patient's signature on a consent form because it can legally be done by any member of staff. That is in fact correct in this situation: there is no requirement for any specific person to witness a signature.

However, it does nothing to address the concerns often raised by nursing and midwifery staff, as the signing of the form often brings about a plethora of questions heretofore unasked. This is where it is important to remember that, if the patient has agreed to come into hospital for treatment, it is usually on the basis of the advice of the medical practitioner. Therefore, as a matter of commonsense and good practice, it is the medical practitioner who should witness the patient's written consent to that treatment, particularly when the procedure is elective.

In hospitals where such a task is still designated to the nursing staff (or indeed administrative staff) the only role that the staff member plays in obtaining the patient's signature is to witness that signature.

Witnessing a patient's signature in no way imposes on the staff member the primary responsibility for informing the patient of the nature and extent of the procedure to which the patient is consenting.

If a nurse or midwife is required to ask a patient to sign a consent form, they should observe these steps. (See also **Box 6.9** for the status of written consent forms.)

- Always ensure that the consent form is completely filled in. A patient should never be asked to sign a blank consent form. It is expected that the admitting medical officer would fill in that information.
- If a patient wishes to alter the consent form in any way by adding or crossing out words, then the nurse or midwife must advise the treating practitioner as soon as possible.
- If a patient starts to ask questions concerning the nature and extent of the procedure to which the patient is consenting, the nurse or midwife should offer to ask the patient's treating doctor to come and talk to the patient. In contacting the treating practitioner, the nurse or midwife should make a relevant entry in the patient's records, as well as noting the practitioner's response to the request.
- If a patient refuses to sign a consent form, the treating practitioner must be advised, and a relevant entry made in the patient's record. In a hospital, the appropriate administrative personnel should also be advised.

Consent Provided by Email, Fax or Electronically. As more and more of our records are being generated electronically and particularly given the growth of virtual consultations during COVID-19, it is to be expected that other documents such as consent forms might also be generated virtually in some way. However, the requirements for a valid consent do not change in any way. It is simply the practicalities of providing the evidence of a valid consent that need to be considered. The New South Wales Ministry of Health policy, *Consent to medical and healthcare treatment manual*, also addresses this issue (as do other contemporary jurisdictional policies):

> *Information provided to a patient as part of obtaining consent must be documented. This can be achieved a number of ways, depending on the electronic medical records program in use — through free text typing by the Health Practitioner, uploading a voice recording of the Health Practitioner advising the patient about the procedures and material risks, or using a pamphlet as part of the information provision and then uploading it or uploading a photo of the pamphlet in the electronic medical record.*
>
> - *If the facilities are available to the Health Service, the patient may be provided with an electronic device and use a compatible instrument to manually sign the device to signify consent. Also, a patient's voice recording giving consent may be uploaded to the Health Record. These recordings must be clearly linked to the treatment the patient is consenting to and must be readily accessible in the patient's Health Record.*
> - *There must be processes in place to verify the identity of the patient or the patient's Person Responsible either through a photo identification or Patient Identifier (including patient identification bands) before consent being recorded. The Health Service must ensure that the electronically recorded consent is as reliable as the hard copy version in terms of security, storage and access. If exceptional circumstances arise whereby the Person Responsible is providing consent over the telephone, there must be a local level policy in place to confirm the identity of the Person Responsible and their connection to the patient. This could include asking standard questions to confirm the Person Responsible's personal information. The details of identity confirmation must be documented in the patient's Health Record.*
> - *The user interface elements must indicate that the Health Practitioner had a discussion around the proposed treatment, material risks and consequences. The act of checking or ticking the user interface element(s) to indicate what was discussed and that valid consent was obtained*

> *must record the user that performed that action in a permanent log, together with time and date stamps.*
> - *A physically signed, hard copy consent form may be uploaded in an appropriate human readable format to form part of the patient's electronic medical record. Examples of electronic formats include jpeg and pdf.*
> - *If subsequent changes to the state or content of any user interface elements or scanned documents are allowed, the user interface must indicate clearly that changes have been made without any action required by the viewer and must log all changes with clear identification of the user making the change and the date and time of each change. Where changes are made to a scanned document and a new version is created, the original scanned copy must be retained for medico-legal reasons.*[37]

Notwithstanding these accommodations, the policy still makes the following caveat:

> *An original consent form should be obtained where possible as it is preferable to a faxed, photocopied or scanned and emailed form. If it is not possible to obtain an original consent form, a faxed, photocopied or scanned version can be retained, provided it is of reasonable quality and it is possible to verify the signature of the patient/Person Responsible. When faxing, copying or scanning consent forms, care should be taken to ensure that double-sided documents are captured in their entirety. The use of a stamp signature or electronic equivalent signature as part of the consent process should be discouraged as they make it difficult to verify whether the Health Practitioner signed the documentation or whether it was stamped by someone else. The use of these methods could be used later to call into question whether the Health Practitioner actually turned their mind to making that decision.*[38]

The Professional Responsibility to Inform. Nursing and midwifery staff members who are not the **primary** treating practitioner still do have a professional responsibility to educate patients and to provide **secondary**

information about a particular treatment, once the course of treatment has been agreed upon and the information necessary to inform that agreement given by the treating practitioner.

Nursing and midwifery staff members are often questioned by patients about the treatment they are undergoing. They are the most frequent source of contact and conversation in a hospital, and patients often relate readily to the nursing and midwifery staff for that reason. It is completely appropriate for them to provide the best advice and information available and to answer patients' questions honestly and helpfully in relation to the agreed treatment, and significant advantages are known to attach to the provision of preoperative information.[39] However, there have been occasions where nurses and midwives have found themselves in the difficult position of caring for a patient whom, they believe, has not received sufficient information concerning the particular treatment they are to undergo or the alternative courses of treatment which may be available to the patient. The most frequent problem for nurses has been in relation to the treatment of patients for various types of cancer, which quite often involves the administration of large doses of cytotoxic drugs and radiotherapy. This type of treatment often results in physically and mentally distressing side effects for the patient, which, if the patient's life expectancy is quite limited, can cause many health professionals to question the efficacy of the treatment. In such a situation the nurse must carefully assess their professional position before seeking to intrude on the patient–doctor relationship.

There have been occasions where nursing or midwifery staff members have become concerned and openly critical about the standard of care being practised by a nursing or medical colleague. The problem becomes particularly difficult when the criticism is directed at a medical practitioner whom the nursing or midwifery staff members believe to be giving unsafe and/or inappropriate medical care to a patient.

If a member of the nursing or midwifery staff is genuinely concerned about the standard of care being delivered by a professional colleague, that concern should first, as a matter of courtesy and commonsense, be dealt with by discussing it directly with the colleague. If those direct discussions do not resolve the problem, it should then be expressed formally to the appropriate administrative personnel.

Sometimes, a nurse or midwife may feel unable to initiate such a conversation, and, if they are genuinely concerned about a matter of safety, it is imperative that they discuss the matter with more senior professional staff who could take the matter up on their behalf. However, it is important that the person has clear information and evidence to support their concern. It may be that the matter can be resolved at that level by discussions between the parties involved. *The Speaking up for safety* program,[40] developed by the Cognitive Institute, has been introduced by most jurisdictions and provides helpful avenues to work through some of these difficulties.

If such approaches are unsuccessful and the criticisms expressed are valid, then there is a mandatory requirement under the *Health Practitioner Regulation National Law Act 2009* (Qld) (discussed in more detail in **Chapter 4**) to report 'notifiable conduct' by a colleague to their relevant professional registration board. **Notifiable conduct** is defined under the Act as meaning that the registered healthcare practitioner has:

a. *practised the practitioner's profession while intoxicated by alcohol or drugs; or*
b. *engaged in sexual misconduct* in connection with the practice of the practitioner's *profession; or*
c. *placed the public at risk of substantial harm* in the practitioner's *practice of the profession because the practitioner has an impairment; or*
d. *placed the public at risk of harm because* the practitioner has practised the profession in a way that constitutes a significant departure from accepted professional standards.[41] *[emphasis added]*

In doing so, criticisms that form the subject of the complaint should be supported by objective and factual documentation. At no time should such professional criticisms become the subject of general gossip, particularly outside the hospital where some people may be only too ready to believe such criticisms. If this happens, then that person's professional reputation may be irreparably damaged, and they would have legitimate resort to an action in defamation.

In recent years, there has been a greater emphasis on a systems approach to problems and errors in healthcare. Human beings make mistakes[42] and health professionals are no exception.[43] The aviation industry developed the concept of 'crew resource management' (CRM), which created the imperative for each member of the aviation team, regardless of status, to speak out strongly if he or she believed there to be a problem.[44] In the healthcare sector, there is now a prevailing view that all health professionals have a responsibility to speak up (appropriately, as discussed above) to avoid adverse incidents occurring and to report adverse events so that they can be analysed and preventive strategies can be implemented. The *Speaking up for safety* program identified above[45] takes these elements of crew resource management and translates them for health professionals, the outcomes of which are set out in **Box 6.10**. The Cognitive Institute describes its program as follows:

> *For every provider of healthcare, Speaking Up for Safety is a critical aspect of achieving a safe and reliable culture. The program teaches a common language, where clinicians support each other by effectively communicating concern to colleagues that unintended harm to patients may be about to occur.*[46]

Therapeutic Privilege

In some limited situations the law will recognise that, although there may well be a general duty to disclose what is reasonable and necessary in the circumstances,

---

BOX 6.10

OUTCOMES OF SPEAKING UP FOR SAFETY PROGRAM[47]

The programme provides healthcare organisations with:
- improved patient safety attributable to greater staff willingness to speak up for patient safety
- respectful, collegiate communication as a first approach to raising a concern when something is not right
- creation of a professional culture embedded with patient safety, where anyone in the organisation is able to raise a concern with another person, thus normalising speaking up
- a positive framework reinforcing that everyone has a role to play in patient safety
- a proactive tool to enable staff to intervene before mistakes happen and unintended patient harm occurs.

---

an exception may arise. The usual situation is where the treating doctor elects to use what is termed **therapeutic privilege** — that is, the doctor chooses not to disclose information to a patient that he or she believes would be detrimental to the patient's best interests, generally for mental health reasons. The NSW Health policy *Consent to medical and health treatment manual* identifies two limited scenarios where it might be acceptable to withhold information. See **Box 6.8**.

To widen the application of therapeutic privilege beyond the circumstances referred to would run counter to the general duty to inform. The issue of therapeutic privilege was also raised in **Chapter 2** in the discussion on ethics.

The Person Giving Consent Has the Legal Capacity to Give Such Consent

The second requirement for a valid consent relates to the capacity of the person to actually be able to agree to the proposed treatment. Legal capacity or competence to give or refuse consent has a number of components, whether it relates to mental capacity or to age. These were identified in the English case of *Re C (Adult: Refusal of Treatment)*, which addressed the question of whether a man who suffered from a mental illness was capable of refusing treatment to amputate a limb which was gangrenous.[48] Here Thorpe J determined that he had capacity, and defined capacity as a sufficient understanding of 'the nature, purpose and effects of the proffered treatment'.[49]

Section 4 of the *Medical Treatment Planning and Decisions Act 2016* (Vic) sets out the requirements for determining decision-making capacity, including advice on strategies to do so; see **Box 6.11**.

The abilities identified here are quite high-level cognitive requirements and readers may be able to recall a number of people who would have struggled to meet all these criteria, and yet were considered capable of providing consent to treatment. However, there are a number of exceptions to the general rule, which are dealt with below.

Adults and Consent

Any person over 18, barring any determination of mental incapacity, can give and withhold consent to treatment. Yet even with adults, situations arise where the issue of consent or otherwise needs to be carefully

---

BOX 6.11

PRINCIPLES FOR ASSESSING DECISION-MAKING CAPACITY

DECISION-MAKING CAPACITY

(1) A person has ***decision-making capacity*** to make a decision to which this Act applies if the person is able to do the following —

   (a) understand the information relevant to the decision and the effect of the decision;

   (b) retain that information to the extent necessary to make the decision;

   (c) use or weigh that information as part of the process of making the decision;

   (d) communicate the decision and the person's views and needs as to the decision in some way, including by speech, gestures or other means.

(2) For the purposes of subsection (1), an adult is presumed to have decision-making capacity unless there is evidence to the contrary.

(3) For the purposes of subsection (1)(a), a person is taken to understand information relevant to a decision if the person understands an explanation of the information given to the person in a way that is appropriate to the person's circumstances, whether by using modified language, visual aids or any other means.

(4) In determining whether or not a person has decision-making capacity, regard must be had to the following —

   (a) a person may have decision-making capacity to make some decisions and not others;

   (b) if a person does not have decision-making capacity for a particular decision, it may be temporary and not permanent;

   (c) it should not be assumed that a person does not have decision-making capacity to make a decision —

     (i) on the basis of the person's appearance; or

     (ii) because the person makes a decision that is, in the opinion of others, unwise;

   (d) a person has decision-making capacity to make a decision if it is possible for the person to make a decision with practicable and appropriate support.

EXAMPLES

Practicable and appropriate support includes the following —

   (a) using information or formats tailored to the particular needs of a person;

   (b) communicating or assisting a person to communicate the person's decision;

   (c) giving a person additional time and discussing the matter with the person;

   (d) using technology that alleviates the effects of a person's disability.

(5) A person who is assessing whether a person has decision-making capacity must take reasonable steps to conduct the assessment at a time and in an environment in which the person's decision-making capacity can be most accurately assessed.

---

considered. The common law and statutory situations that may arise for consideration in the provision of healthcare services to adults where consent may need to be obtained from a third party, or may not be necessary to obtain, are now examined.

Intellectual Capacity to Make a Decision. The disability rights movement of the 1960s brought recognition for groups of people who may lack the capacity to make decisions for themselves, yet who need access to the same services and opportunities as everyone else in the community. Over the ensuing 20 years, each jurisdiction in Australia enacted legislation to protect the rights of adults who, for whatever reason, lacked the full capacity to make their own decisions.[50] In addition, the United Nations' Convention on the Rights of Persons with Disabilities (CRPD) and its Optional Protocol were adopted at the United Nations

Headquarters in New York on 13 December 2006, and entered into force internationally on 3 May 2008.

The Intellectual Disability Rights Service (IDRS) explains that Australia was one of the first countries to ratify the CRPD, on 17 July 2008. Its purpose is to 'promote, protect and ensure the full and equal enjoyment of all human rights and fundamental freedoms for all persons with disabilities, and to promote respect for their inherent dignity'.[51] A number of the Articles are identified by the IDRS as bearing on the fundamental principles of autonomy, personal decision-making and self-determination and they include:

- *equality and non-discrimination (Art 5);*
- *equal recognition before the law (Art 12);*
- *access to justice (Art 13);*
- *freedom from exploitation, violence and abuse (Art 16);*

- *protecting the integrity of the person (Art 17);*
- *freedom of expression and opinion, and access to information (Art 21).*[52]

When the *National Disability Insurance Scheme Act 2014* (Cth) (NDIS Act) was passed the principles under s 4 of the NDIS Act went to the heart of the right of people living with a disability to exercise decision-making:

- *people with disability should be supported to participate in and contribute to social and economic life to the extent of their ability;*
- *people with disability should be supported to exercise choice, including in relation to taking reasonable risks, in the pursuit of their goals and the planning and delivery of their support;*
- *people with disability have the same right as other members of Australian society to be able to determine their own best interests, including the right to exercise choice and control, and to engage as equal partners in decisions that will affect their lives, to the full extent of their capacity;*
- *people with disability should be supported in all their dealings and communications with the Agency so that their capacity to exercise choice and control is maximised in a way that is appropriate to their circumstances and cultural needs;*
- *the role of families, carers and other significant persons in the lives of people with disability is to be acknowledged and respected.*[53]

To help make decisions for people, where their full understanding of the nature and consequences of the decision may be absent or less than optimal, a statutory guardianship framework has been developed to ensure that they receive the best support and that the best possible decisions are made with or for them. *Australian Guardianship Law* is an excellent website that provides a time-defined range of case law and clear explanations about guardianship law in Australia, as it is generally poorly understood.[54]

The decision-making requirements for an adult are complex and important and include such aspects as accommodation, healthcare and health services, and medical and dental treatment. Usually, financial decisions and management are subject to more intensive and/or circumscribed scrutiny. An example of such scrutiny can be found in section 4(2) of the *Guardianship and Management of Property Act 1991* (ACT), which identifies a set of principles to be followed by a decision-maker acting for a protected person:

*4(2) The **decision-making principles** to be followed by the decision-maker are the following:*

(a) the decision-maker must provide or facilitate, as far as practicable, support necessary for the protected person to understand the decision to be made, participate in decision-making and communicate their wishes;

(b) the protected person's wishes, as far as they can be worked out, must be given effect to, unless making the decision in accordance with the wishes is likely to significantly adversely affect the protected person's interests;

(c) if giving effect to the protected person's wishes is likely to significantly adversely affect the person's interests—the decision-maker must give effect to the protected person's wishes as far as possible without significantly adversely affecting the protected person's interests;

(d) if the protected person's wishes cannot be worked out or given effect to at all — the interests of the protected person must be promoted;

(e) the protected person's life (including the person's lifestyle) must be interfered with to the smallest extent necessary;

(f) the protected person must be encouraged to look after himself or herself as far as possible;

(g) the protected person must be encouraged to live in the general community, and take part in community activities, as far as possible.

For the purposes of this chapter, the most important aspect of the guardianship framework is the ability of another person to consent to medical and dental treatment on behalf of the adult who is unable to make the decisions. This consent is known as a '**substitute consent**' and occurs in the following context:

Where a person or agency other than the patient gives consent for medical or dental treatment, it is called 'substitute consent'. This can only occur in accordance with the legislation or an order of the Tasmanian Civil and Administrative Tribunal — Guardianship Stream (Tribunal).[55]

To administer this substitute consent decision-making framework, each jurisdiction has legislation that sets out the rules and parameters for the decision-making. Although all have similar elements, the details of the legislation do vary between jurisdictions, and nurses will need to acquaint themselves with government policy in relation to guardianship provisions in their own state or territory. The various statutes for each jurisdiction are shown in **Table 6.1**.

Some statutes set out the objectives of the Act, and this enables the reader to understand why parliament enacted the legislation. Some go even further and outline how these objectives are to be implemented. For example, section 4(2) of the *Guardianship and Administration Act 1986* (Vic) states that:

1. *It is the intention of Parliament that the provisions of this Act be interpreted and that every function, power, authority, discretion, jurisdiction and duty conferred or imposed by this Act is to be exercised or performed so that —*
   a. *the means which is the least restrictive of a person's freedom of decision and action as is possible in the circumstances is adopted; and*

TABLE 6.1
Legislation Applying to Guardianship Decision-Making Framework

State or Territory	Statute
ACT	*Guardianship and Management of Property Act 1991*
NSW	*Guardianship Act 1987* *Guardianship of Infants Act 1916*
NT	*Guardianship of Adults Act 2016* *Guardianship of Infants Act 1972*
Qld	*Powers of Attorney Act 1998* *Public Guardian Act 2014* *Guardianship and Administration Act 2000*
SA	*Guardianship and Administration Act 1993* *Guardianship of Infants Act 1940*
Tas	*Guardianship and Administration Act 1995* *Guardianship and Custody of Infants Act 1934*
Vic	*Guardianship and Administration Act 2019* *Medical Treatment Planning and Decisions Act 2016*
WA	*Guardianship and Administration Act 1990*

b. *the best interests of a person with a disability are promoted; and*
c. *the wishes of a person with a disability are wherever possible given effect to. [emphasis added]*

Almost all of the statutes contain such a set of principles for administering a decision-making framework. Section 5 of the *Guardianship and Administration Act 1993* (SA), reproduced in **Box 6.12**, provides another good example.

In relation to consent to medical or dental treatment, the concept of treatment itself is broken up into a range of different degrees of seriousness of consequences, and thus the people who are able to give consent on behalf of the individual also vary. For example, the *Guardianship and Administration Act 2000* (Qld) identifies the categories of urgent healthcare (s 63), life-sustaining measures in an acute emergency (s 63A), minor, uncontroversial healthcare (s 64) and special healthcare (s 68 et seq.).

Provision is made under section 63 that:

1. *Health care, other than special health care, of an adult may be carried out without consent if the adult's health provider reasonably considers —*
   a. *the adult has impaired capacity for the health matter concerned; and*
   b. *either —*
      i. *the health care should be carried out urgently to meet imminent risk to the adult's life or health; or*
      ii. *the health care should be carried out urgently to prevent significant pain or distress to the adult and it is not reasonably practicable to get consent from a person who may give it under this Act or the Powers of Attorney Act 1998. [emphasis added]*

However, section 63A also provides:

1. *A life-sustaining measure may be withheld or withdrawn for an adult without consent if the adult's health provider reasonably considers —*
   a. *the adult has impaired capacity for the health matter concerned; and*
   b. *the commencement or continuation of the measure for the adult would be inconsistent with good medical practice; and*

BOX 6.12
**EXAMPLE OF BEST INTEREST PROVISIONS, GUARDIANSHIP
AND ADMINISTRATION ACT 1993 (SA), S 5**

Where a guardian, an administrator, the Public Advocate, the Tribunal or any court or other person, body or authority makes any decision or order in relation to a person or a person's estate pursuant to this Act or pursuant to powers conferred by or under this Act —

a. consideration (and this will be the paramount consideration) must be given to what would, in the opinion of the decision-maker, be the wishes of the person in the matter if he or she were not mentally incapacitated, but only so far as there is reasonably ascertainable evidence on which to base such an opinion; and

b. the present wishes of the person should, unless it is not possible or reasonably practicable to do so,

be sought in respect of the matter and consideration must be given to those wishes; and

c. consideration must, in the case of the making or affirming of a guardianship or administration order, be given to the adequacy of existing informal arrangements for the care of the person or the management of his or her financial affairs and to the desirability of not disturbing those arrangements; and

d. the decision or order made must be the one that is the least restrictive of the person's *rights and personal autonomy as is consistent with his or her proper care and protection.* [emphasis added]

---

c. consistent with good medical practice, the decision to withhold or withdraw the measure must be taken immediately. [emphasis added]

Neither of these provisions apply if there is an advance directive to the contrary. Artificial nutrition and hydration are defined as life-sustaining measures for the purpose of Schedule 2, section 5A of the Act, but not within this section, thereby limiting the range of decisions the healthcare provider can make without reference to the Tribunal.

Provision is further made that 'minor, uncontroversial health care' (s 64) may also be given to an adult patient without their consent if the healthcare provider reasonably considers that the patient lacks capacity and that the care promotes the patient's health and wellbeing and is minor and uncontroversial. Examples given in section 64 include administering a tetanus injection and an antibiotic requiring a prescription.

Provisions throughout the Queensland statute prevent patients being treated if they are known to object to the treatment, unless that treatment would cause minimal distress and the person has limited understanding of what the treatment would entail (s 67). However, the objection would still prevail in the event of tissue donation or engagement in research. The consent of a tribunal is required for special healthcare, which includes such interventions as sterilisation, but does not include such treatments as electroconvulsive

therapy or psychosurgery under section 68. Most statutes make specific provision for consent to sterilisation. Other special treatments mentioned in other statutes include termination of pregnancy, treatment with particular groups of medications, tissue donation and participation in medical research. These treatments are not necessarily forbidden; it is just that great care is taken to be transparent and rigorous in making decisions to give consent to them.

Usually there is a hierarchy of people who can give substitute consent. Several statutes use the term 'person responsible' to describe who might give consent. For example, under section 33A(4) of the *Guardianship Act 1987* (NSW), the person responsible is defined in a hierarchy of descending order as follows:

a. the person's guardian, if any, but only if the order or instrument appointing the guardian provides for the guardian to exercise the function of giving consent to the carrying out of medical or dental treatment on the person,

b. the spouse of the person, if any, if:
  i. the relationship between the person and the spouse is close and continuing, and
  ii. the spouse is not a person under guardianship,

c. a person who has the care of the person,

d. a close friend or relative of the person. [emphasis added]

If a formal guardian is appointed, their powers are usually quite specific and often valid for only a limited time, so that there is little risk of the guardian overstepping their boundaries when making decisions on the person's behalf.

Over and above a formal guardian being appointed, where there is no one to be either a person responsible or a formal guardian (also known as an 'enduring guardian'), then a Public Guardian may be appointed to give consent and make decisions on behalf of the person. Where any 'special' treatment or healthcare (also referred to as 'prescribed treatment') is required, this may need to be decided by a Guardianship Tribunal or even, in some cases, by the Supreme Court in the exercise of its *parens patriae* jurisdiction. Although most statutes differ slightly in the determination of special treatment and the consent requirements, there is a significant degree of similarity in the intent of the statutes in relation to these hierarchies.

Where there is less certainty is in relation to the withdrawal of life-sustaining treatment. Some jurisdictions allow for consent to withholding or withdrawing life-sustaining treatment. For example, the *Guardianship and Administration Act 2000* (Qld) makes specific provision for withholding or withdrawing life-sustaining treatment, under section 63A (extracted above), providing the adult's health provider reasonably considers that the 'commencement or continuation of the measure for the adult would be inconsistent with good medical practice' and 'the decision to withhold or withdraw the measure must be taken immediately'.

A decision to withhold artificial nutrition and hydration was allowed by the New South Wales Guardianship and Administration Tribunal in the case of *Re QAN*,[56] as summarised in **Case example 6.2**.

CASE EXAMPLE 6.2

Re QAN [2008] NSWGT 16

Mr QAN, a 49-year-old plumber with insulin dependent diabetes, had severe hypoglycaemic encephalopathy, having been found unconscious with an unrecordable blood sugar level. Mr QAN was not able to respond to commands and had become blind. The results of an MRI brain scan and EEG were compatible with severe encephalopathy and were poor prognostic indicators. His treating doctors believed

---

CASE EXAMPLE 6.2

Re QAN [2008] NSWGT 16 (Continued)

he was a clear candidate for a nursing home, as he had no terminal illness, but considered that the removal of feeding and insulin, as requested by members of his family, might be interpreted as euthanasia. They wished to insert a PEG tube, but his family did not want this.

Very many of Mr QAN's friends and relatives had written to the Tribunal before the hearing, expressing the view that Mr QAN would not wish to be kept alive if he were to be so physically incapacitated as to be unable to care for himself. Some of these letters indicated that Mr QAN had expressed the view that he did not wish to be alive if one of his limbs required amputation as a result of his diabetic condition.

The Tribunal was satisfied on the evidence before it that it was in the best interests of Mr QAN that his guardian be given an end-of-life healthcare function. For these reasons, the Tribunal determined to give Mr QAN's guardian that function. Accordingly, the guardian has the authority to make end-of-life healthcare decisions, including advance care planning decisions, for Mr QAN.

Mr QAN's mother told the Tribunal that she wished to be appointed as his guardian. His sisters strongly supported the appointment of their mother to be their brother's guardian. Ms O, a friend of Mr QAN who attended the hearing, also supported the appointment of his mother as the guardian.

An Involuntary Patient in a Psychiatric Hospital. There are essentially two types of patients who are admitted to psychiatric hospitals: voluntary patients and involuntary patients (deemed to be mentally ill in accordance with the relevant state or territory mental health legislation).

The **voluntary patient** presents himself or herself for treatment and professional care and retains the right to give and withhold consent to treatment and leave hospital at any time.

The **involuntary patient** is admitted for treatment against their wishes and, in some circumstances as set out in the legislation, has no legal capacity to give or withhold consent to treatment. There are legislative safeguards in the Acts to protect the patient's interests, while at the same time permitting hospital authorities to carry out therapeutic procedures on such patients if considered necessary. This matter is discussed at length in **Chapter 10**.

Emergency Situations. No consent is required where the patient is unconscious or seriously ill and the situation calls for immediate intervention to save the person's life. The overriding duty of care which arises in such emergency situations negates the need for consent on the grounds of the doctrine of emergency or necessity. However, the treatment must be an urgent treatment required to save life or prevent severe and long-lasting deterioration to the patient. The *WA Health consent to treatment policy* states that:

> *In an emergency where a person is incapable of giving consent, treatment may be provided without consent, i.e., where treatment is necessary to save a person's life or prevent serious injury to the person's health.*

> *The treatment in these cases is that which is:*
> - *reasonably required to meet the emergency*
> - *in the patient's best interests*
> - *the least restrictive of the patient's future choices.*

> *In these situations, the completion of a consent form is not required, but the circumstances that constitute the medical emergency and the patient's inability to consent must be clearly documented in the patient's medical record.*

> *The emergency exception (to the requirement to obtain consent prior to treatment) only applies where a person:*
> - *is unable to give consent*
> - *does not have an Advance Health Directive (AHD) or common law directive that is known, immediately available and applicable in the circumstances*
> - *does not have a substitute decision-maker who can be readily identified and immediately available to consider consent.*[57]

Blood Transfusions and Other Treatments. Problems can arise where the adult patient is conscious and refusing treatment. The situation that occasionally occurs

is where a patient refuses blood transfusions on the grounds of religious beliefs. In common law, an adult has the right to refuse such treatment, and hospitals have no authority to override that decision. An example of that situation is the case referred to earlier in this chapter (see **Case example 6.1**) of the Jehovah's Witness patient (Mrs Malette) who sued the treating doctor for battery on the grounds that he had overridden her express objections in the form of a printed signed card carried in her purse which stated that, because of her religious convictions, she did not want any blood transfusions.[58] In upholding Mrs Malette's claim for damages for battery the appeal court stated, in part, as follows:

> *While the law may disregard the absence of consent in limited emergency circumstances, it otherwise supports the right of competent adults to make decisions concerning their own healthcare by imposing civil liability on those who perform medical treatment without consent.*

> *…To transfuse a Jehovah's Witness in the face of her explicit instructions to the contrary would, in my opinion, violate her right to control her own body and show disrespect for the religious values by which she has chosen to live her life.*[59]

And further:

> *…the state may in certain cases require that citizens submit to medical procedures in order to eliminate a health threat to the community or it may prohibit citizens from engaging in activities which are inherently dangerous to their lives. But this interest does not prevent a competent adult from refusing life preserving medical treatment in general or blood transfusions in particular.*[60]

The only way a hospital could seek to override an adult patient's wishes in such a matter would be to seek the intervention of either the Supreme Court of the state or territory or to seek advice from the Guardianship Board as to whether consent to a blood transfusion may be granted. There have been two Australian cases determined by Guardianship Boards that, on the interventions of their families, overturned the express wishes of the patients not to receive blood transfusions.[61] In the 1998 Victorian case of *Qumsieh* (or *Q's case*) the decision was made very narrowly on the specific facts of the case and does not set out clear legal principles. The decision in *Q's case* has been criticised as it seems to disregard some of the provisions of the Victorian *Medical Treatment Act 1988*. The second decision, made in 2004 in New South Wales, *In AB*, was also unusual, based on the family's desire for the man to receive a transfusion in disregard of his express written wish not to receive one.[62] A more recent Victorian case is that of *Mercy Hospitals Ltd v D1*[63] where the Victorian Supreme Court made an order permitting practitioners employed by Mercy Hospitals Ltd to administer blood products, or a blood transfusion, to a pregnant 17-year-old Jehovah's Witness (D1), over her objections and the objections of her mother. The primary issue before the court was whether there was any legal authority that permitted the practitioners to administer blood products to a child (D1) in the absence of her, and her mother's consent. Macaulay J held that the Supreme Court's welfare jurisdiction permitted the court to authorise the administration of blood products. The judge took into account the jurisdiction of the Supreme Court of Victoria, and the provisions of the *Human Tissue Act 1982* (Vic) and the *Medical Treatment Planning and Decisions Act 2016* (Vic). It was reported that D1 was only in the early stages of her studies to become a Jehovah's Witness and was keen to please her mother and her friend. Her obstetrician was concerned that she had a large baby and, being a first pregnancy, it would be preferable for her to consent to blood transfusion. She was also assessed by a child psychiatrist, who felt that she had a stronger understanding of the requirements of her faith than she did of the risks of childbirth. Macaulay J stated that:

> I am not satisfied D1 does have a sufficient understanding of the consequences of her choice. I am not convinced she has based her choice on a maturely formed and entrenched religious conviction. Put another way, I am not convinced that overriding her expressed choice would so rob her of her essential self as to outweigh the loss she would suffer through losing her life or sustaining a catastrophic injury. In summary, I do not consider that allowing her, in effect, to choose to die or only

> survive with serious injury is in her best interests taking into account a holistic view of her welfare (physical, spiritual and otherwise).[64]

Treatment of a Spouse or De Facto Partner. There is no legal provision requiring hospitals to obtain the consent of the spouse or *de facto* partner where the spouse or partner undergoes treatment or an operation of any sort. The type of operation which generally attracted this requirement in hospitals was when the female partner was having a tubal ligation, laparoscopic sterilisation or termination of pregnancy. Equally, where the male partner was admitted for a vasectomy, the same requirement applied. It is to be hoped that when a spouse or partner chooses to have such an operation, they will discuss it between themselves. However, should a spouse or partner refuse or fail to discuss medical treatment with their spouse, he or she is quite able to give valid consent to such treatment.

The only situations where the consent of a spouse, partner, relative or guardian may be legally required are provided for in legislation, for example:

- guardianship or mental health legislation, which allows for an appointed guardian to consent to medical treatment where the person lacks legal capacity;
- human tissue legislation (the *Human Tissue Acts*) of all the states and territories, which provides that the 'nearest available next of kin' or similar phrase is able to consent to the removal of organs from a deceased person if the deceased person's wishes are unknown or unable to be ascertained;
- in vitro fertilisation programs provided for by legislation require the consent of both parents to participate in the program; and
- adoption legislation, which provides that the consent of both partners to a marriage must agree to adopt a child.

Statutory Provisions

The Commonwealth and some states and territories have imposed laws which enable certain authorities to treat adults without their consent. As an example, section 47I of the *Road Traffic Act 1961* (SA) provides for the taking of blood and oral fluids for analysis from a person who is involved in a motor vehicle accident. If that person is admitted to hospital as a result of the motor vehicle accident, there is an obligation on the treating doctor or the doctor's agent (generally a nurse) to take a blood sample without the patient's consent.

Temporary Factors that Might Impair Capacity

Although the normal assumption is that adults are considered to have capacity to give consent except in unusual circumstances, in a number of older cases the courts have decided that a person's capacity was temporarily impaired. In *Re T*, a woman who was a Jehovah's Witness was given a blood transfusion while ventilated following a postpartum haemorrhage despite her express wishes to the contrary.[65] However, she had been given incorrect information about the alternative treatments available. It was held that it would not be unlawful to give her a blood transfusion because her decision to refuse one had been based on incorrect information. In the course of his judgment, Lord Donaldson, while making it clear that a person of capacity has the right to refuse treatment, described *obiter dictum* a number of other possible scenarios where a temporary loss of capacity might occur, as follows:

> *However, the presumption of capacity to decide, which stems from the fact that the patient is an adult, is rebuttable. An adult patient may be deprived of his capacity to decide either by long-term mental incapacity or retarded development or by temporary factors such as unconsciousness or confusion or the effects of fatigue, shock, pain or drugs.[66]*

Findings of temporary loss of capacity have been made in two older cases where pregnant women were 'needle phobic' and refused to have the anaesthetic needle for caesarean section.[67] In *Re L*, Kirkwood J found that the patient, who was in obstructed labour, had an extreme needle phobia which:

> *…amounted to an involuntary compulsion that disabled L from weighing treatment information in the balance to make a choice. Indeed, it was an affliction of a psychological nature that compelled L against medical advice with such force that her own life would be in serious peril.[68]*

These situations would not be the norm, but it is worth noting that there have been situations where the courts have found that it was acceptable to administer treatment against the patient's expressed wishes because it was believed they had temporarily lost the capacity to make a rational decision. Notwithstanding these issues, the question of the way in which consent is managed in labour is currently under scrutiny as the rights of women in labour are seen as a matter of concern.[69]

Minors and Consent

Traditionally, the legal definition of a minor was a person below 18 years of age, and the term 'minor' was used in legislation dealing with legal matters relating to people of that age.[70] Where legislation was designed for more protective purposes, the term 'children' has tended to be used.[71] More recently a distinction has been drawn between children and young people. The *Children and Young People Act 2008* (ACT) Div.1.3.1 defines a 'child' as a person under the age of 12 (s 11) and a 'young person' as a person aged 12 or older but not yet an adult (s 12).

In New South Wales, under section 3 of the *Children and Young Persons (Care and Protection) Act 1998*, a 'child' is defined (except for the purposes of employment) as a person under 16 years of age and a 'young person' as someone aged 16 or over but under 18. However, not all legislation makes the distinction even when it uses both terms. In the Victorian *Children, Youth and Families Act 2005* (s 3) the term 'child' is defined as:

> a. …in the case of a person who is alleged to have committed an offence, a person who at the time of the alleged commission of the offence was under the age of 18 years but of or above the age of 10 years but does not include any person who is of or above the age of 19 years when a proceeding for the offence is commenced in the court; and
>
> b. in any other case, a person who is under the age of 17 years or, if a protection order, a child protection order within the meaning of Schedule 1 or an interim order within the meaning of that Schedule continues in force in respect of him or her, a person who is under the age of 18 years.

It should be noted that several additional definitions for the term 'child' can also be found under section 3 covering specific circumstances, such as where a child is to be proceeded against by summons. The term 'young person' is not defined.

The current situation with the common law is that a child or young person is legally competent to give valid consent to treatment if the child is capable of understanding the nature and consequences of the proposed treatment. This was confirmed in the High Court in a case usually referred to as *Marion's case*, where the question was whether the parents of a 14-year-old girl with severe intellectual and physical handicap could give consent for her to be sterilised, or whether this could only be given by the court.[72] The High Court recognised that, despite this concept of parental power diminishing as the authority of the minor to meet the above test increases, it 'lack[s] the certainty of a fixed age rule, [it] accords with experience and with psychology'. They went on to say that this 'should be followed in this country as part of the common law'.[73]

In the case of *Gillick v West Norfolk & Wisbech Health Authority*,[74] when determining whether minors aged under 16 could consent to treatment at all, Lord Scarman (reflecting the majority judgment) declared that:

> *a minor's capacity to make their own decision depends on the minor having sufficient understanding and intelligence to make the decision and is not to be determined by reference to any judicially fixed age limit.*[75]

Note that the level of understanding for minors at common law is therefore currently higher than that for adults. Adults are required to understand only 'in broad terms', whereas minors are required to 'understand fully' what is proposed.

In some jurisdictions this has been incorporated into statute. For example, section 12 of the South Australian *Consent to Medical Treatment and Palliative Care Act 1995* makes provision for a medical practitioner to administer medical treatment to a child if:

(a) the parent or guardian consents; or
(b) the child consents and—
  (i) the medical practitioner who is to administer the treatment is of the opinion that

the child is capable of understanding the nature, consequences and risks of the treatment and that the treatment is in the best interest of the child's health and wellbeing; and
(ii) that opinion is supported by the written opinion of at least one other medical practitioner who personally examines the child before the treatment is commenced. [emphasis added]

Although the common law does not apply a specific age cut-off point, some statutes still adopt 14 years as an accepted age for such purposes. For example, in New South Wales, the age of 14 has been formally accepted by its insertion into section 49(2) of the *Minors (Property and Contracts) Act 1970*, as far as a child's ability to consent to medical and dental treatment is concerned. Similarly, in South Australia, section 6 of the *Consent to Medical Treatment and Palliative Care Act 1995* permits a young person of 16 years of age or over to consent to medical treatment. However, government policies are beginning to apply an amalgam of common law and statute law to assist health professionals in the difficult task of determining how to manage the ability of minors to consent to treatment. For example, in section 8.3 of the New South Wales Ministry of Health policy directive *Consent to medical treatment and health care treatment manual* the question is asked, 'What is a mature minor and when can they consent to non-emergency treatment?' The answer is both detailed and nuanced.

> *Generally, a Minor is capable of independently consenting to or refusing their medical treatment when they achieve a sufficient level of understanding and intelligence to enable them to understand fully what is proposed. This means that there is no set age at which a child or young person is capable of giving consent.*
>
> *Health Practitioners must decide on a case-by-case basis whether a Minor has sufficient understanding and intelligence to enable them to fully understand what is proposed.*
>
> *The legal position relating to a Minor's capacity to consent was established by an English case known as Gillick. Gillick was approved by the High Court*

of Australia in a case known as Marion's case. The Gillick case holds that a child's capacity increases as they approach maturity or in other words, the authority of a parent decreases as their child's capacity increases.

The significance of the proposed treatment will be a relevant factor in assessing whether a Minor has capacity to consent. For example, it may be likely that a 15-year-old would be assessed as having the capacity to consent to receive contraceptive treatment, but less likely that she would be assessed as having the capacity to consent to a heart transplant. The child's capacity to consent will need to be assessed carefully in relation to each decision to be made. If a Medical Practitioner assesses a Minor as Gillick competent (also known as a Mature Minor) and the Minor can give valid consent, then the consent of the parent or guardian will not be required. However, where the Minor agrees, it is good practice to involve the family in the decision-making process where appropriate.[76]

Issues of conflict between children (particularly adolescents) and their parents have come to light in recent years due to some 'gender dysphoria' cases where young people have wanted to have either hormone or surgical treatment because they wished to have gender reassignment. Ouliaris states:

The laws governing consent for the treatment of gender dysphoria are distinct from that for routine medical procedures, where a child who is Gillick competent may consent to their own treatment; or special medical procedures, where court authorisation is required in all cases. Currently, all three stages of treatment for gender dysphoria in children and adolescents require consent from all parties with parental responsibility. This applies even when a young person is Gillick competent and consents to their own treatment. If there is any dispute between treating medical practitioners or parents regarding a young person's Gillick competence and/or diagnosis or treatment, a court application is required.[77]

An example of where the wishes of a parent or guardian in relation to children have been overturned by the courts occurred in Western Australia in the case of *Director Clinical Services, Child & Adolescent Health Services v Kiszko* [2016] FCWA 19, 34 and 75.[78] The relevant facts are set out in **Case example 6.3**.

CASE EXAMPLE 6.3[79]

Director Clinical Services, Child & Adolescent Health Services v Kiszko [2016] FCWA 19, 34 and 75

The initial decision was made by the Western Australian Family court in relation to a child with a brain tumour, whose parents were resistant to his being treated with chemotherapy and radiotherapy by reason of their commitment to natural therapies, and their belief at an early stage after his diagnosis that orthodox medical treatment should be abandoned in favour of palliative care. A treating doctor took legal action after the parents refused to allow the treatment. The Family Court Chief Justice Thackray J said that while the parents tried to approach the matter on the basis of the best interests of their child, medical evidence could not be ignored. In the decision the judge stated that parental power was to be exercised in the best interests of the child and was 'not unlimited'. He explained that the evidence was that Oshin would die within a few months if nothing was done, but that there was a 30 per cent chance of survival at five years if he started chemotherapy immediately, and about a 50 per cent chance if he had chemotherapy and radiotherapy.

Judicial approval is usually required in relation to what are referred to as special procedures or treatments which include research involvement, procedures such as sterilisation, termination of pregnancy and medications such as hormonal treatment for long-term contraception, psychotropic medications in out-of-home situations and long-term administration of drugs of addiction. For example, section 175 of the *Children and Young Persons (Care and Protection) Act 1998* (NSW) sets the penalty for carrying out 'special medical treatment' otherwise than in accordance with the section as 7 years imprisonment.

Under the section a medical practitioner may carry out special medical treatment on a child only if either, they believe it is necessary, as a matter of urgency, to save the child's life or to prevent serious damage to the child's health, or if the Guardianship Tribunal consents to the treatment being carried out.

The Guardianship Tribunal can give consent to the carrying out of special medical treatment on a child only if it is satisfied that such treatment is necessary to save the child's life or to prevent serious damage to the child's psychological or physical health. The definitions of 'medical treatment' and 'special medical treatment' (s 175(5)) are reproduced in **Box 6.13**.

Many young people aged between 14 and 18 years seek medical treatment that they do not wish their parents to know about. In such circumstances, a young person can give valid consent to treatment, subject to the legislative and common law principles already stated. The question of confidentiality in these situations is quite complex and does create significant dilemmas for health professionals. Family Planning NSW makes this statement:

Confidentiality is an important part of your relationship with the staff at Family Planning NSW because it means that:
- *You will feel comfortable seeking help to deal with the issues worrying you*
- *You will be able to share information that will help our staff give you the best advice*
- *You will be able to discuss issues openly and make the best decisions*[80]

However, even within these parameters, Family Planning reserves the right to 'contact authorities' if they believe the young person to be 'at risk'.[81]

BOX 6.13

DEFINITIONS OF 'MEDICAL TREATMENT' AND 'SPECIAL MEDICAL TREATMENT', *CHILDREN AND YOUNG PERSONS (CARE AND PROTECTION) ACT 1998* (NSW) S 175(5)

5. IN THIS SECTION:

medical treatment includes:
(a) any medical procedure, operation or examination, and
(b) any treatment, procedure, operation or examination that is declared by the regulations to be medical treatment for the purposes of this section.

special medical treatment means:
5(a) any medical treatment that is intended, or is reasonably likely, to have the effect of rendering permanently infertile the person on whom it is carried out, not being medical treatment —
  (i) that is intended to remediate a life-threatening condition, and
  (ii) from which permanent infertility, or the likelihood of permanent infertility, is an unwanted consequence, or
(b) any medical treatment for the purpose of contraception or menstrual regulation declared by the regulations to be a special medical treatment for the purposes of this section, or
(c) any medical treatment in the nature of a vasectomy or tubal occlusion, or
  (c1) any medical treatment that involves the administration of a drug of addiction within the meaning of the *Poisons and Therapeutic Goods Act 1966* over a period or periods totalling more than 10 days in any period of 30 days, or
  Note: A drug of addiction is a substance specified in Schedule Eight of the Poisons List proclaimed under the *Poisons and Therapeutic Goods Act 1966*. The Poisons List adopts by reference, with certain modifications, Schedules 1–8 of the Poisons Standard under the Therapeutic Goods Act 1989 of the Commonwealth. See also the Poisons List information available at www.health.nsw.gov.au/resources/publichealth/pharmaceutical/poisons_list_pdf.asp.
  (c2) any medical treatment that involves an experimental procedure that does not conform to the document entitled *National Statement on Ethical Conduct in Human Research 2007* published by the National Health and Medical Research Council in 2007 and updated in 2013, or
  Note: A copy of the National Statement on Ethical Conduct in Human Research 2007 can be found at www.nhmrc.gov.au/guidelines/publications/e72.
(d) any other medical treatment that is declared by the regulations to be special medical treatment for the purposes of this section.

As with adults, there are certain situations where consent is not required or, specifically with children, where parental refusal to consent to treatment for a child can be overridden or is not required. These situations are examined below.

Emergency Situations. No parental consent is required where the child is unconscious or seriously ill and the situation calls for immediate intervention to save the child's life. The overriding duty of care that arises in such emergency situations negates the need for parental consent. For example, if a child with severe injuries were brought into casualty following a motor vehicle accident, the obvious duty to treat that child as quickly as possible would operate as a defence against a suggestion of battery.

The Administration of Blood Transfusions Without Parental Consent. Each state and territory makes such provision in differently named Acts, but each allows a legally qualified medical practitioner to give a blood transfusion to a child without the consent of the parent or guardian if it can be shown that a blood transfusion is a reasonable and proper form of treatment and is necessary to save the child's life. Section 21 of the *Human Tissue and Transplant Act 1982* (WA) provides a good example of the types of situations in which medical practitioners may need to administer a blood transfusion to a child in the absence of parental consent:

(1) *A medical practitioner may perform a blood transfusion upon a child without the consent of any person who is legally entitled to authorise the blood transfusion if —*
  (a) *such person —*
    (i) *fails or refuses to so authorise the blood transfusion when requested to do so; or*
    (ii) *cannot be found after such search and enquiry as is reasonably practicable in the circumstances of the case; and*
  (b) *the medical practitioner and another medical practitioner agree —*
    (i) *as to the condition from which the child is suffering; and*
    (ii) *that the blood transfusion is a reasonable and proper treatment for that condition;*

and (iii) that without a blood transfusion the child is likely to die; and
  (c) *the medical practitioner who performs the blood transfusion on the child —*
    (i) *has had previous experience in performing blood transfusions; and*
    (ii) *has, before commencing the transfusion, assured himself that the blood to be transfused is suitable for the child.*

The individual state and territory provisions are shown in **Table 6.2**.

Children Under the Care of the State. Consent for the treatment of children who are the subject of care and protection orders has to be given by the minister or secretary of the relevant government department empowered with the guardianship of such children. In most states and territories, that is the Minister for Youth and Community Services. The names of the relevant Acts vary; for example, in Western Australia it is the *Children and Community Services Act 2004*, and

TABLE 6.2
Statutory Provisions Concerning Situations in Which Parental Consent to Blood Transfusions is Not Required, or Parental Refusal to Give Consent May Be Overridden

State or Territory	Statute
ACT	*Transplantation and Anatomy Act 1978* section 23
NSW	*Children and Young Persons (Care and Protection) Act 1998* section 174
NT	*Emergency Medical Operations Act 1973* section 3
Qld	*Transplantation and Anatomy Act 1979* section 20
SA	*Consent to Medical Treatment and Palliative Care Act 1995* section 13(5)
Tas	*Human Tissue Act 1985* section 21
Vic	*Human Tissue Act 1982* section 24
WA	*Human Tissue and Transplant Act 1982* section 21

in Tasmania the *Children, Young Persons and Their Families Act 1997*.

Reporting, Examining and Treating Children at Risk Without Parental Consent. It has now been recognised that there are occasions when it is necessary, for the protection of the child, to remove a child from the parents without their consent and to detain a child in hospital for examination and treatment without parental consent. Such steps are generally required when instances of child neglect or child abuse become suspected or known. All states and territories have now made specific provision to deal with these issues, while at the same time making sure that appropriate protection against defamation or other civil actions is afforded to those persons required to report such incidents to the relevant authorities. These statutory provisions are shown in **Table 6.3**.

The precise wording of the statutory requirements varies, but, as is usual, the major provisions are the same and have been summarised in **Box 6.14**.

TABLE 6.3	
Statutory Provision for Removal of a Child and Detaining a Child in Hospital Without Parental Consent	
State or Territory	**Statute**
ACT	*Children and Young People Act 2008*
NSW	*Children and Young Persons (Care and Protection) Act 1998*
NT	*Care and Protection of Children Act 2007*
Qld	*Child Protection Act 1999*
SA	*Children's Protection Act 1993*
Tas	*Children, Young Persons and Their Families Act 1997*
Vic	*Children Youth and Families Act 2005*
WA	*Children and Community Services Act 2004*

BOX 6.14
SUMMARY OF STATUTORY REQUIREMENTS FOR REPORTING CHILD ABUSE AND NEGLECT[82]

DEFINING CHILD ABUSE AND NEGLECT

Child abuse and neglect refers to any behaviour or treatment by parents, caregivers, other adults or older adolescents that results in the actual and/or likelihood of causing physical or emotional harm to a child or young person. Such behaviours may be intentional or unintentional and can include acts of omission (i.e. neglect) and commission (i.e. abuse) (CFCA, 2018).

Child abuse and neglect is commonly divided into five subtypes:

- physical abuse
- emotional abuse
- neglect
- sexual abuse
- exposure to family violence.

WHO HAS TO REPORT?

Mandatory reporting legislation generally contains lists of particular occupations that are mandated to report cases of suspected child abuse and neglect. The groups of people mandated to report range from persons in a limited number of occupations (Qld) to a more extensive list (Vic and WA), to a very extensive list (ACT, NSW, SA and Tas), through to every adult (NT). The occupations most commonly named as mandated reporters are those who deal frequently with children in the course of their work: teachers, early childhood education and care practitioners, doctors, nurses and police.

WHAT PROTECTIONS ARE GIVEN TO MANDATORY REPORTERS?

In all jurisdictions, the legislation protects the mandatory reporter's identity from disclosure. In addition, the legislation provides that as long as the report is made in good faith, the reporter cannot be liable in any civil, criminal or administrative proceedings.

HOW DOES MANDATORY REPORTING LEGISLATION DEFINE A CHILD?

Legislation in all jurisdictions except New South Wales and Victoria requires mandatory reporting in relation to all young people up to the age of 18 years. In New South Wales, the duty only applies to situations involving children aged under 16 years. In Victoria, the duty only applies to situations involving children under 17 years of age.

THE RIGHT TO WITHHOLD CONSENT TO TREATMENT

In addition to the need to obtain a patient's consent to medical treatment, there is also the related right of a person to withhold their consent. This has been a somewhat controversial topic over the years, both at law and in practice, as health professionals have taken some time to accommodate and acknowledge it, since it can clash with their professional culture of intervention to save life. When this professional culture is coupled with the overriding legal obligation, particularly in a hospital environment, of doing all that can be done to save life and preserve health, it is understandable that some health professionals find refusal of consent to treatment so difficult.

Concerns about being able to determine the course of treatment, particularly in the face of medical futility at the end of life, have arisen owing to the increasing ability to extend life. The challenge has been to decide whether, just because it was *possible* to do more to keep a person alive, it was *appropriate* to do so, if the burden of the proposed therapy outweighed the benefits. As treatment and cure have developed throughout the twentieth century, healthcare practitioners have found it increasingly difficult to discontinue life-prolonging treatment and, therefore, have frequently provided aggressive therapy until the point of death, in some instances depriving the patient of the opportunity for appropriate palliative care. Indeed, a recent, comprehensive Australian study has demonstrated that there are significant increases in healthcare costs in the last 6 months of life, but that these are by no means demonstrated to be of value to lead to increased patient and carer satisfaction or even to be of equal quality. Reeve, Srasuebkul, Langton, Haas, Viney and Pearson conclude:

> *The results suggest differences in end-of-life care pathways dependent on patient factors, with younger, community-dwelling patients and those with a history of cancer incurring significantly greater costs. There is a need to examine whether the investment in end-of-life care meets patient and societal needs.*[83]

At the same time, some of those advocating for and those opposing euthanasia have brought the debate about the potential for and problems with end-of-life care into the mainstream, even if the public does not necessarily agree with the goals of either group.[84] A significant recent development has been that, since the initial legislation in the Victorian Parliament in November 2017, every state in Australia has passed legislation on voluntary assisted dying, under which there is the ability to voluntarily terminate one's own life, and to enable an individual with a terminal illness to obtain a lethal drug to do so. These legislative changes will be discussed in detail later in this chapter.

It is important to understand that, despite the outcome for a person in some instances clearly being the same, the (now) limited legislated right to obtain assistance to die and the right to refuse treatment, which may incidentally hasten the dying process, are considered to be significantly different issues in law. The right to withhold consent to treatment, as much as the right to give consent to treatment, is a fundamental common law right of all patients of full legal capacity.

This has been confirmed in the 2010 South Australian case of *H Ltd v J*.[85] J was a 73-year-old woman who was suffering from post-polio syndrome and diabetes. She was partially paralysed and confined to a wheelchair. She resided in a nursing home owned by H Ltd. J decided to end her life by refusing to eat and drink. She also refused insulin. J made an advance directive in accordance with South Australian legislation and refused artificial nutrition and hydration. The nursing home approached the court for directions as to the lawfulness of J's decision. Kourakis J held that there was no common law duty imposed on J to eat and drink. Furthermore, it was not suicide for her to die from self-starvation, and there was no duty on the part of the nursing home to force-feed her or to give her insulin.

In essence, therefore, such a right to refuse treatment requires no legislative prescription to sustain it. Despite this, the need for legislation to enshrine the right to withhold consent to treatment, particularly in cases of terminal illness, has been perceived as necessary in most states and territories. Others have simply developed policy, to help clarify and implement the existing common law. The major argument in support of the need for legislation is to ensure protection from any potential civil and criminal liability on the part of a healthcare practitioner who acts in good faith and in accordance with the expressed wishes of a fully informed, competent patient who refuses medical treatment.

To date, the majority of legislation passed has been merely a statutory reflection of the common law position, where a person has the right to refuse medical treatment. This type of legislation enables competent adults in certain specified situations to direct medical treatment to be withdrawn or withheld. People may feel that legislative status perhaps offers clearer protection to those with terminal or incurable illnesses, or health professionals who treat them, from potential criminal or civil liability, but a policy document provides similar clarity of the current legal situation. However, one of the important aspects of codifying the common law is that it has the potential to make mainstream some relatively new practices, such as the development and acknowledgment of advance directives.

Advance Directives, Advance Care Planning and Proxy Decision-Making

A critical aspect of a patient's right to refuse treatment is whether that right can be assured if they lack capacity. The development of advance directives,[86] or 'living wills' as they are sometimes known, is one way that people can ensure that their wishes to refuse treatment are known even if they are no longer able to communicate at the time that that treatment is under consideration. Advance directives are considered to be of particular importance for patients with dementia, as the prognosis of incapacity is clear from the outset of the disease, and it is thus possible to ascertain the patient's wishes about an almost certain future scenario.[87] There is a new emphasis on planning ahead, or advance care planning, as much more of an iterative conversation that all adults need to undertake to ensure they feel comfortable about their financial, physical and mental wellbeing into the future.[88]

The level of proof required to ascertain what the patient's wishes would be in relation to their treatment was explained in the Supreme Court of the United States in the case of *Cruzan v Director, Missouri Department of Health*,[89] which identified the requirement for 'clear and convincing evidence'. Advance directives are one way of obtaining 'clear and convincing evidence' of a patient's wishes about future treatment. An 'advance care directive' is described by Advance Care Planning Australia as:

> ... *documenting your preferences for future care yourself. It can include your values, life goals and preferred outcomes, and directions about care and treatments. You can also formally appoint a substitute decision-maker in an advance care directive. The process of creating an advance care directive and the names of the required documents varies between states and territories. Advance care directives are legally binding and the preferences for health care that you document must be followed.*[90]

A possible problem of not having a statutory framework for advance directives may be that many issues, such as duration of effect, liability for health professionals, questions of what may or may not be excluded, management of relatives and drafting provisions could still be left as both discretionary and optional issues. The only place for legal resolution would then be through the common law, which means that some parties will have been sufficiently dissatisfied with the clinical process of decision-making that they needed to seek resolution from the courts. Concerns about misinterpretation and applicability to future events[91, 92] are acknowledged as being problems with advance directives. However, it seems apparent that the value of clear and convincing evidence of pre-determined wishes in relation to treatment outweighs any disadvantages.

Australia has legislated for advance directives in some states and territories but not others, and the types of medical treatment that can be refused in advance also varies from state to state and territory. Victoria, which has long had the most permissive legislation in relation to what treatments might be refused and in what circumstances, recently enacted the *Medical Treatment Planning and Decisions Act 2016* (Vic) to replace the *Medical Treatment Act 1988* (Vic). The new Act introduced provisions governing advance care directives to clarify their position under Victorian law.[93]

The different approaches to refusal of treatment taken by the states and territories are set out in **Table 6.4**.

TABLE 6.4
Different Approaches to Refusal of Treatment[94]

State or Territory	Provision Made	Key Features
ACT	*Medical Treatment (Health Directions) Act 2006* section 7(1)	(1) An adult can make a direction (a *health direction*) to refuse, or require the withdrawal of, medical treatment generally or a particular kind of medical treatment.
NT	*Advance Personal Planning Act 2013* (NT) section 8	(1) An adult who has planning capacity may, by making an *advance personal plan*, do one or more of the following: (a) make consent decisions about future health care action for the adult (*advance consent decisions*); (b) set out the adult's views, wishes and beliefs as the basis on which he or she wants anyone to act if they make decisions for him or her (*advance care statements*); (c) appoint one or more persons to make decisions for the adult if he or she loses decision-making capacity (*decision-makers*). (2) The decisions mentioned in subsection (1)(b) and (c) may be about all or any aspect of the adult's care and welfare (including healthcare) and property and financial affairs.
Qld	*Powers of Attorney Act 1998* section 35(1)	(1) By an *advance health directive*, an adult principal may — (a) give directions, about health matters and special health matters, for his or her future healthcare; and (b) give information about his or her directions; and (c) appoint 1 or more persons who are eligible attorneys to exercise power for a health matter for the principal in the event the directions prove inadequate; and (d) provide terms or information about exercising the power. (2) Without limiting subsection (1), by an advance health directive the principal may give a direction — (a) consenting, in the circumstances specified, to particular future healthcare of the principal when necessary and despite objection by the principal when the healthcare is provided; and (b) requiring, in the circumstances specified, a life-sustaining measure to be withheld or withdrawn; and (c) authorising an attorney to physically restrain, move or manage the principal, or have the principal physically restrained, moved or managed, for the purpose of healthcare when necessary and despite objection by the principal when the restraint, movement or management is provided. (3) A direction in an advance health directive has priority over a general or specific power for health matters given to any attorney. (4) An advance health directive is not revoked by the principal becoming a person with impaired capacity.
SA	*Consent to Medical Treatment and Palliative Care Act 1995* section 3; *Advance Care Directives Act 2013* (SA) sections 9, 11 and 21	*Consent to Medical Treatment and Palliative Care Act 1995* The objects of this Act are — … b. to provide for the medical treatment of people who have impaired decision-making capacity; and c. to allow for the provision of palliative care, in accordance with proper standards, to people who are dying and to protect them from medical treatment that is intrusive, burdensome and futile. *Advance Care Directives Act 2013*: ■ s 9 Objects ■ s 11 Giving advance care directives ■ s 21 Requirements in relation to appointment of substitute decision-makers.

Continued on following page

TABLE 6.4

Different Approaches to Refusal of Treatment *(Continued)*

State or Territory	Provision Made	Key Features
Tas	*Guardianship and Administration Act 1995,* Part 5A Advance Care Directives	The objects of this Part include the following: (a) to enable persons with decision-making ability to give directions about their future healthcare; (b) to enable persons with decision-making ability to express their preferences and values in respect of their future healthcare, including by specifying outcomes or interventions they wish to avoid; (c) to ensure, as far as is reasonably practicable and appropriate, that healthcare that is provided to a person who has given an *advance care directive* accords with the person's directions, preferences and values; (d) to protect health practitioners and others giving effect to the directions, preferences and values of a person who has given an advance care directive; (e) to provide mechanisms for the resolution of disputes in relation to advance care directives.

Vic	*Medical Treatment Planning and Decisions Act 2016* (Vic) section 1	The main purposes of this Act are—
		(a) to provide for a person to execute in advance a directive that gives binding instructions or expresses the person's preferences and values in relation to the person's future medical treatment;
		(b) to provide for the making of medical treatment decisions on behalf of persons who do not have decision-making capacity;
		(c) to provide for a person to appoint—
		  (i) another person to make medical treatment decisions on behalf of the person when the person does not have decision-making capacity;
		  (ii) another person to support the person and represent the interests of the person in making medical treatment decisions;
		(d) to provide for a process for obtaining approval and consent for medical research procedures to be administered to a person who does not have decision-making capacity;
		(e) to repeal the *Medical Treatment Act 1988*;
		(f) to amend the *Mental Health Act 2014* in relation to approval procedures for electroconvulsive treatment of adults who do not have capacity.

WA	*Guardianship and Administration Act 1990* Part 9B Advance Health Directives	S.110P A person who has reached 18 years of age and has full legal capacity may make an *advance health directive* containing treatment decisions in respect of the person's future treatment.
		S.110S operation generally
		(1) A treatment decision in an advance health directive operates in respect of the treatment to which it applies —
		  (a) at any time the maker of the directive is unable to make reasonable judgments in respect of that treatment; and
		  (b) as if —
		    (i) the treatment decision had been made by the maker at that time; and
		    (ii) the maker were of full legal capacity.
		(2) Subject to subsection (3), a treatment decision in an advance health directive operates only in the circumstances specified in the directive.
		(3) Subject to subsection (4), a treatment decision in an advance health directive does not operate if circumstances exist or have arisen that —
		  (a) the maker of that directive would not have reasonably anticipated at the time of making the directive; and
		  (b) would have caused a reasonable person in the maker's position to have changed his or her mind about the treatment decision.

	TABLE 6.4	
	Different Approaches to Refusal of Treatment (*Continued*)	
State or Territory	**Provision Made**	**Key Features**
		(4) In determining whether or not subsection (3) applies in relation to a treatment decision that is in an advance health directive, the matters that must be taken into account include the following —
		(a) the maker's age at the time the directive was made and at the time the treatment decision would otherwise operate;
		(b) the period that has elapsed between those times;
		(c) whether the maker reviewed the treatment decision at any time during that period and, if so, the period that has elapsed between the time of the last such review and the time at which the treatment decision would otherwise operate;
		(d) the nature of the condition for which the maker needs treatment, the nature of that treatment and the consequences of providing and not providing that treatment.
		(5) For the purpose of determining whether or not subsection (3) applies in relation to a treatment decision that is in an advance health directive, subject to the terms of the directive, any of the following persons may be consulted —
		(a) if the maker has an enduring guardian — the enduring guardian;
		(b) if the maker has a guardian — the guardian;
		(c) a person who has a relationship with the maker described in section 110ZD(3)(a) to (d);
		(d) any other person considered appropriate in the circumstances.

THE RIGHT TO REQUEST ASSISTANCE TO END YOUR LIFE

Section 9 of the *Voluntary Assisted Dying Act 2017* (Vic) sets out the eligibility criteria for access to voluntary assisted dying. This reads as follows:

(1) For a person to be eligible for access to voluntary assisted dying —

  a. the person must be aged 18 years or more; and

  b. the person must —

    i. be an Australian citizen or permanent resident; and

    ii. be ordinarily resident in Victoria; and

    iii. at the time of making a first request, have been ordinarily resident in Victoria for at least 12 months; and

  c. the person must have decision-making capacity in relation to voluntary assisted dying; and

  d. the person must be diagnosed with a disease, illness or medical condition that —

    i. is incurable; and

    ii. is advanced, progressive and will cause death; and

    iii. is expected to cause death within weeks or months, not exceeding 6 months; and

    iv. is causing suffering to the person that cannot be relieved in a manner that the person considers tolerable.

There are a number of exceptions to eligibility also, such as having *only* a mental illness or disability (ss 9 (2) and 9 (3)).

At the time of writing, all states in Australia have enacted voluntary assisted dying (VAD) legislation (ACT and NT have not at this stage, although there is discussion in both jurisdictions). All have now gone live with their legislation, with NSW the last state to do so on 28 November 2023. The relevant legislation for each jurisdiction is set out in **Table 6.5**. Although each statute varies slightly, overall, there are significant consistent requirements in each statute. For example, the principles of the legislation for each jurisdiction are very similar. For example, s 5 of the *Voluntary Assisted Dying Act 2021* (Qld) states:

The principles that underpin this Act are —
(a) human life is of fundamental importance; and

TABLE 6.5		
Voluntary Assisted Dying Legislation		
State or territory		Name of statute
NSW		*Voluntary Assisted Dying Act 2022*
Qld		*Voluntary Assisted Dying Act 2021*
SA		*Voluntary Assisted Dying Act 2021*
Tas		*End-of-Life choices (Voluntary Assisted Dying) Act 2021*
Vic		*Voluntary Assisted Dying Act 2017*
WA		*Voluntary Assisted Dying Act 2019*

(b) *every person has inherent dignity and should be treated equally and with compassion and respect; and*

(c) *a person's autonomy, including autonomy in relation to end-of-life choices, should be respected; and*

(d) *every person approaching the end of life should be provided with high quality care and treatment, including palliative care, to minimise the person's suffering and maximise the person's quality of life; and*

(e) *access to voluntary assisted dying and other end-of-life choices should be available regardless of where a person lives in Queensland; and*

(f) *a person should be supported in making informed decisions about end-of-life choices; and*

(g) *a person who is vulnerable should be protected from coercion and exploitation; and*

(h) *a person's freedom of thought, conscience, religion and belief and enjoyment of their culture should be respected.*

Every other statute has similar principles, not necessarily in the same order and not necessarily with identical wording but close enough for there to be no doubt that VAD is to be seen as an optional part of end-of-life care, not a substitute for end-of-life care and that it is to be available to all residents of the state regardless of location.

The legislation is limited to people who have decision-making capacity, which is defined tightly under all of the legislation, and they are required to have decision-making capacity until the moment of VAD.

The *Voluntary Assisted Dying Act 2022* (NSW) s 6 defines decision-making capacity as follows:

(1) *For the purposes of this Act, a patient has **"decision-making capacity"** in relation to voluntary assisted dying if the patient has the capacity to —*

   (a) *understand information or advice about a voluntary assisted dying decision required under this Act to be provided to the patient, and*

   (b) *remember the information or advice referred to in paragraph (a) to the extent necessary to make a voluntary assisted dying decision, and*

   (c) *understand the matters involved in a voluntary assisted dying decision, and*

   (d) *understand the effect of a voluntary assisted dying decision, and*

   (e) *weigh up the factors referred to in paragraphs (a), (c) and (d) for the purposes of making a voluntary assisted dying decision, and*

   (f) *communicate a voluntary assisted dying decision in some way.*

(2) *For the purposes of this Act, a patient is —*

   (a) *presumed to have the capacity to understand information or advice about voluntary assisted dying if it reasonably appears the patient is able to understand an explanation of the consequences of making the decision, and*

   (b) *presumed to have decision-making capacity in relation to voluntary assisted dying unless the patient is shown not to have the capacity.*

Who can request VAD is also limited, as can be seen in s 9 of the *Voluntary Assisted Dying Act 2017* (Vic) above. Again, there are some slight variations, but what is clear is that the person's death must be imminent (at least within the next 12 months), their suffering must be intolerable, and they must have capacity. So, there is no possibility of making an advance care directive for VAD, nor could a person in early-stage dementia make a request for VAD, unless they were likely to die from the disease within the next 12 months.

This is a significant development in Australian healthcare and, although there was a significant groundswell of support in Australian society, nevertheless it is a very serious thing to assist a person to die and all legislation has the facility for conscientious objection. For example, s 6 of the *Voluntary Assisted Dying Act 2021* (SA) states:

> *A registered health practitioner who has a conscientious objection to voluntary assisted dying has the right to refuse to do any of the following:*
> *(a) to provide information about voluntary assisted dying;*
> *(b) to participate in the request and assessment process;*
> *(c) to apply for a voluntary assisted dying permit;*
> *(d) to supply, prescribe or administer a voluntary assisted dying substance;*
> *(e) to be present at the time of administration of a voluntary assisted dying substance;*
> *(f) to dispense a prescription for a voluntary assisted dying substance.*

However, in order to comply with the principle that VAD will be available to all, there are provisions under all the statutes to ensure that patients are referred on after they have made a request. There is also a strict requirement that it is the patient who must make the request. It cannot be suggested by the treating practitioner. Practitioners who wish to be involved in the scheme in any jurisdiction are required to undergo education. Both medical practitioners and nurse practitioners can be involved in VAD but the extent of involvement for nurse practitioners varies between the jurisdictions. As with all legislation, it is important that nurses and midwives familiarise themselves with the relevant legislation for their state.

THE RIGHT TO RESTRAIN OR DETAIN PATIENTS WITHOUT THEIR CONSENT

The right of a hospital or nursing home to restrain patients against their wishes is of genuine concern to nursing staff who often have to deal with violent, aggressive or demented patients or residents, or patients whose particular medical condition makes them physically or mentally temporarily unstable and very threatening. Also, some patients who are ill and require continuing care demand to be discharged.

In most circumstances all competent adults have a legal right not to be restrained or detained — doing so is the third in the trio of trespasses to the person mentioned at the beginning of this chapter. Having said that, the legal right of hospitals and nursing homes to restrain patients or residents without their consent and the right of hospitals to detain patients against their wishes does exist in particular circumstances. Before those circumstances are outlined, it is important to examine the legal context in which these issues arise — and that requires consideration of the elements that constitute the civil wrong of false imprisonment. False imprisonment, like assault and battery and negligence, can be both a civil wrong and a criminal offence. However, as far as nursing staff members are concerned, false imprisonment, also like assault and battery and negligence, has greater significance as a civil wrong.

What is False Imprisonment?

In essence, **false imprisonment** is the wrongful and intentional application of restraint on a person, restricting the person's freedom to move from a particular place or causing the person to be confined to a particular place against their will. The 'wrongful' aspect of the restraint means that it is not, expressly or impliedly, authorised by the law. By implication then, there are a number of situations where the law does permit people to be detained against their will — the most common example being the detention of people in prison for criminal offences. Putting aside this most obvious example, other situations relevant to nursing staff are now discussed.

How is False Imprisonment Committed?

Apart from the obvious steps of locking a person in a room without any means of escape and against their will, it is quite possible to commit the civil wrong of false imprisonment without imprisoning a person as the term is commonly understood. In fact, neither physical contact nor anything resembling a prison is necessary to constitute false imprisonment.

For example, if a lecturer locked the classroom door after the final lecture of the day and there was no other means of escape for the students inside, that would constitute false imprisonment, even though the lecturer had not physically touched the students and they were not being confined in a prison cell.

In addition, it is not necessary to confine a person physically to constitute false imprisonment. It is sufficient if a person believes he or she is not free to go because of some fear or apprehension that has been created in the person's mind and which acts as a constraint on the person's will.

As another example, a male patient attends the accident and emergency department of a hospital for treatment for a badly gashed arm. After the treatment, he is about to leave when the ward clerk presents him with a bill for $50 for the treatment received. The patient states he has only $5 on him and will pay the bill later. He is told that he is not permitted to leave the hospital until the bill is paid and that he had better make arrangements to do so, otherwise the police will be called. Believing this to be correct, the patient then spends hours in the waiting room phoning friends and relatives to find someone to come to the hospital with the required money. Six hours after the patient was originally ready to leave, a friend arrives with the money and the ward clerk says the patient is now free to leave.

Although nobody has laid a hand on him or locked him in a room, the patient has been falsely imprisoned. A situation was created in which he genuinely believed he was not free to go and that the police would be called if he should attempt to do so. In fact, as far as paying accounts is concerned, no organisation, hospital or department store can detain a person for failing to pay their debts. What it can do is litigate through the appropriate court to recover the money owed.

Restraint Must Be Intentional and Complete

What this means is that the restraint must not only be intended, but also be complete, in that there is no means of escape. Referring to the earlier example of the lecturer locking the classroom door, if the classroom were on the ground floor and there were plenty of open windows through which the students could climb, then the restraint might have been intentional, but it would not have been complete. Alternatively, if the classroom were on the tenth floor, then any number of open windows would have been to no avail and the restraint would have been complete. At the same time, if a person has the means to escape but does not know it, such a situation would still be false imprisonment, unless it could be shown that a reasonable person would have realised there was a means of escape available.

An interesting example occurred in the case of *Sayers v Harlow Urban District Council*[95] where the courts held that the restraint was total but not intentional. The relevant facts are set out in **Case example 6.4**.

CASE EXAMPLE 6.4
Sayers v Harlow Urban District Council

Mrs Sayers went to a toilet cubicle in the council's public rest rooms. The toilets were coin-operated and, after entering the toilet, Mrs Sayers was unable to leave because of a problem with the door handle. She was unable to attract anybody's attention so, using her initiative, Mrs Sayers attempted to climb over the top of the toilet cubicle. To do so, Mrs Sayers placed her weight on the toilet roll fitting on the wall of the cubicle. The fitting gave way under her weight, and she slipped and fell to the floor injuring herself. Mrs Sayers brought an action against the council for false imprisonment and negligence. The court dismissed Mrs Sayers' claim of false imprisonment on the basis that the restraint had been complete, but not intentional. The court upheld Mrs Sayers' claim of negligence against the council because of the faulty door handle. However, the court reduced her damages by 25% on the grounds of contributory negligence, in that she should not have relied on the toilet roll fitting to carry her weight while attempting to escape.

In the New South Wales case of *Hart v Herron*, the plaintiff, Mr Hart, successfully sued Dr Herron for, among other things, wrongful imprisonment when he was admitted to Chelmsford Private Hospital and administered narcosis therapy and electroconvulsive therapy (ECT) without his consent.[96] It was held that the restraint amounted to wrongful imprisonment even though he had no recollection of it happening.

Defences to an Action Alleging False Imprisonment
Reasonable Condition

It is not false imprisonment to prevent a person from leaving a particular premises because he or she does not wish to fulfil a reasonable condition subject to which the person entered them. The matter of *Herd v Weardale Steel Co*[97] provides an example of this situation. The relevant facts are set out in **Case example 6.5**.

CASE EXAMPLE 6.5

Herd v Weardale Steel Co

Mr Herd was employed as an underground miner. On reporting for duty at a particular time, the workmen would be taken by lift down the mineshaft, where they would work their shift. It was understood that, except in certain emergencies, the workmen would remain down the mineshaft until the completion of their shift and would then be brought to the surface by lift. Mr Herd was taken down the mineshaft, assigned to a job, which he then refused to do, and demanded to be taken to the surface. The management refused to do so until the normal lift time some hours later. Mr Herd brought an action against his employers for false imprisonment. His claim failed on the basis that Mr Herd entered the lift to go down the mineshaft on the reasonable condition that he would undertake a particular job and be returned to the surface at a particular time. In doing so, Mr Herd had submitted to a restriction on his liberty and the employers were not liable.

Lawful Arrest in Relation to Criminal Offences

A lawful arrest is not false imprisonment. Accordingly, for example, a police officer or other authorised person who arrests another person, pursuant to the issue of a valid warrant for that person's arrest, cannot be sued for false imprisonment.

Specific Defences in Relation to Hospitals and Healthcare Generally

The right of hospitals and health centres to detain or restrain patients arises by the operation of statutory or common law as follows.

Detention of Patients

- The relevant mental health legislation in each state and territory gives health authorities limited power to detain those people, against their will, who come within the provisions of the legislation. The power to admit, treat and detain involuntary patients under the provisions of the mental health legislation is fully covered in **Chapter 10**.
- Relevant legislation in each state and territory gives health and welfare authorities the power to detain a child in hospital or an appropriate place without parental consent for the purposes of examination and treatment in the case of suspected child abuse. This matter was covered earlier in this chapter (see 'Reporting, examining and treating children at risk without parental consent').
- Specific provision under public health legislation may provide for the detention and treatment of persons with particular diseases in the interests of public health or safety, or obligatory notification by medical practitioners to health authorities of persons with 'proclaimed' notifiable diseases. For example, the Commonwealth *Biosecurity Act 2015* empowers health authorities to detain people attempting to enter Australia with suspected infectious diseases. They can be detained onboard ship or in a quarantine station. There have been numerous examples of the quarantine powers being exercised during the COVID-19 pandemic, although there were concerns expressed about the impact on those with mental illness and disability[98] and those detained in hotel quarantine.[99]

Apart from any statutory powers to detain, which have already been referred to, there is no common law power to detain a person in hospital against that person's wishes, no matter how ill the person may be. In situations where a patient of full legal capacity insists on leaving hospital against all medical advice, he or she must be allowed to do so. As a matter of policy, most healthcare facilities will have a standard voluntary discharge form, which the patient should be asked to sign, indicating that he or she is leaving the hospital against medical advice (often called a discharge against medical advice or DAMA form). If the patient refuses to sign such a form the patient must still be permitted to leave and the appropriate entry made in the patient's notes, detailing the events surrounding the patient's departure from hospital. The patient's relatives or carers should be advised as soon as possible of the patient's intentions.

Restraint of Patients. There are occasions in hospitals and nursing homes when patients become violent, aggressive and extremely difficult to control and care for properly. The reasons for this aggression are many and varied, and a 2020 NSW report has demonstrated the extent of injury to nurses and midwives, in addition to providing a range of recommendations to address the issue.[100] However, if strategies to de-escalate the violence or aggression fail, or if for some other clinical reason the patient is a danger to themselves or others, nursing staff may need to restrain a patient to protect:

- the patient from injury — particularly if the patient is a child;
- other patients who may be at risk;
- themselves from unnecessary risk or harm, but remembering that such restraint is for the protection and not for the convenience of staff.

As far as nursing staff are concerned, the application of any restraint to a patient or resident against their wishes must be done only following a careful consideration of the issues involved, consultation with the patient's medical practitioner and, where possible, the patient's relatives. Every hospital and healthcare organisation should have a clear policy on this issue, which should be known to all nursing staff.

In the aged care sector, following the Royal Commission into Aged Care established in 2018, significant changes have been made in relation to the use of restraint. Since 1 July 2021, under the *Aged Care Act 1997* (Cth) and the *Quality of Care Principles 2014,* there are now specific responsibilities for aged care providers relating to the use of any restrictive practice in residential aged care.

The *Quality of Care Principles* require providers to satisfy a number of conditions before and during the use of any restrictive practice:

- Providers are required to document the alternatives to restrictive practices that have been considered and used, and why they have not been successful.

- Where any restrictive practices are used, the consumer must be regularly monitored for signs of distress or harm, side effects and adverse events, and changes in wellbeing, as well as independent functions or ability to undertake activities of daily living.
- The use of the restrictive practice must be regularly reviewed by the provider with a view to removing it as soon as possible or practicable.
- Providers are required to develop and implement a behaviour support plan for every consumer who exhibits behaviours of concern, or changed behaviours, or who has restrictive practices considered, applied or used as part of their care.[101]

A range of tools and resources are provided for guidance that assist care providers in managing the problems that might lead to the need for restraint in the elderly. Providers are required to have a clinical governance framework in place that is intended to reduce the use of restrictive practices. However, where restrictive practices are used, such a framework will ensure that requirements such as informed consent are in place. The principles also set up the concept of *Behaviour support plans* that are required to be in place for consumers who need them.[102]

There is also a significant body of work occurring in both the mental health sector[103] and the acute care sector[104] to reduce the reliance on restraint as a management strategy.

CONCLUSION

The question of giving and refusing consent to treatment is of considerable importance for nurses. However, despite the level of concern which the question of consent generates, in reality the essence of this area of law relates to respect for people's integrity and care and diligence in the communication of information. Many health organisations in Australia at national, state and local level, in addition to many consumer groups, have undertaken a lot of work and produced valuable aids to assist health professionals and consumers alike to understand their rights and responsibilities.

CHAPTER 6 REVIEW QUESTIONS

Following your reading of **Chapter 6**, consider these questions in reaching the objectives of this chapter. Guidance on which part of the chapter will assist you in answering the questions can be found at http://evolve.elsevier.com/AU/Staunton/law/. You may, of course, consider other sources as part of your considerations.

1. What is the purpose of the tort of trespass to the person, and why is consent so critical to the clinical practice of health professionals?

2. What are the elements required for a valid consent, and how would you know that a person has actually consented to treatment, minor or major?

3. In what circumstances does a person have the right to refuse consent?

4. How does the use of advance directives help a person to manage their healthcare?

5. How does the tort of false imprisonment impact on the use of restraint in clinical practice?

ENDNOTES

Note: all links were last accessed by 23 April 2023.

1. Kennedy I, 'The patient on the Clapham Omnibus', (1984) MLR 47:454, 460.
2. Hall D, Prochazka A and Fink A, 'Informed consent for medical treatment', *Canadian Medical Association Journal*, (2012) 184(5):533–40; https://www.ncbi.nlm.nih.gov/pmc/articles/PMC3307558/.
3. Ibid.
4. *Schloendorff v Society of New York Hospital* (1914) 211 Ny 125, 129; 105, NE 92, 93.
5. *Crimes Act 1900* (NSW) s 61J.
6. *Malette v Shulman* (1991) 2 Med LR at 165.
7. Ibid, at 162.
8. Ibid, at 163.
9. Australian Commission on Safety and Quality in Health Care, *Implementing and practising open disclosure: a guide for health service managers*, 2013, p 35, https://www.safetyandquality.gov.au/publications-and-resources/resource-library/implementing-and-practising open-disclosure-guide-health-service-managers.
10. *Rogers v Whitaker* [1992] HCA 58; (1992) 175 CLR 479 at 484.
11. Ibid, at 490. This was reiterated in *Rosenberg v Percival* [2001] HCA 18, and also more recently in *Jambrovic v Day* [2017] NSWSC 1468.
12. *Malette v Shulman* (1991), op. cit., at 163.
13. Ibid.
14. Two Australian cases since Malette determined by Guardianship Boards overturned the express wishes of the patients not to receive blood transfusions at the requests of their families — *Qumsieh v Guardianship and Administration Board* (1998) 14 VAR 46 and *In AB (application for consent to medical treatment)* (NSWGT, 2004/1867, 6 April 2004, unreported). See also *The Hospital v T and Anor [2015] QSC 185*. For a useful account of how to care for a Jehovah's Witness patient refusing blood see Lawson T and Ralph C, 'Perioperative Jehovah's Witnesses: a review', (2015) *British Journal of Anaesthesia* 115(5):676–87. https://www.bjanaesthesia.org/article/S0007-0912(17)31069-3/fulltext

15. *X v The Sydney Children's Hospitals Network* (2013) 85 NSWLR 294.
16. Ibid at 308, para 60.
17. *The Hospital v T and Anor* [2015] QSC 185.
18. Ibid at 192, para 24.
19. National Health and Medical Research Council, *National statement on ethical conduct in human research*, updated 2018, https://www.nhmrc.gov.au/about-us/publications/national-statement-ethical-conduct-human-research-2007-updated-2018.
20. Ibid at p 16.
21. Government of Western Australia, Department of Health, *WA Health consent to treatment policy*, 2016, https://www.health.wa.gov.au/-/media/Files/Corporate/Policy-Frameworks/Clinical-Governance-Safety-and-Quality/Policy/WA-Health-Consent-to-Treatment-Policy/OD657-WA-Health-Consent-to-Treatment-Policy.pdf; New South Wales Health, *Consent to medical and health care treatment manual*, 2020, https://www.health.nsw.gov.au/policies/manuals/Pages/consent-manual.aspx.
22. Canberra Health Literacy, *Informed consent*, 2023, https://cbrhl.org.au/consumers-carers/making-decisions-about-health-care/informed-consent-for-consumers/.
23. *healthdirect*, Health topics, *Informed consent*, 2020, https://www.healthdirect.gov.au/informed-consent.
24. *Hart v Herron* [1984] *Aust Torts Report* 80–201.
25. Government of Western Australia, Department of Health, *WA Health consent to treatment policy*, 2016, pp 5–6, https://www.health.wa.gov.au/-/media/Files/Corporate/Policy-Frameworks/Clinical-Governance-Safety-and-Quality/Policy/WA-Health-Consent-to-Treatment-Policy/OD657-WA-Health-Consent-to-Treatment-Policy.pdf.
26. NSW Health. Consent to Medical and Healthcare Treatment Manual. https://www.health.nsw.gov.au/policies/manuals/Documents/consent-section-4.pdf
27. The Hon. Wootton J H, QC, *Report of the Royal Commission into Deep Sleep Therapy*, vol 6, 1990, p 76.
28. *Rogers v Whitaker* [1992] HCA 58; (1992) 175 CLR 479 at 484.
29. These early American decisions acknowledged: 'a patient needed adequate information about the nature of proposed treatment, its risks and feasible alternatives in order to make an

intelligent choice about whether or not to undergo it', in Teff H, 'Consent to medical procedures: paternalism, self-determination or therapeutic alliance', (1985) LQR 101, at 432.

30. *Rogers v Whitaker* [1992] HCA 58; (1992) 175 CLR 479 at 490.

31. Ibid.

32. NSW Health, *Consent to medical and health treatment manual,* s 4 Consent, 2020, pp 18–19, https://www.health.nsw.gov.au/policies/manuals/Documents/consent-section-4.pdf.

33. Ibid.

34. Ibid, p 22.

35. Ibid, p 25.

36. Ibid, p 23.

37. Ibid, p 23.

38. Ibid, p 24.

39. Jaensson M, Dahlberg K and Nilsson U, 'Factors influencing day surgery patients' quality of postoperative recovery and satisfaction with recovery: a narrative review', (2019) *Perioperative Medicine*, 8 (3), https://doi.org/10.1186/s13741-019-0115-1.

40. Cognitive Institute, *Speaking up for safety program*, 2023, https://www.cognitiveinstitute.org/healthcare-courses/speaking-up-for-safety-programme/.

41. *Health Practitioner Regulation National Law Act 2009* (Qld) Part 8, section 140.

42. Institute of Medicine, *To Err Is Human: Building A Safer Health System*, National Academies Press, Washington DC (US), 2000, https://pubmed.ncbi.nlm.nih.gov/25077248/.

43. Scott I and Crock C, 'Diagnostic error: incidence, impacts, causes and preventive strategies', (2020) *Medical Journal of Australia,* 213 (7), https://doi.org/10.5694/mja2.50771.

44. Civil Aviation Academy of Australasia, *Crew resource management/ Aviation decision making course*, 2020, https://www.caaa.com.au/crew-resource-management/.

45. Cognitive Institute, *Speaking up for safety program,* 2023, https://www.cognitiveinstitute.org/healthcare-courses/speaking-up-for-safety-programme/.

46. Ibid.

47. Ibid.

48. *Re C (Adult: Refusal of Treatment)* [1994] 1 WLR 290.

49. Ibid, at 295.

50. People with Disability Australia (PWD), *History of disability rights movement in Australia*, 2023, https://pwd.org.au/about-us/our-history/history-of-disability-rights-movement-in-australia/. This web page contains a link to key pieces of legislation (home/about us/about disability/key disability legislation/and other useful information).

51. Australian Government Australian Law Reform Commission (ALRC), *Equality, capacity and disability in Commonwealth laws*, Discussion paper 81, May 2014, p 28, https://www.alrc.gov.au/publication/equality-capacity-and-disability-in-common-wealth-laws-dp-81/, quoting the United Nations' Convention on the Rights of Persons with Disabilities, opened for signature 30 March 2007, 999 UNTS 3 (entered into force 3 May 2008), Art 1.

52. United Nations Department of Economic and Social Affairs, *Convention on the rights of persons with disabilities,* https://www.un.org/development/desa/disabilities/convention-on-the-rights-of-persons-with-disabilities/convention-on-the-rights-of-persons-with-disabilities-2.html.

53. Australian Law Reform Commission, *Equality, capacity and disability in Commonwealth Laws: The NDIS Objects and Principles*, 2023, https://www.alrc.gov.au/publication/equality-capacity-and-disability-in-commonwealth-laws-dp-81/5-the-national-disability-insurance-scheme/objects-and-principles/.

54. Stewart C, McLoughlin K, McGrath C and Christie E, *Discovering Australian guardianship law*, 2023, http://www.austguardianshiplaw.org/.

55. Tasmanian Government Protective Division Guardianship Stream fact sheet *Consent to medical or dental treatment,* https://www.tascat.tas.gov.au/__data/assets/pdf_file/0006/684123/4.-Consent-to-Medical-or-Dental-Treatment.pdf.

56. *Re QAN* [2008] NSWGT 16 (23 September 2008), https://www.austlii.edu.au/cgi-bin/viewdoc/au/cases/nsw/NSWGT/2008/19.html.

57. Government of Western Australia, Department of Health, *WA Health consent to treatment policy*, 2016, https://www.health.wa.gov.au/-/media/Files/Corporate/Policy-Frameworks/Clinical-Governance-Safety-and-Quality/Policy/WA-Health-Consent-to-Treatment-Policy/OD657-WA-Health-Consent-to-Treatment-Policy.pdf: p 13.

58. *Malette v Shulman* (1991), op. cit., at 162.

59. Ibid, at 165.

60. Ibid, at 166.

61. *Qumsieh v Guardianship and Administration Board* (1998) 14 VAR 46; *Qumsieh v Guardianship and Administration Board & Pilgrim* [1998] VSCA 45; (Winnecke P, Brooking and Ormiston JJA, 17 September 1988, unreported).

62. *In AB (application for consent to medical treatment)* (NSWGT, 2004/1867, 6 April 2004, unreported).

63. *Mercy Hospitals Ltd v D1 & Anor* [2018] VSC 519, http://www8.austlii.edu.au/cgi-bin/viewdoc/au/cases/vic/VSC/2018/519.html.

64. Ibid, at para 76

65. *Re T* [1993] Fam 95.

66. Ibid, at 95.

67. *Re MB* [1997] EWCA Civ 1361; *Re L* (Fam Div, Kirkwood J, 5 December 1996, unreported).

68. *Re L* (Fam Div, Kirkwood J, 5 December 1996, unreported) at 837.

69. van der Pilj M, Verhoeven C, Hollander M, de Jonge A and Kingma E, 'The ethics of consent during labour and birth: episiotomies', (2023) *Journal of Medical Ethics* 30 January 2023, doi: 10.1136/jme-2022-108601.

70. For example, *Minors (Property and Contracts) Act 1970* (NSW), *Minors Contracts Act 1988* (Tas).

71. For example, *Child Protection Act 1999* (Qld), *Child Wellbeing and Safety Act 2005* (Vic).

72. *Department of Health and Community Services (NT) v JWB (Marion's case)* (1992) 175 CLR 218.

73. Ibid, 237–8.

74. *Gillick v West Norfolk & Wisbech Health Authority and another* [1986] 1 AC 112 (HL).

75. Ibid, at 188.

76. NSW Health, (2020) *Consent to medical and healthcare treatment manual*, https://www.health.nsw.gov.au/policies/manuals/Documents/consent-section-8.pdf, p 43.

77. Ouliaris C, 'Consent for treatment of gender dysphoria in minors: evolving clinical and legal frameworks', (2022) *Medical Journal of Australia* 216(5):230–233, doi: 10.5694/mja2.51357.

78. *Director Clinical Services, Child & Adolescent Health Services v Kiszko* [2016] FCWA 19, 34 and 75.

79. For a full discussion on the sum of decisions made in relation to this child, see Freckleton I, 'Parents' opposition to potentially life-saving treatment for minors: learning from the Oshin Kiszko litigation', (2016) *Journal of Law and Medicine* 24(1):61–71.

80. Family Planning NSW, *Confidentiality and privacy for young people*, undated, https://www.fpnsw.org.au/health-information/under-25s/confidentiality-and-privacy-young-people.

81. Ibid.

82. Australian Institute for Family Studies, *Reporting child abuse and neglect resource sheets*, 2023, https://aifs.gov.au/resources/resource-sheets/reporting-child-abuse-and-neglect.

83. Reeve R, Srasuebkul P, Langton J, Haas M, Viney R and Pearson S-A, 'Health care use and costs at the end of life: a comparison of elderly Australian decedents with and without a cancer history', (2017) *BMC Palliative Care* 17(1):1, https://www.ncbi.nlm.nih.gov/pmc/articles/PMC5480123/.

84. See, for example, a range of useful publications: McGee A, Purser K, Stackpoole C, White B, Willmott L and Davis J, 'Informing the euthanasia debate: perceptions of Australian politicians', (2018) *University of New South Wales Law Journal* 41(4):1368–1417.

85. *H Ltd v J* [2010] 107 SASR 352.

86. Also known as advance care directives and advance health directives.

87. Harrison Dening K, Sampson EL and De Vries K, 'Advance care planning in dementia: recommendations for healthcare professionals', (2019) *Palliative Care*. Feb 27;12, https://www.ncbi.nlm.nih.gov/pmc/articles/PMC6393818/.

88. See, for example, the NSW Government website that incorporates a range of documents, policies, legislation and general advice for planning ahead, https://www.health.nsw.gov.au/patients/acp/Pages/more-info.aspx.

89. *Cruzan v Director, Missouri Department of Health* 497 US 261 (1990).

90. Advance Care Planning Australia, *Advance care planning explained*, 2021, https://www.advancecareplanning.org.au/understand-advance-care-planning/advance-care-planning-explained.

91. Bernard C, Tan A, Slaven M, Elston D, Heyland DK and Howard M, 'Exploring patient-reported barriers to advance care planning in family practice', (2020) *BMC Fam Pract* 21, 94, https://doi.org/10.1186/s12875-020-01167-0.

92. Silveira M, Advance care planning and advance directives, (2023) *Up to date*, https://www.uptodate.com/contents/advance-care-planning-and-advance-directives.

93. *Medical Treatment Planning and Decisions Act 2016* (Vic), Part 2.

94. See also NSW Health, *Advance care planning*, 2023, https://www.health.nsw.gov.au/patients/acp/Pages/default.aspx and NSW Health, *Making an advance care directive*, 2022, https://www.health.nsw.gov.au/patients/acp/Publications/acd-form-info-book.pdf.

95. *Sayers v Harlow Urban District Council* [1958] 1 WLR 623.

96. *Hart v Herron* [1984] Aust Torts Reports 80-201, Fisher J.

97. *Herd v Weardale Steel Co* [1915] AC 67.

98. Wilson K, 'The COVID-19 pandemic and the human rights of persons with mental and cognitive impairments subject to coercive powers in Australia', (2020) *International Journal of Law and Psychiatry* Nov–Dec;73, https://www.ncbi.nlm.nih.gov/pmc/articles/PMC7318936/.

99. Williams J, Gilbert G, Dawson A, Kaldor J Hendrickx D and Haire B, 'Uncertainty and agency in COVID-19 hotel quarantine in Australia', (2022) *Qualitative Research in Health 2*, https://www.sciencedirect.com/science/article/pii/S2667321521000342.

100. Pich J, *Violence in nursing and midwifery in NSW: study report*, NSWNS/UTS, Sydney, 2019, https://www.nswnma.asn.au/wp-content/uploads/2019/02/Violence-in-Nursing-and-Midwifery-in-NSW.pdf.

101. Australian Government Aged Care Quality and Safety Commission, *Minimising the use of restrictive practices*, 2023, https://www.agedcarequality.gov.au/minimising-restrictive-practices.

102. Australian Government Aged Care Quality and Safety Commission, *Guidance resources*, 2023, https://www.agedcarequality.gov.au/providers/standards/guidance-resources.

103. Royal Australian and New Zealand College of Psychiatrists, *Position statement 61: minimising and, where possible, eliminating the use of seclusion and restraint in people with mental illness*, 2021, https://www.ranzcp.org/news-policy/policy-and-advocacy/position-statements/minimising-use-of-seclusion-and-restraint.

104. Acevedo-Nuevo M, González-Gil MT and Martin-Arribas MC, 'Physical restraint use in intensive care units: exploring the decision-making process and new proposals: a multi-method study', (2021) *International Journal of Environmental Research and Public Health* 18(22), https://www.ncbi.nlm.nih.gov/pmc/articles/PMC8623552/.

PROFESSIONAL NEGLIGENCE

LEARNING OBJECTIVES

In this chapter, you will:

- gain an understanding of professional negligence as a civil wrong
- identify the legal principles that must be established if and when an allegation of professional negligence is made
- learn, in particular, how the law determines the duty and standard of care expected of registered and enrolled nurses and midwives in the delivery of their professional services
- gain awareness of the legal and professional consequences that may flow from a professionally negligent act that occurs in the course and scope of your employment
- examine the different legal outcomes that may arise as a consequence of performing a professionally negligent act in the delivery of professional services as an independent contractor as distinct from an employee
- understand the legal provisions relating to the role of acting as a 'good samaritan'.

INTRODUCTION

In the context of the delivery of healthcare services, an allegation of professional negligence is part of civil law. When such an allegation is made, the central complaint is that, in the delivery of a particular health service, the health professional delivering the service has been negligent in a particular respect causing the complainant to suffer damage and loss. When that occurs this area of the law permits patients, the relatives of patients or other persons to bring claims against hospitals, health authorities, medical practitioners, nurses, midwives and other health professionals, seeking financial compensation as a result of an alleged negligent act that has caused damage and financial loss, as well as pain and suffering.

When such claims are made, the civil law principles that arise for consideration and the professional and legal consequences that may arise if they are established require all health professionals to be aware of those principles, how they apply to their professional practice and what their professional obligations are in relation to them.

In a civil claim, the party bringing the claim for compensation is known as the **plaintiff** and the party defending the claim is known as the **defendant**. The plaintiff bears the onus of proof and must establish his or her claim according to the standard of proof for civil law matters — that is, on the balance of probabilities.

THE DEVELOPMENT OF COMMON LAW PRINCIPLES IN RELATION TO ALLEGATIONS OF PROFESSIONAL NEGLIGENCE AND LEGISLATIVE CHANGES AFFECTING THEM

As **Chapter 1** explains (in the section 'The Development of the Common Law'), the development of common law principles in Australia has its origin in the development of the common law of England dating from the 12th century. Over time, the established common law principles have been significantly added to or replaced by laws passed by parliament and known as

TABLE 7.1	
Legislation Relevant to a Claim Alleging Professional Negligence	
Australian Capital Territory	*Civil Law (Wrongs) Act 2002*
New South Wales	*Civil Liability Act 2002*
Northern Territory	*Personal Injuries (Liabilities and Damages) Act 2003*
Queensland	*Civil Liability Act 2003*
South Australia	*Civil Liability Act 1936*
Tasmania	*Civil Liability Act 2002*
Victoria	*Wrongs Act 1958*
Western Australia	*Civil Liability Act 2002*

parliamentary law or legislation. In Australia, since 2002, legislative changes have impacted on the law applicable to civil negligence and professional negligence in particular. The end result has seen an amalgam of common law principles embedded within the legislation that has reaffirmed those principles and, in some cases, extended or replaced them.

The title of the legislation in each state and territory relevant to considerations of professional negligence is set out in **Table 7.1**. There are differences of approach between the states and territories. Those sections of the legislation relevant to the delivery of your professional services are set out further in this chapter. Only the more significant differences between the states and territories in relation to professional negligence are referred to.

Although relevant legislation has been put in place, the courts still use common law principles determined in previously decided cases to assist them in interpreting and applying the legislative provisions now in place relating to professional negligence.

PROFESSIONAL NEGLIGENCE IN A HEALTHCARE CONTEXT

In the healthcare system, the great majority of court cases involving allegations of professional negligence are against members of the medical profession. Given the major role that medical practitioners play in diagnosing, determining and delivering the healthcare to

be given to a patient, this is not surprising. As a consequence, the case law developed by the courts, particularly the High Court, in determining the standard of care expected in the delivery of health services is made up of cases concerning the actions of medical practitioners in specific clinical circumstances. Notwithstanding the focus on medical practitioners, the legal principles that have emerged from these cases are relevant to all health professionals, including nurses and midwives involved in delivering healthcare and/or providing advice and information about proposed healthcare.

The Legal Principles of Professional Negligence

In bringing a claim alleging professional negligence, the plaintiff must prove, on the balance of probabilities, that:

- the defendant owed the plaintiff a duty of care; **and**
- the defendant was in breach of the duty of care owed to the plaintiff by failing to deliver his or her professional services according to the standard expected; **and**
- as a result of the defendant's negligent act, the plaintiff suffered damage and loss (factual causation); **and**
- the damage and loss the plaintiff is complaining of was a reasonably foreseeable consequence of the defendant's negligent act (the scope of the defendant's liability).

Each of these principles is examined below, with particular reference to nurses and midwives acting in their professional capacity.

THE PRINCIPLE OF DUTY OF CARE AS IT APPLIES TO A NURSE OR MIDWIFE

The first principle in professional negligence is that the defendant owed the plaintiff a duty of care.

It has been a long-established common law principle that, in carrying out your professional services, a duty of care is owed to your patients, your fellow employees and potentially other persons. That principle was laid down in 1932 by the English House of Lords (then a superior court of appeal whose decisions bound Australian courts) in *Donoghue v Stevenson*. That decision determined the now well-established common law principle concerning the existence and scope of one's duty of care in an action alleging civil negligence.[1]

In determining the extent and the existence of a duty of care generally, the court stated that each of us owed a duty of care, in law, to our neighbour. In response to the question, 'Who, in law, is my neighbour?', the answer given in the decision of the court was:

> *... persons who are so closely and directly affected by my act that I ought reasonably to have had them in my contemplation as being likely to be damaged when I set out to do the acts or omissions which are now being complained of.*[2]

The common law principle established from that case is that a duty of care is owed when it is reasonable to foresee harm occurring in relation to the particular activity being undertaken.

Consider that principle in relation to your work in the delivery of your professional services. In carrying out your work as a nurse or midwife, your professional activities closely and directly affect your patients, your fellow employees and potentially other persons. Accordingly it can reasonably be foreseen that, should you undertake your professional activities below the standard that would be expected or fail to perform a service that would have been expected, one or all of those categories of people may be injured. Therefore, those people are your 'neighbours in law' and a duty of care exists in relation to them.

A good example of how the scope or extent of one's professional duty of care can extend beyond the patient or fellow employee to a third party is the decision of the New South Wales Supreme Court in the case known as *BT v Oei*[3] set out in **Case example 7.1**.

Comment and Relevant Considerations Relating to *BT v Oei*

Relying on that case, nurses and midwives should, in carrying out their professional activities, be mindful that their duty of care may, depending on the facts and circumstances, extend much wider than it first appears.

CASE EXAMPLE 7.1

BT v Oei

FACTS

Dr Oei was a general practitioner. AT was his patient. In late 1991, Dr Oei first saw AT and treated him for a flu-like illness. In early 1992, AT was again seen by Dr Oei as his earlier symptoms had not settled. Tests taken at that time revealed a urinary tract infection and hepatitis. Dr Oei did ask AT at that time about his sexual activities and whether he was an intravenous drug user. AT denied any history of drug-taking and referred to 'casual sexual exploits' as a possible source of hepatitis B. At that time, Dr Oei gave AT a number of pamphlets about hepatitis B and safe sex practices but, despite the evidence of hepatitis, Dr Oei did not recommend that AT have an HIV test. As a result AT was unaware of his HIV status, which was positive. AT subsequently formed a sexual relationship with BT. They had unprotected sex on a number of occasions, and AT passed the virus to BT who subsequently became ill. BT sued Dr Oei for professional negligence. BT claimed that Dr Oei, who owed a duty of care to AT as his patient, should have suspected an HIV infection and advised AT to have an HIV test when he first presented. BT argued, and the court agreed, that if Dr Oei had done so then AT's HIV status would have been detected early enough for him to have practised safe sex with BT and, as a consequence, BT would not have contracted the HIV infection.

In coming to its decision in relation to Dr Oei, the court considered the obligation imposed on medical practitioners under the *Public Health Act 1991* (NSW).[4] Under that Act, a doctor who reasonably believes a patient may have an HIV infection is required to inform the patient of the danger that he or she poses to others, including sexual partners in particular, and the measures the patient should take to protect others from infection.

What is the Position Outside of Work?

Outside of your work as a nurse or midwife, there are obviously circumstances where a legal duty of care to other people arises. For example, if you are driving your motor vehicle on a public highway, it is 'reasonably foreseeable' that if you fail to drive in accordance with the road rules then somebody may get hurt. That 'somebody' would be any other user of the highway, be they another driver or a pedestrian. It follows, therefore, that when you drive a motor vehicle you owe to all the other users of the road a duty of care to drive in accordance with the road rules. In such an activity, it is the 'reasonable foreseeability' of harm that determines that a duty of care arises.

In the legislation listed in **Table 7.1** most of the states and territories (except the Northern Territory) have enshrined the common law principle of a 'reasonable foreseeability of harm' test to determine whether a duty of care arises in relation to any activity or undertaking. For example, section 5B of the *Civil Liability Act 2002* (NSW) provides that a person is **not** negligent in failing to take precautions against a risk of harm unless:

(a) the risk was foreseeable (that is, it is a risk of which the person knew or ought to have known), and
(b) the risk was not insignificant, and
(c) in the circumstances, a reasonable person in the person's position would have taken those precautions.

Further, in determining whether a reasonable person would have taken precautions against a risk or harm, the court is to consider (amongst other relevant things):

(a) the probability that the harm would occur if care were not taken;
(b) the likely seriousness of the harm;
(c) the burden of taking precautions to avoid the risk of harm;
(d) the social utility of the activity that creates the risk of harm.

The other states and territories (with the exception of the Northern Territory) have similar provisions. See the *Civil Law (Wrongs) Act 2002* (ACT) sections 42 and 43, *Civil Liability Act 2003* (Qld) section 9, *Civil Liability Act 1936* (SA) section 32, *Civil Liability Act 2002* (Tas) section 11, *Wrongs Act 1958* (Vic) section 48, and *Civil Liability Act 2002* (WA) section 5B.

Relevantly, in a majority of the states and territories, the legislation identifies categories of activities where,

it is said, *liability will not automatically arise*. Such provisions, where applicable, intentionally negate the notion of a duty of care arising in relation to the nominated categories of activity as follows.

The *first category* where liability is conditional is where a person is engaged in activities that may be considered socially valuable. These include:

■ public authorities, particularly those that provide or manage services for the general benefit of the community, or exercise regulatory functions;
■ 'good samaritans' who provide assistance in emergencies (the obligation imposed on health professionals including nurses and midwives as 'good samaritans' is discussed in more detail later in this chapter);
■ volunteers involved in carrying out work for a community organisation.

The *second category* where liability may not arise is where the plaintiff is engaged in a particular activity where it is considered the plaintiff should bear the risks associated with that activity, for example:

■ an activity that involves inherent and/or obvious risks;
■ an activity referred to as a 'dangerous recreational' activity;
■ the consumption of alcohol or other drugs;
■ criminal activity, including where the defendant acts in self-defence.

As an example, section 5K of the *Civil Liability Act 2002* (NSW) defines 'dangerous recreational activity' as a 'recreational activity that involves a significant risk of physical harm' and 'recreational activity' includes:

a. *any sport (whether or not the sport is an organised activity), and*
b. *any pursuit or activity engaged in for enjoyment, relaxation or leisure, and*
c. *any pursuit or activity engaged in at a place (such as a beach, park or other public open space) where people ordinarily engage in sport or in any pursuit or activity for enjoyment, relaxation or leisure.*

The effect of these provisions is that, outside one's professional activities as a nurse or midwife, whether a duty of care is owed would depend, in the first instance, on the facts and circumstances of the activity giving rise to the allegation of negligence and whether it meets the test to determine whether a duty of care arises. As well, it would be necessary to consider whether the facts and circumstances of the activity complained of fell into one of the above categories where the relevant civil liability legislation now provides that liability generally does not arise.

SECOND PRINCIPLE IN A CIVIL ACTION ALLEGING PROFESSIONAL NEGLIGENCE: DETERMINING THE STANDARD OF CARE EXPECTED OF HEALTH PROFESSIONALS

The second principle of professional negligence is that the defendant breached the duty of care owed to the plaintiff by failing to deliver his or her professional services according to the standard that would have been expected.

Since 1992 in Australia, the principal court cases involved in determining the standard of care expected of health professionals have centred around two important aspects of their work:

■ the standard of care expected in the actual performance of their work — that is, the actual delivery of treatment; and

■ the standard of care expected in giving patients information and advice, disclosing material risks inherent in the treatment being recommended and providing relevant warnings — that is the giving of information and advice as a prerequisite to obtaining the patient's consent to the treatment being proposed.

The Common Law Principle that Determined the Standard of Care in the Delivery of Professional Services

The standard of care expected of medical practitioners, nurses and midwives in the actual performance of their work has long been expressed in the common law principle that, in the performance of his or her work, a health professional should exercise a level of skill and care that, at the time the service was delivered, would be accepted by 'peer professional opinion' to be 'competent professional practice'.

In 1992 the High Court of Australia handed down its decision in the case of *Rogers v Whitaker*[5] that reaffirmed that common law principle by stating:

In Australia, it has been accepted that the standard of care to be observed by a person with some special skill or competence is that of the ordinary skilled person exercising and professing to have that special skill.[6]

The relevant facts of that case are set out in **Case example 7.2.**

CASE EXAMPLE 7.2

Rogers v Whitaker

FACTS

In 1946, when Mrs Whitaker was only 9 years old, she suffered a penetrating injury to her right eye. As a result she became almost totally blind in that eye. However, she retained normal vision in her left eye. Despite this handicap Mrs Whitaker was able to lead a normal life. She completed her schooling and after leaving school worked in a variety of occupations. She married and had four children. In between having children she continued to work.

Mrs Whitaker ceased employment in 1980 but in 1983 she decided to return to work and with employment in mind she set out to obtain an eye 'check-up'. She was referred by her general practitioner to Dr Rogers, an ophthalmologist, for possible surgery on her right eye; in the words of the referral 'if you think she would benefit, even cosmetically'.

Following his examination of Mrs Whitaker at the initial consultation, Dr Rogers told her that he could operate on her right eye to remove the scar tissue. This would improve the appearance of the eye and at the same time would probably restore significant sight to that eye.

At the second consultation Mrs Whitaker agreed to submit to surgery on her right eye and the procedure was carried out later that year. Subsequently, complications developed in the right eye and then in the left eye, although that eye had not been interfered with during the operation. This was the result of a rare condition known as 'sympathetic ophthalmia'.

Rogers v Whitaker (Continued)

This is a serious complication of eye surgery involving inflammation in the treated eye and sympathetic inflammation in the untreated eye. It carries with it a serious risk of blindness. Ultimately Mrs Whitaker lost the sight in her left eye, becoming virtually blind as her right eye remained visually impaired.

Mrs Whitaker brought an action against Dr Rogers for professional negligence claiming he had performed the procedure negligently and also that he had failed to properly inform her of the possibility of the complication of sympathetic ophthalmia.

Comment and Relevant Considerations Relating to *Rogers v Whitaker*

Essentially, in *Rogers v Whitaker* the High Court reaffirmed the common law principle that the standard of care expected of a person exercising a special skill or competence such as Dr Rogers should, at the time the service was delivered, be determined by reference to what would be the level of skill and expertise accepted by a responsible body of peer opinion as being competent professional practice. Specifically in relation to Dr Rogers, the High Court determined he had performed the operation with requisite care and skill.

The Determination of the Test to Determine the Standard of Care Expected in Giving Advice and Information to a Patient about Proposed Treatment

In bringing her claim against Dr Rogers, Mrs Whitaker alleged Dr Rogers had performed the procedure on her right eye negligently — a claim the High Court dismissed. However, Mrs Whitaker also claimed Dr Rogers had failed to provide her with sufficient information and advice in relation to the risk of sympathetic ophthalmia arising in carrying out the procedure on her right eye and stated, if he had, she would not have had the surgery. In his defence Dr Rogers acknowledged he had not advised Mrs Whitaker about the risk of sympathetic ophthalmia because, he argued, the risk of such a complication was remote (1:15 000) and in carrying out such a procedure, the ordinary reasonable ophthalmic surgeon would not have done so. Evidence was given by other ophthalmic surgeons that supported Dr Rogers' position. On that point the High Court rejected the 'ordinary reasonable competent surgeon' test and determined, in giving information and advice to a patient about proposed treatment, a patient was entitled to make informed decisions about the procedure being recommended and should therefore be informed of 'material risks' in the proposed treatment. Further the court said, a risk was 'material' if a reasonable person in the patient's position was likely to attach significance to it. In the case of Mrs Whitaker, with one good eye, it was entirely reasonable she would be concerned about the possibility of injury to it particularly as the procedure was elective. Given the circumstances the court determined Dr Rogers had been professionally negligent in failing to advise Mrs Whitaker about the risk of sympathetic ophthalmia arising from the procedure.

Essentially, the decision of the High Court in *Rogers v Whitaker* determined, in relation to the giving of advice to a patient about proposed treatment, the 'ordinary reasonable competent/peer professional opinion' test should not be followed. Instead, the court determined, the question whether a risk is relevant to a patient, and one about which they should be warned, requires a different approach, and courts are able to determine this question themselves.

The decision of the High Court in *Rogers v Whitaker* was a very significant one in the field of professional negligence litigation for health professionals concerning the approach to be taken in determining the standard of care expected in giving information and advice to patients about proposed treatment. It shifted the test from what a doctor may believe to be sufficient information and advice about proposed treatment, to what a patient, in his or her particular circumstances, would consider sufficient. On that issue, the High Court stated relevantly:

> *Further, and more importantly, particularly in the field of non-disclosure of risk and the provision of advice and information, ... the courts have adopted the principle that, while evidence of acceptable medical practice is a useful guide for the courts, it is for the courts to adjudicate on what is the appropriate standard of care after giving weight to 'the paramount consideration that a person is entitled to make his own decisions about his life'.*[7]

The High Court stated further:

> ... except in cases of emergency or necessity, all
> medical treatment is preceded by the patient's
> choice to undergo it. In legal terms, the patient's
> consent to the treatment may be valid once he or
> she is informed in broad terms of the nature of the
> procedure which is intended. But the choice is, in
> reality, meaningless unless it is made on the basis
> of relevant information and advice. Because the
> choice to be made calls for a decision by the patient
> on information known to the medical practitioner
> but not to the patient, it would be illogical to hold
> that the amount of information to be provided by
> the medical practitioner can be determined from
> the perspective of the practitioner alone or, for that
> matter, of the medical profession.[8]

The above principle established in *Rogers v Whitaker* has been reaffirmed by the High Court in later decisions.[9] In one of the later cases, the High Court said relevantly that 'a doctor has a duty to warn a patient of a material risk inherent in the proposed treatment'.[10] In the same case, the High Court also said that 'a risk was material' if:

> ... in the circumstances of the particular case,
> a reasonable person in the patient's condition,
> if warned of the risk, would be likely to attach
> significance to it or if the medical practitioner is
> or should reasonably be aware that the particular
> patient, if warned of the risk, would be likely to
> attach significance to it.[11]

Those decisions make it clear that the standard of care that health professionals owe to their patients includes an obligation not only to treat them competently according to professional standards but also to inform, advise and warn them about risks associated with the proposed treatment, to answer their questions candidly and to respect their rights (including, where they so choose, to postpone medical procedures and go elsewhere for treatment).

Following the High Court decision in *Rogers v Whitaker*, the National Health and Medical Research Council issued *general guidelines about this topic that are reviewed and updated from time to time*.[12]

This important issue is canvassed more extensively in **Chapter 6** relating to consent to treatment and it is relevant to all health professionals including nurses and midwives.

Legislative Provisions Requiring Health Professionals to Warn of Risks in Treatment

In addition to the case law determined by the courts, the civil liability legislation in some of the states and territories has made specific provision for a medical practitioner to warn patients of 'risks in treatment' whereas in other states there is no duty to disclose 'obvious risks' except in some circumstances. Queensland and Tasmania provide for what is described as a proactive and reactive duty of a medical practitioner to warn of risks. For example, section 21 of the *Civil Liability Act 2003* (Qld) states:

> 1. A doctor does not breach a duty owed to a patient
>   to warn of risk, before the patient undergoes any
>   medical treatment (or at the time of being given
>   medical advice) that will involve a risk of personal
>   injury to the patient, unless the doctor at that time
>   fails to give or arrange to be given to the patient
>   the following information about the risk —
>   a. information that a reasonable person in the
>   patient's position would, in the circumstances,
>   require to enable the person to make a reasonably informed decision about whether to
>   undergo the treatment or follow the advice;
>   b. information that the doctor knows or ought
>   reasonably to know the patient wants to be
>   given before making the decision about whether
>   to undergo the treatment or follow the advice.

Section 21 of the Tasmanian *Civil Liability Act 2002* is in similar terms except that the above obligations are exempted in emergency circumstances where it is necessary to save life and/or where the patient is unable to be consulted or advised because of prevailing circumstances.

In Victoria the obligation to warn of risk is not confined to doctors and, in our view, simply restates the common law position determined in *Rogers v Whitaker*. Section 50 of the *Wrongs Act 1958* states:

> A person (the **defendant**) who owes a duty of care
> to another person (the **plaintiff**) to give a warning

*or other information to the plaintiff in respect of
a risk or other matter, satisfies that duty of care if
the defendant takes reasonable care in giving that
warning or other information.*

In New South Wales, South Australia and Western
Australia, there is no duty to warn of 'obvious risks' but
in most of the states there are limits to such a provision
relevant to health professionals. For example, section
5H of the *Civil Liability Act 2002* (NSW) states:

1. *A person (**the defendant**) does not owe a duty of
   care to another person (**the plaintiff**) to warn of
   an obvious risk to the plaintiff.*
2. *This section does not apply if:*
   a. *the plaintiff has requested advice or informa-
      tion about the risk from the defendant, or*
   b. *the defendant is required by a written law to
      warn the plaintiff of the risk, or*
   c. *the defendant is a professional and the risk is
      a risk of the death of or personal injury to the
      plaintiff from the provision of a professional
      service by the defendant.*
3. *Subsection (2) does not give rise to a presumption of a duty to warn of a risk in the circumstances referred to in that subsection.*

As a proper reading of that section confirms, health
professionals would almost invariably not be exempted
from a duty to warn of an 'obvious risk' as they are generally in the business of responding to a request from a
patient or client for advice or information about proposed treatment, and the person asking for advice or
information faces a risk of death or personal injury
arising from the services provided by that professional.

Similar provisions apply in these states: *Civil Liability
Act 2003* (Qld) sections 13–15, *Civil Liability Act 1936*
(SA) sections 36–8, *Civil Liability Act 2002* (Tas)
sections 15–17, *Wrongs Act 1958* (Vic) sections 53, 54 and
56, and *Civil Liability Act 2002* (WA) sections 5M–5O.

There are no such provisions in the Australian Capital Territory or the Northern Territory, in which case
the approach enunciated by the High Court in *Rogers v
Whitaker* would apply — that is, that the information
and advice to be given to a patient would be what the
ordinary reasonable person, in the patient's position,
would want to know.

Legislative Provisions Relevant to Determining the Standard of Care in the Delivery of a Professional Service

Each of the states and territories introduced the civil
liability legislation listed in **Table 7.1**. That legislation,
among other things, effectively embedded the com-
mon law test enunciated by the High Court in *Rogers
v Whitaker* as to the standard of care expected of professionals delivering their services as well as making
specific legislative provisions in relation to the obligation or otherwise on a professional to give a warning,
advice or other information to a person.

As a consequence, it is necessary as a nurse or midwife to know the standard of care provisions that apply
to health professionals in your respective state or territory legislation.

With the exception of the Northern Territory, each
state and territory has made specific provisions in their
civil liability legislation for the standard of care expected
of 'professionals' or, in the case of Western Australia,
specifically of 'health professionals'. The Australian Capital Territory legislation refers simply to the standard of
care expected of a 'reasonable person in the defendant's
position'. Because of the absence of uniformity of approach on this issue, it is important for nurses and midwives to be aware of those differences depending on the
particular state or territory in which they are practising.
The relevant legislative provisions of each state and
territory are set out below.

Australian Capital Territory. Section 42 of the *Civil
Law (Wrongs) Act 2002* provides for the standard of
care for professionals as follows:

*For deciding whether a person (the defendant) was
negligent, the standard of care required of the defendant
is that of a reasonable person in the defendant's position
who was in possession of all the information that the
defendant either had, or ought reasonably to have had,
at the time of the incident out of which the harm arose.*

New South Wales. Section 5O (i.e. capital O) and section
5P of the *Civil Liability Act 2002* provide as follows.
Section 5O states:

1. *A person practising a profession (**a professional**)
   does not incur a liability in negligence arising*

from the provision of a professional service if it is established that the professional acted in a manner that (at the time the service was provided) was widely accepted in Australia by peer professional opinion as competent professional practice.

2. *However, peer professional opinion cannot be relied on for the purposes of this section if the court considers that the opinion is irrational.*

3. *The fact that there are differing peer professional opinions widely accepted in Australia concerning a matter does not prevent any one or more (or all) of those opinions being relied on for the purposes of this section.*

4. *Peer professional opinion does not have to be universally accepted to be considered widely accepted.*

Section 5P provides:

This Division (incorporating section 5O and section 5P) does not apply to liability arising in connection with the giving of (or the failure to give) a warning, advice or other information in respect of the risk or death or of injury to a person associated with the provision by a professional of a professional service.

Queensland. Section 22 of the *Civil Liability Act 2003* provides as follows:

1. *A professional does not breach a duty arising from the provision of a professional service if it is established that the professional acted in a way that (at the time the service was provided) was widely accepted by peer professional opinion by a significant number of respected practitioners in the field as competent professional practice.*

2. *However, peer professional opinion can not be relied on for the purposes of this section if the court considers that the opinion is irrational or contrary to a written law.*

3. *The fact that there are differing peer professional opinions widely accepted by a significant number of respected practitioners in the field concerning a matter does not prevent any 1 or more (or all) of the opinions being relied on for the purposes of this section.*

4. *Peer professional opinion does not have to be universally accepted to be considered widely accepted.*

5. *This section does not apply to liability arising in connection with the giving of (or the failure to give) a warning, advice or other information, in relation to the risk of harm to a person, that is associated with the provision by a professional of a professional service.*

South Australia. Section 41 of the *Civil Liability Act 1936* provides as follows:

1. *A person who provides a professional service incurs no liability in negligence arising from the service if it is established that the provider acted in a manner that (at the time the service was provided) was widely accepted in Australia by members of the same profession as competent professional practice.*

2. *However, professional opinion cannot be relied on for the purposes of this section if the court considers that the opinion is irrational.*

3. *The fact that there are differing professional opinions widely accepted in Australia by members of the same profession does not prevent any one or more (or all) of those opinions being relied on for the purposes of this section.*

4. *Professional opinion does not have to be universally accepted to be considered widely accepted.*

5. *This section does not apply to liability arising in connection with the giving of (or the failure to give) a warning, advice or other information in respect of a risk of death of or [sic] injury associated with the provision of a health care service.*

Tasmania. Section 22 of the *Civil Liability Act 2002* provides as follows:

1. *A person practising a profession ('a professional') does not breach a duty arising from the provision of a professional service if it is established that the professional acted in a manner that (at the time the service was provided) was widely accepted in Australia by peer professional opinion as competent professional practice.*

2. *Peer professional opinion cannot be relied on for the purpose of this section if the court considers that the opinion is irrational.*

3. *The fact that there are differing peer professional opinions widely accepted in Australia concerning*

a matter does not prevent any one or more (or all) of those opinions being relied on for the purpose of subsection (1).

4. Peer professional opinion does not have to be universally accepted to be considered widely accepted.

5. This section does not apply to liability arising in connection with the giving of (or the failure to give) a warning, advice or other information in relation to the risk of harm associated with the provision by a professional of a professional service to a person.

Victoria. Sections 58 and 59 of the *Wrongs Act 1958* provide as follows.

Section 58:

In a case involving an allegation of negligence against a person (the defendant) who holds himself or herself out as possessing a particular skill, the standard to be applied by a court in determining whether the defendant acted with due care is, subject to this Division, to be determined by reference to —

a. what could reasonably be expected of a person possessing that skill; and

b. the relevant circumstances as at the date of the alleged negligence and not a later date.

Section 59:

1. A professional is not negligent in providing a professional service if it is established that the professional acted in a manner that (at the time the service was provided) was widely accepted in Australia by a significant number of respected practitioners in the field (peer professional opinion) as competent professional practice in the circumstances.

2. However, peer professional opinion cannot be relied on for the purposes of this section if the court determines that the opinion is unreasonable.

3. The fact that there are differing peer professional opinions widely accepted in Australia by a significant number of respected practitioners in the field concerning a matter does not prevent any one or more (or all) of those opinions being relied on for the purposes of this section.

4. Peer professional opinion does not have to be universally accepted to be considered widely accepted.

5. If, under this section, a court determines peer professional opinion to be unreasonable, it must specify in writing the reasons for that determination.

6. Subsection (5) does not apply if a jury determines the matter.

Western Australia. Western Australia is the only state to have a specific standard of care for health professionals. Section 5PB of the *Civil Liability Act 2002* provides as follows:

1. An act or omission of a health professional is not a negligent act or omission if it is in accordance with a practice that, at the time of the act or omission, is widely accepted by the health professional's peers as competent professional practice.

2. Subsection (1) does not apply to an act or omission of a health professional in relation to informing a person of a risk of injury or death associated with —
   a. the treatment proposed for a patient or a foetus being carried by a pregnant patient; or
   b. a procedure proposed to be conducted for the purpose of diagnosing a condition of a patient or a foetus carried by a pregnant patient.

3. Subsection (1) applies even if another practice that is widely accepted by the health professional's peers as competent professional practice differs from or conflicts with the practice in accordance with which the health professional acted or omitted to do something.

4. Nothing in subsection (1) prevents a health professional from being liable for negligence if the practice in accordance with which the health professional acted or omitted to do something is, in the circumstances of the particular case, so unreasonable that no reasonable health professional in the health professional's position could have acted or omitted to do something in accordance with the practice.

5. A practice does not have to be universally accepted as competent professional practice to be considered widely accepted as competent professional practice.

6. In determining liability for damages for harm caused by the fault of a health professional, the plaintiff always bears the onus of proving, on the

balance of probabilities, that the applicable standard of care (whether under this section or any other law) was breached by the defendant.

Northern Territory. The Northern Territory has enacted the *Personal Injuries (Liabilities and Damages) Act 2003* but it does not make provision for any test to determine the standard of care expected in relation to professional practice. In the absence of any such provision, the determination of the standard of care where professional negligence is alleged would be determined by reference to the common law tests enunciated in *Rogers v Whitaker*.

Note: section 42 of the Australian Capital Territory legislation set out above does not refer to persons practising as 'professionals' *or* to persons holding 'himself or herself out as possessing a particular skill'. Consequently it is of wider application than the legislation of the other jurisdictions and would apply to any defendant in a civil negligence action.

DETERMINING THE STANDARD OF CARE EXPECTED OF NURSES AND MIDWIVES

When determining the appropriate standard of care expected of a nurse or midwife in any particular professional practice situation, consideration would first be given to whether the standard of care expected had arisen as an issue in the actual delivery of professional services or in relation to the professional advice and information given to a patient to obtain the patient's consent to a proposed treatment.

To determine the standard of care expected in the delivery of professional services by a nurse or midwife, it is necessary to consider the relevant provisions in the civil liability legislation of your state or territory as set out above having regard to what 'peer professional opinion' would consider 'competent professional practice' in the clinical situation being reviewed.

If, however, the allegation was that the nurse or midwife in question failed to give the patient sufficient information and advice about the possible risks of a proposed treatment as a prerequisite to obtaining their consent to undergo the proposed treatment, that issue would be determined by the court having regard to the specific facts and circumstances and, given those facts

and circumstances, what the patient in his or her particular position would have considered a 'material risk' and would have wanted to know.

Is There a Different Standard Expected of a Registered Nurse and an Enrolled Nurse?

Remember, the test to be applied when determining the standard of care expected when delivering a professional service is whether the professional in question delivered the particular service in a manner that was widely accepted by 'peer professional opinion' to be 'competent professional practice'. Accordingly, where an incident arose involving the professional actions of an enrolled nurse, his or her actions would be determined by reference to 'peer professional opinion' evidence from an enrolled nurse 'expert' as to whether what was done or not done was considered 'competent professional practice' for an enrolled nurse in the situation under review. Likewise if the incident involved a registered nurse, reference would be made to 'peer professional opinion' evidence from a registered nurse 'expert' as to whether what was done or not done was considered 'competent professional practice' for a registered nurse in the situation under review. In short, each would be judged by their professional peers.

Given the differing educational preparation between a registered and enrolled nurse, it could be presumed on initial consideration that in the same clinical situation, the level of skill, knowledge and expertise expected of a registered nurse would be different than that expected of an enrolled nurse. That initial presumption is reinforced by the *Enrolled nurse standards for practice*[13] issued by the Nursing and Midwifery Board of Australia. Amongst other matters, those standards reinforce the requirement for an enrolled nurse to work under the supervision of a registered nurse. For example, Standard 3.1 states that an enrolled nurse 'Accepts accountability and responsibility for own actions', specifically identifying the following relevant Indicators:

3.3 *Recognises the RN as the person responsible to assist EN decision-making and provision of nursing care.*

3.4 *Collaborates with the RN to ensure delegated responsibilities are commensurate with own scope of practice.*

3.5 Clarifies own role and responsibilities with supervising RN in the context of the healthcare setting within which they practice.

3.6 Consults with the RN and other members of the multidisciplinary healthcare team to facilitate the provision of accurate information, and enable informed decisions by others.

3.7 Provides care within scope of practice as part of multidisciplinary healthcare team, and with supervision of a RN.

Also, Standard 5 states that the enrolled nurse 'Collaborates with the RN, the person receiving care and the healthcare team when developing plans of care' and specifically at Indicator 5.5 the enrolled nurse 'Clarifies orders for nursing care with the RN when unclear'.

In the main, the above Standards clearly indicate the expectation that an enrolled nurse works under the overall supervision of, and collaboratively with, a registered nurse in the delivery of patient care. As always, each case would have to be determined by reference to its own particular facts and circumstances. For example, the standard of care expected of a registered nurse and an enrolled nurse in taking and recording a patient's temperature and blood pressure would generally be identical. Also, if an enrolled nurse was endorsed to administer medication within his or her scope of practice, the standard of care expected would be identical to that of a registered nurse in the same clinical situation. However, if an enrolled nurse did not have such an endorsement and went beyond his or her scope of practice and administered medication without the knowledge and supervision of a registered nurse, and the patient suffered harm as a result it would be argued that the enrolled nurse had gone beyond their scope of practice and did not have the requisite skills, knowledge and expertise to undertake the particular procedure that should generally be undertaken by a registered nurse.

Peer Professional Opinion

Peer professional opinion is the expert opinion expressed by one's professional peers following consideration by the expert of the facts and circumstances of a particular incident. In short, an expert is asked to express an opinion about what should or should not have been done in a specific situation. When that expert is asked to give that evidence to a court, it is regarded as expert opinion evidence.

Notwithstanding the minor differences in the respective state and territory legislation, the common approach to determining the requisite professional standard in any particular clinical situation requires evidence of a professional standard that is 'widely accepted' by 'peer professional opinion' as being 'competent professional practice'. The majority of the states (New South Wales, South Australia, Tasmania and Victoria) provide that the professional standard be widely accepted 'in Australia' whereas Queensland and Western Australia provide no such limitation, which would allow evidence of a professional standard to be obtained from overseas nursing and midwifery experts.

Remember also that the Northern Territory makes no legislative provision for determining the requisite standard of care in a professional situation; therefore, the common law principle established in *Rogers v Whitaker* would apply and evidence would be elicited from one's professional peers to determine what would have been expected of the 'professionally competent' nurse or midwife in a specific clinical situation. Likewise the case in the Australian Capital Territory.

Expert evidence is obtained from a professional peer working in the relevant clinical area who is recognised as an expert in their field of practice based on academic knowledge and, in particular, extensive clinical experience. Therefore, if an incident occurred in an operating theatre where the actions of a nurse were alleged to have been negligent, evidence would be called from a nurse with extensive clinical experience in operating theatre practice who would be regarded as an expert in that area by her or his peers. That nurse would be asked to give an opinion, on the basis of the known facts, about what was considered to be widely accepted competent professional practice in such circumstances — that is, what would have been the professional standard expected of a nurse in the particular clinical situation under scrutiny. It is quite possible, of course, that his or her evidence may be rejected or disputed by other nursing experts in the field who give evidence in the matter. The ultimate decision as to whether expert opinion evidence is accepted or rejected ultimately rests with the court.

The operating theatre example is paralleled in other areas. For example, if it were necessary to establish what was competent professional practice in the area of midwifery, expert evidence would be elicited from a midwife considered to be an expert in the field. Likewise if it was necessary to determine what was competent professional practice for an endorsed enrolled nurse in a particular clinical situation, evidence would be obtained from an endorsed enrolled nurse considered to be an expert in the particular field of professional practice.

The critical point to remember is that it is the profession itself, through the development of skills and knowledge and the application of professional standards, that determines what is or is not competent professional practice in any given clinical situation where one's professional competence is called into question.

Identifying a nurse or midwife who would be considered an expert in their field of practice is relatively straightforward. Usually, the relevant special interest nursing or midwifery group is asked to identify a number of nurses or midwives who would be considered experts practising in the particular area of clinical practice under consideration.

Other Potential Sources of Evidence

The major additional sources of evidence that assist the courts in determining standards of practice in a particular clinical situation are:

- professional practice standards and guidelines;
- legislative obligations;
- departmental guidelines and/or employers' policy and procedural directives;
- academic texts and publications;
- the patient's medical records.

Professional Practice Standards and Guidelines

Nurses and midwives, like many other professional groups within the health industry, have addressed the need for the development of professional standards covering a wide range of their professional activities and responsibilities. The development of such standards is to be applauded and encouraged, as long as they are subject to regular professional peer review

and assessment and they are generally recognised by the profession as appropriate for the professional activity to which they refer. Like the departmental and employer policy and procedural directives, professional standards documents would, where relevant, provide objective evidence of an expected and competent standard of professional conduct in a given clinical situation.

The courts in Australia and overseas have, on occasions, specifically referred to documented practice and procedure standards as evidence to assist them in determining the standard of care expected of a nurse or midwife in a given situation. For example, the Court of Appeal of the Supreme Court of Queensland relied on a professional standards document in the case of *Langley v Glandore Pty Ltd*[14] (see **Case example 7.8** for the relevant facts of that matter).

That matter involved, among other things, the standard expected of nursing staff in operating theatres when counting sponges. In commenting on that issue, the court said:

> *The relevant established standard for counting of sponges, swabs, instruments and needles is called the 'ACORN' standard and it supports the description of the duties that has been outlined. Importantly, there was no dissent at the trial concerning its applicability.*[15]

Nurses who work in operating theatres would know that ACORN refers to the standards adopted by the Australian Council of Operating Room Nurses (ACORN).

More recently, in 2014, the New South Wales Coroner's Court referred to the Australian College of Midwives' *Guidelines for consultation and referral* when inquiring into the manner and cause of death of a baby following an attempted homebirth overseen by an independent midwife.[16] The relevant facts of that matter are set out in **Case example 7.10**.

As well, a Canadian case used the standing orders of an emergency room as the standard against which medical and nursing practice should be measured.[17] In another Canadian case, an entire section of the procedure manual was reproduced in the judgment as it was considered crucial to determining the question of whether the practice under review had fallen below the standard of care which could reasonably have been expected.[18]

Closer to home, the Supreme Court of South Australia has made specific reference to professional standards in dealing with an appeal against a finding of a disciplinary tribunal of the Nurses Board of South Australia in these terms:

It may be seen that the Board in reaching its decision that the Appellant had been guilty of unprofessional conduct, had regard to the various standards of nursing practice which had been laid down by its own guidelines, the policy of the nursing home, regulations, the International Council of Nursing's Code of Ethics and what it describes as the ANRAC competencies. It may be accepted that those standards are well recognised and accepted in the nursing profession.[19]

What is critical in developing professional practice standards is that they should quite properly reflect the way in which the work is done, and able to be done, day to day, in the delivery of care. Professional practice standards that take little or no account of the day-to-day clinical environment in which nurses and midwives work render such standards unattainable and may be considered to have limited evidentiary assistance to the court.

Professional practice standards should become the foundation for all professionals, including nurses and midwives, to develop good professional habits in the way they deliver services.

Legislative Obligations

There are often clear legislative (also known as statutory) obligations on nurses, midwives and other health professionals to undertake specific actions in the delivery of clinical care. For example, the *Poisons Acts* and *Regulations* of the states and territories provide that a registered nurse or midwife is required to check a dangerous drug (generally referred to as a Schedule 8 drug) with another nurse or midwife before administering it. A failure to do so, without reasonable cause and which results in an incorrect drug being administered and the patient suffering harm as a result, would be deemed to be a breach of the nurse's or midwife's obligations under the *Poisons Acts* and *Regulations*.

This would be in addition to a breach of his or her general duty of care to the patient by failing to observe proper professional standards of care and safety in administering a dangerous drug.

Likewise, in the area of mental health care and treatment, the decision to utilise seclusion or restraint in relation to a patient is accompanied by clear legislative or mandatory policy obligations on nursing staff. (See details of those provisions in **Chapter 10.**) A failure to abide by those provisions would be considered a breach of the nurse's duty of care to the patient pursuant to the provision in the mental health legislation of the state or territory or, in the case of New South Wales and South Australia, pursuant to the mandated policy of the employer.

Another example of where a breach of a legislative obligation by a medical practitioner was relied on to support an allegation of professional negligence was the case of *BT v Oei* (see **Case example 7.1**). One of the specific failures alleged by the plaintiff against Dr Oei was that he was in breach of the *Public Health Act 1991* (NSW)[20] and *Public Health (General) Regulation 2002* (NSW).[21] On that point the judge agreed, stating relevantly in the following paragraphs as follows:

[92] The Public Health Act 1991 *s 12(1)*[22] *requires a medical practitioner who believes on reasonable grounds that his or her partner is suffering from a sexually transmissible medical condition to provide the patient with such information as required by the Regulations of the Act.*

Regulation 4[23] *of the Public Health Act sets out the categories of information to be supplied:*
a. *the means of minimising the risk of infecting other people with the condition;*
b. *the public health implications of the condition;*
c. *the responsibilities under s 11*[24] *of the Act including any precautions considered reasonable;*
d. *responsibilities under s 13*[25] *of the Act;*
e. *diagnosis and treatment;*
f. *treatment options.*

[93] Section 13[26] *of the Public Health Act makes it an offence for a person who knows that he or she suffers from a sexually transmissible medical condition to have sexual intercourse with another*

person unless, before the intercourse takes place, the other person has been informed of the risk of contracting a sexually transmissible medical condition and has voluntarily agreed to accept that risk.

[94] The scheme of the Public Health Act thus requires a medical practitioner who reasonably believes his or her patient to have HIV to inform the patient of the public health implications of the condition and the means of protecting others. The practitioner must inform the patient of the patient's statutory responsibility to warn prospective sexual partners of his or her condition.[27]

In finding Dr Oei negligent, the judge agreed that Dr Oei had, among other matters, failed to discharge his legislative obligation to properly advise his patient, AT, of the need to be HIV tested, and, as a result and at the relevant time, AT had unprotected sex with BT who contracted HIV.

Departmental Guidelines and/or Employers' Policy and Procedural Directives

More often than not, the respective state, territory and Commonwealth departments of health issue numerous policy circulars, many of which are directly relevant to nurses and midwives in their day-to-day work. Such policy circulars very often lay down procedures and practices to be observed and enforced in given clinical situations and are generally issued as a clear indication of the standards to be observed in such situations.

In addition, employers in the health industry put in place a large number of policy and procedural directives designed to ensure that employees follow a safe and recognised standard of clinical practice. Accreditation standards documents are often another source of expected professional clinical standards. Often a plaintiff alleging failure by a nurse or midwife to abide by a particular policy or procedural directive may provide supportive evidence of the standard of care expected in a given situation by referring to such documents.

For example, if a hospital procedure manual laid down the strict procedure to be followed in adding prescribed drugs to a patient's intravenous (IV) fluid line, or in the administration of a blood transfusion, then an unreasonable failure or refusal to abide by such procedural directives, with consequent adverse effects on the patient, would place the nurse or midwife in breach of the proper and generally recognised safety standards laid down by the employer. It would also place the nurse or midwife in breach of his or her overall duty of care to the patient because he or she failed to observe proper standards of care and safety in carrying out professional activities. The employer's policy and procedural directive would be used as evidence of what constituted competent professional practice, against which the conduct of the nurse or midwife would be judged.

Academic Texts and Publications

Recognised academic texts relevant to the particular area of healthcare and professional practice under scrutiny may provide the foundation for establishing evidence of widely accepted and competent professional practice.

The Patient's Medical Records

Although the patient's medical records are not documents that, of and by themselves, would be referred to for determining the standard of care expected in a given clinical situation, we mention them in relation to this issue because the patient's medical records will invariably disclose whether the clinical care given to the patient did or did not accord with competent professional practice.

When 'peer professional opinion' evidence is elicited and policy and professional practice standards documents are subpoenaed and read, the patient's medical records will be scrutinised to ascertain whether the staff involved in the care of the patient, by their actions or omissions, did or did not abide by the expected standard of care expressed by peer professional opinion or found in policy and procedural directives of the employer or health service.

A patient's medical records contain critical evidence of what treatment, care or advice was given to the patient — or not, as the case may be. For example, all treatment notes, medication order sheets, observation charts, pathology results, radiological reports and other documents relating to the patient's care will be located in the patient's medical records. Those records will often be a valuable source of evidence for a health professional to demonstrate that the treatment and care given was of a 'professionally competent' standard. Alternatively, they can be a source of evidence for a plaintiff's lawyers who may point to entries in such documents (or the absence thereof) as evidence in support of their allegation of professional negligence. As a consequence, the importance of documentation in the delivery of healthcare is a critical factor of which nurses and midwives should be ever mindful. This subject is addressed in detail in **Chapter 9**.

Examples of Cases Highlighting the Standard of Care Expected in Specific Clinical Situations

This section examines nine cases determined by courts in Australia involving nurses and midwives to highlight the standard of care expected in particular clinical situations. Following these **Case examples 7.3–7.11** are comments, relevant findings and critical thinking questions for your reflection.

The best way to understand how the courts approach the determination of the standard of care expected of nurses and midwives in a professional setting is by examining the outcomes of cases, specifically those that have come before the courts where the professional standards of those involved had been highlighted with regard to the performance of their work.

Some of the cases that follow arise from a formal finding of civil negligence by a relevant civil court or from a Coroner's Court following an inquest into the death of a patient. In the case of the Coroner's Court, there is no formal finding of civil or criminal negligence, but often the coroner will make adverse and critical comments concerning the actions of the nursing staff, among others, leading to the manner and cause of death of the patient. Also, where a coroner makes adverse findings about a health professional in an inquest, he or she may refer the matter to the relevant professional registration board for consideration of professional disciplinary proceedings and possible de-registration. For that reason, coroners' inquest reports are a valuable source of guidance in understanding the standard of care expected of nurses and midwives in clinical situations.

The majority of the cases arose before the introduction of the civil liability legislation setting out the provisions relevant to determining the standard of care for health professionals (among others). That legislative approach does not negate the following case reports being practical examples that would still be relevant in determining whether the standard of care provided in a given situation was 'widely accepted' by 'peer professional opinion' as being 'competent professional practice' or otherwise.

CASE EXAMPLE 7.3

Coroner's Inquest into the Death of Paul Lau[28]

Highlights issues of concern in the use of electronic medical records; nurses working in the recovery room and postoperative ward; failure to confirm written postoperative medication orders on transfer to recovery and failure to question postoperative medication orders; and failure of critical thinking by nursing staff.

FACTS

Mr Lau was admitted for day surgery to undergo an anterior cruciate ligament reconstruction in June 2015. At the time of his admission, the hospital was using TrakCare, a complete medical records system that managed all aspects of the patient's stay in hospital including managing admission, prescription and administering of medication, managing laboratory results and managing documentation and forms. At the time of Mr Lau's death, the TrakCare system had been in place since the beginning of May 2015. The staff members were provided with training about the new system and, as of June 2015, although there had been some errors detected in the system, none had caused the death of a patient or any adverse outcomes for patients.

At the time of Mr Lau's death, TrakCare contained the complete medical record of a patient detailing all medications administered within the hospital including the operating theatres. In short, TrakCare allowed a pharmacist to review a patient's medication history online in the pharmacy. The role of the

Continued

designated dispensing pharmacist on a day-to-day basis was to ensure that the prescribed medication was appropriate for the patient in light of the patient's known demographics, reason for admission, known allergies and current medication profile.

During Mr Lau's operation, and in accordance with usual practice, the anaesthetist charted Mr Lau's postoperative medications. These included an antiemetic, a further antibiotic, pain relief including acetaminophen and oral oxycodone 5–10 mg every 4 hours and an anti-inflammatory. They were considered routine and at appropriate dosages given the procedure Mr Lau had undergone. The medications were charted by the anaesthetist during Mr Lau's surgery using a combination of 'one-touch' and longhand prescribing in TrakCare. The latter procedure was described by the coroner as follows:

> *Longhand prescribing required the anaesthetist to select medication from a drop down box, type further information regarding the administration of the medication, click 'update' to add the medication to a 'shopping cart' on the right hand side of the screen and then enter his personal TrakCare passcode before clicking 'submit'.*[29]

Mr Lau's operation was uneventful and he was transferred to the recovery unit. At approximately 1.25 pm, the anaesthetist handed over the care of Mr Lau to the registered nurse in recovery and returned to the theatre to anaesthetise the next patient on the list (GS), that operation getting underway at approximately 1.35 pm.

At the time of his transfer, Mr Lau's TrakCare record had been transferred online to identify him as being in recovery.

No review of Mr Lau's postoperative medications was undertaken between the anaesthetist and the registered nurse as part of the handover and the registered nurse did not consult Mr Lau's medication orders in TrakCare during the handover.

During the operation on the next patient GS, the anaesthetist clicked onto Mr Lau's TrakCare chart to prescribe a small amount of fluids necessary to 'keep the line open' for intravenous antibiotics. As he was completing this task, the anaesthetist's attention was drawn back to the clinical needs of the patient GS, who was still being operated on.

In due course at approximately 1.55 pm, and in accordance with his usual practice, the anaesthetist commenced to chart the postoperative medication for the patient GS. In doing so, the anaesthetist failed to realise he still had Mr Lau's TrakCare record open. As a consequence, the anaesthetist charted the postoperative medications for the patient GS into Mr Lau's TrakCare record. Those medications were significantly different from those initially entered for Mr Lau's postoperative care as the patient GS had a history of long-term chronic pain and had previously been prescribed fentanyl patches.

The postoperative medications for GS included a fentanyl infusion 20 mcg/mL, 60 mL as a fentanyl patient-controlled analgesia (PCA) as well as a fentanyl 100 mcg/h transdermal patch, one patch every 3 days with a total of five patches.

In the course of making those entries, 22 different alerts were triggered by the TrakCare system and were overridden by the anaesthetist.

The anaesthetist's postoperative medication orders for the patient GS entered in error into Mr Lau's TrakCare records were noted by the dispensing pharmacist in the hospital pharmacy, who believed them to be for Mr Lau. Despite knowing the fentanyl 100 mcg patch was the strongest fentanyl patch available and that there was nothing in Mr Lau's TrakCare record to suggest he had ever taken opioids before, the pharmacist dispensed the fentanyl 100 mcg patch to the ward for Mr Lau.

At or about 2 pm, the medication orders for fentanyl PCA and fentanyl patch appeared in Mr Lau's TrakCare record in the recovery unit. Notwithstanding what must have appeared to be an abnormal amount of pain relief medication having been ordered for a relatively minor procedure, one of the recovery room registered nurses commenced the fentanyl PCA. That particular registered nurse had taken over Mr Lau's care at about 2 pm for a short period while her colleague was on a meal break. Mr Lau's observations were stable at this time. No query was raised with the anaesthetist by that registered nurse in recovery about the orders for the fentanyl for Mr Lau in addition to

Coroner's Inquest into the Death of Paul Lau (Continued)

the oral pain relief that had already been ordered and no mention of fentanyl had been made by her colleague when she took over Mr Lau's care.

The patient GS was ultimately transferred to the recovery unit and handed over to the nursing staff by the anaesthetist. During this handover there was no review of the postoperative medication orders on the TrakCare system for GS and it was not until the anaesthetist had left the hospital that the nursing staff noted that no pain relief or other medication had been charted for that patient. When the anaesthetist was contacted by phone about that, he 'assumed he had closed GS's electronic patient file incorrectly and that TrakCare had not saved the medication orders'. He verbally stated the medications GS was to receive and they were subsequently charted by the medical officer on duty at the hospital.

In the meantime, Mr Lau had been transferred to the ward. The registered nurses on the ward noted the order for the fentanyl patch and applied it some 4 hours after his surgery had been completed and in spite of the fentanyl PCA also being administered at the same time.

The anaesthetist made a return visit to the hospital later in the evening to check the postoperative patients, including Mr Lau. At that time neither he nor the nursing staff reviewed Mr Lau's medication orders. Also, the nursing staff raised no concerns about the amount of high-dose opioid medication Mr Lau had been ordered, although he had no history of prior opioid use and the procedure he had had would not normally warrant such a high dose of fentanyl.

The anaesthetist agreed that when he saw Mr Lau that evening he noticed the fentanyl PCA and the fentanyl patch but assumed they must have been ordered by the surgeon or the medical officer. He made no inquiries or raised any concerns.

During the evening Mr Lau had routine observations taken every 2 hours. By the time the night duty shift appeared at about 10 pm, Mr Lau was noted to still be 'alert and orientated'. His care was assigned to an assistant in nursing (AIN). The night duty registered nurse was aware of Mr Lau's fentanyl patch but did not inquire as to the dosage.

Mr Lau was checked for his 2-hourly observations just after midnight by the assistant in nursing. He initially did not respond but then did so briefly when roused. The AIN moved the PCA away from his hand 'because he was so drowsy'. The nurse noted his breathing 'seemed a little off'. The AIN asked the registered nurse to come and check Mr Lau as 'his breathing rhythm seemed a little odd'. The registered nurse was busy at the time and by the time she reached the room, Mr Lau was not breathing and no pulse was evident. The Code Blue alarm was triggered but Mr Lau could not be revived.

During the inquest that followed, toxicological examination found a potentially fatal level of fentanyl in Mr Lau's blood. His cause of death was found to be aspiration pneumonia caused by multiple drug toxicity.

Comment and Relevant Considerations Relating to the Coroner's Inquest into the Death of Paul Lau

This case highlights a number of important issues for health professionals, particularly nursing staff in postoperative recovery care. It also highlights the dangers to be aware of in the use of electronic medical records. As the coroner noted, the expert opinion evidence in relation to safe anaesthetic practice observed that:

… there are benefits to electronic medical records, however the introduction of e-prescribing presents new risks and challenges. While TrakCare did not cause Paul's death, the initial prescription error was made easier due to a function of TrakCare of great utility — the ability to open and close different patient records from a single terminal. Prior to the introduction of electronic medical records, it was much more difficult to chart medication on the wrong patient file.[30]

As the facts of the matter disclose, significant clinical errors were made by the anaesthetist, the dispensing pharmacist and a number of the nursing staff. Central to those respective professional errors was a failure in critical thinking throughout the sequence of events leading to Mr Lau's death.

In relation to the anaesthetist, the coroner was satisfied that he 'failed to exercise proper care, diligence and caution when prescribing medication erroneously'[31] into Mr Lau's TrakCare record compounded by the fact that he overrode 22 alerts presented to him by the TrakCare system. Further, when he was contacted by nursing staff advising that he had not charted any postoperative medication for the patient GS, the coroner stated that call should have alerted him to the possibility that the medication had been incorrectly charted for another patient. He had the opportunity to check that when he returned to the hospital and he failed to do so notwithstanding that he saw the fentanyl PCA and a fentanyl patch in place when he checked Mr Lau, which he would have known he had not ordered for him. When asked, the anaesthetist stated he 'assumed' the fentanyl had been ordered by the surgeon or the hospital's medical officer — an explanation the coroner referred to as 'a series of untenable assumptions'. The anaesthetist's conduct was referred to the Health Care Complaints Commission, which referred him in turn to his professional body.

In relation to the dispensing pharmacist, the coroner found she was aware that the fentanyl 100 mcg patch was the strongest available fentanyl patch and there was nothing in Mr Lau's TrakCare record to suggest he had ever taken opioids before. The pharmacist's actions were reviewed by the Pharmacy Council and she was found to have engaged in 'unsatisfactory professional conduct' in that the medication order should have been confirmed with the anaesthetist as it was unusual for an 'opioid-naïve patient' to be prescribed the strongest dose of a fentanyl patch and patches were not regularly prescribed for patients postoperatively.

The actions of the nursing staff in the recovery unit and the ward were the subject of consideration by an identified nursing expert who had over 30 years' experience working with multidisciplinary care teams, particularly in the perioperative environment. She provided expert opinion reports to the court and gave additional oral evidence at the hearing. Having regard to all the known facts and circumstances, she identified the following professional clinical failures by the nursing staff both in recovery and in the ward following Mr Lau's transfer from theatre:

- The handover of Mr Lau by the anaesthetist to the recovery room registered nurse should have included clearer and more complete communication including details of the postoperative medications ordered for Mr Lau. The registered nurse should have consulted the TrakCare record for charted medications and confirmed them with the anaesthetist during the handover. Remember, as the facts disclose, the registered nurse who took the handover of Mr Lau from the anaesthetist did not check the postoperative medications on the TrakCare system at that time. If she had, she would have noted there was no fentanyl prescribed for him at that time and that would have alerted her to confirm the fentanyl orders with the anaesthetist when they did appear on his record knowing it had not initially been prescribed.

- The registered nurse in recovery who took over Mr Lau's care from the first registered nurse failed to clarify the fentanyl PCA order with the anaesthetist or her colleague. No mention had been made of the need for fentanyl PCA as part of the handover. Remember, the erroneous entry for the fentanyl was made into Mr Lau's TrakCare record at approximately 1.55–2 pm, which was about the same time as the handover registered nurse was relieved by her registered nurse colleague.

- The handover by the anaesthetist of the patient GS to the recovery unit registered nurse did not include a review of the medication chart of GS. However, the anaesthetist did mention to the registered nurse that GS was to have a further 200 mcg of fentanyl in divided doses as a fentanyl PCA for postoperative pain and that GS had chronic pain and was on a fentanyl patch, which should be recommenced. As the handover did not involve any review of the patient's TrakCare file for confirmation of her postoperative orders, the absence of any charted medication was not detected.

- Mr Lau was transferred to the ward at 3 pm. During the clinical handover the registered nurses did not consult Mr Lau's TrakCare record to confirm his postoperative medication orders. That should have been done and, in the opinion of the nursing expert, 'the prescription of both the fentanyl PCA and fentanyl patch should have alerted nurses of their experience of the need to clarify the medication order with the anaesthetist as the order was very unusual for a patient in Mr Lau's circumstances'.

- The registered nurse caring for Mr Lau in the ward should have clarified the TrakCare order for the fentanyl PCA and fentanyl patch with the anaesthetist, given that she had already had cause to check with him about the duplication of orders for paracetamol and cephazolin that had been recorded in Mr Lau's TrakCare record. Also, the policy of the hospital at the time in relation to PCA stated that 'supplementary sedatives and/or opioids must not be administered while PCA is in progress unless authorised by medical officer, anaesthetist, intensivist or their registrars as these medications can lead to oversedation and respiratory distress'.

- Notwithstanding the above policy, the registered nurses in the ward checked the drug with a registered nurse colleague and applied the fentanyl patch. When asked, she said she administered the fentanyl patch instead of the oral analgesia that had been prescribed for Mr Lau 'as she was focused on the danger of combining oral opioids with a fentanyl PCA'. The opinion of the nursing expert was that the registered nurses 'had displayed a lack of knowledge regarding high-risk medications and a limited capacity for critical thinking by failing to recognise the potential effects and consequences of such a large volume of fentanyl in Mr Lau's system following a general anaesthetic'. Further, that the 'knowledge of the standard dosing range and routes of administration of fentanyl' should have prompted the nurses to 'consult a reputable pharmacology resource or clarify the order with the anaesthetist'.

- The registered nurse on the evening shift did not increase the frequency of Mr Lau's observations despite him receiving high doses of opiates. Also, when the evening shift came on at 10 pm, the registered nurse in charge of the night duty shift was told of Mr Lau's fentanyl patch but did not ask the dosage of the patch. The expert nursing report stated she should have taken steps to ascertain the active ingredient and dosage of the patch as this was an important piece of information that was necessary for her to make appropriate care plans or make safe delegations to the nurses she was leading on the shift. As a result of this failure, an assistant in nursing with insufficient expertise to monitor a patient receiving Mr Lau's level of opioids was allocated to Mr Lau's care and his observations were maintained at 2-hourly instead of hourly visual inspection checks and checks of his level of sedation.

In addition to the above specific failures on the part of the nursing staff, the expert nursing report also identified a number of systemic issues including a 'persistent failure of critical thinking' by all those involved in Mr Lau's care and a number of deficiencies in handover practices by the nursing staff.

Poor handover practices were identified including reference to a failure to review a patient's TrakCare records at the time of handover resulting in missed opportunities to detect the prescribing error. Also, most of the registered nurses in recovery and on the ward displayed 'a lack of opioid awareness' resulting in a failure to question the fentanyl order given the minimally invasive nature of his surgery as well as poor patient allocation decisions. Overall, it was stated, a 'rote, rather than critical, approach to patient observations was displayed throughout' Mr Lau's care.[32]

CASE EXAMPLE 7.4

Sha Cheng Wang v Central Sydney Area Health Service[33]

Highlights the issue of the adequacy of observation and advice to be given to a patient by nurses working as triage nurses in an accident and emergency department.

FACTS

The plaintiff, Sha Cheng Wang, was left seriously and permanently disabled by irreversible brain damage as a result of an assault perpetrated upon him as he was walking from the railway station to his home. He was struck from behind by a heavy object and fell to the ground and may have been unconscious for a short period.

He managed to walk to his home, and two of his friends there took him by taxi to the Royal Prince Alfred Hospital arriving at approximately 9.20 pm.

Continued

Sha Cheng Wang v Central Sydney Area Health Service (Continued)

Mr Wang was seen on arrival by the triage nurse, a registered nurse, who obtained a brief history and undertook a brief physical examination of him. Her entry in the patient notes read simply 'assaulted ?LOC' and she explained the expression '?LOC' meant a possible loss of consciousness. There was no other notation of any other neurological observations made by her although she gave evidence that, as part of her initial examination of Mr Wang, 'He walked into my office unaided and appeared to be alert. She had him squeeze her fingers to test his hand grip, which she found to be firm and equal. She checked his pupils by having him close his eyes and open them quickly, and they appeared to be equal and reacting to light'. It should be noted at this point that the judge hearing the matter concluded that he found the evidence of the triage nurse 'unreliable in certain respects'.[34]

In any event, the triage nurse advised Mr Wang and his companions that the emergency department was busy and they would have to wait. There was evidence that Mr Wang's companions later approached the triage nurse on two occasions expressing their concern about him.

At about 10.00 pm the triage nurse was relieved by another registered nurse. Evidence was given that one of Mr Wang's companions approached her to ask how much longer he would have to wait to be treated. He was told the department was busy and that a lot of people were waiting. About 15 minutes later he asked her if they could go somewhere else for treatment, perhaps at a private hospital, and she said that they were free to do so. As he put it, she said that 'we can do whatever we want to'.[35]

A decision was taken to leave the hospital and seek treatment elsewhere. Mr Wang and his friends left at about 11.00 pm and the registered nurse wrote in the notes 'did not wait to be seen'.

Mr Wang and his friends went to the city super-clinic not far from the hospital. On arrival Mr Wang was immediately seen by the doctor on duty. There was no adverse finding as to the treatment given by the doctor to Mr Wang, as recorded by his clinical notes at the time. That is:

- The doctor obtained a full history of the assault.
- He examined Mr Wang and took the full range of neurological tests. He found no abnormal signs.
- He examined, cleaned and sutured the head wound and administered a tetanus toxoid injection.
- He advised Mr Wang he should return to the hospital for an X-ray. This was rejected because of the displeasure at what had occurred earlier.
- He gave them a 'head injury advice form' and went on to explain what it said, using gestures to ensure he was understood. He said that an ambulance should be called immediately in the event of vomiting or convulsion, if the patient became drowsy or unrousable, or if they observed weakness in one or more of his limbs or inequality in the size of his pupils. He told them the patient should not be left alone. He advised them to take him to a Chinese-speaking doctor the next morning to arrange for an X-ray and for any ongoing care that might be necessary.

Mr Wang went home to the flat he shared with his friends. During the night Mr Wang started vomiting and convulsing and became unconscious. An ambulance was called and Mr Wang arrived back at the hospital by 4.00 am and underwent surgery but was left with irreversible brain damage.

Comment and Relevant Considerations Relating to Sha Cheng Wang v Central Sydney Area Health Service

Mr Wang's case against the hospital was put on two alternative bases. First, it was alleged that the examination undertaken by the first registered nurse (as triage nurse) was inadequate and superficial and that no notice was taken of his friends' insistence that Mr Wang needed urgent attention. As a result, it was alleged Mr Wang was not afforded the priority which his clinical condition deserved. Alternatively, accepting that his priority was appropriately assessed, the initial triage nurse should have consulted a doctor about him before she went off duty, and the second registered nurse (as triage nurse) should have done so before the plaintiff left the hospital. In either event, it was said, some attempt should have been made to dissuade Mr Wang from leaving before he had been seen by a doctor.

The judge was critical of the actions of both nurses in the terms as expressed above — particularly the second registered nurse, who did not give any evidence. On the role of the triage nurse the judge made the following comment:

> … it is clear that her task as triage sister was to make a primary assessment of him with a view to assessing the urgency of his need for the treatment. That assessment had to be made in the light of the other demands upon the Department at the time and the available professional resources … (her) other responsibility was to keep the plaintiff under observation in the waiting area in case his condition worsened.[36]

The evidence was that the first registered nurse gave an oral report to the second registered nurse at the end of her shift. Mr Wang's friends continued to request that he be seen by a doctor only to be met by the statement of both of the registered nurses that the emergency department was busy and they would have to wait. Eventually one of Mr Wang's friends, a Mr Ng, inquired as to whether they should seek treatment elsewhere. On that issue, the judge stated:

> I turn, then, to the question which has troubled me most. Should hospital staff have attempted to dissuade the plaintiff from leaving? I have referred (at par 21) to the unchallenged evidence of David Ng about his inquiry whether they might seek treatment elsewhere. I am satisfied that that inquiry was directed to Sister Smith and that she did not advise them to wait. It is true that some further time elapsed before they left, and counsel for the hospital submitted that the staff might have not been aware of their departure. However, if appropriate observation of the plaintiff in the waiting area were being maintained, they should have been.

> It was common ground that the plaintiff was free to leave and the hospital staff had no power to restrain him. However, varying views were expressed by the experts about how the situation should have been handled. It was said that normally staff would attempt to persuade a patient from leaving and would find out how soon a doctor might be available, informing the medical staff that the patient was becoming restless.[37]

Another expert medical witness accepted by the judge gave evidence that:

> … when patients decide to leave an emergency department without treatment, staff should attempt to discourage them from doing so. Failing that, they should try to ensure that they seek alternative medical care. The practice in the hospital where he worked was that, if it was clear that a patient could not be persuaded to wait, he or she would be given the names of medical clinics in the area … the approach of staff to the situation must be flexible and would depend on a number of variables, including the clinical presentation of the patient, where the patient intended to go upon leaving, the demands upon the resources of the department at the time, the availability of other medical services in the area and their capacity to deal with the patient's condition.[38]

In considering the circumstances in which Mr Wang left the emergency department, the judge came to the conclusion that the Central Sydney Area Health Service was liable for Mr Wang's permanent damage because of the failure of the triage nurses in the emergency department of the hospital to properly observe him and advise him against leaving the hospital. In determining that liability the judge concluded:

> Given the unpredictable effects of head injuries, it was clearly in the plaintiff's best interests to remain at the hospital, where there were the resources to observe and respond to any deterioration of his condition. I am satisfied that, if he had, he would not be in his present predicament.

> … Sister Smith did not ask Mr Ng where they intended to go, and did not offer any advice about alternative sources of treatment suitable for the plaintiff's condition, should it deteriorate. Indeed

there is no evidence that there was any suitable source at that time of night other than a public hospital. Sister Smith should have counselled the plaintiff to remain at the hospital, explaining why it was in his interests to do so.

… Clearly, the primary duty which the hospital owed to the plaintiff was to assign him his appropriate priority through the triage system and to observe him in the waiting area in case his condition deteriorated.

The Central Sydney Area Health Service, which administers the hospital, is a statutory authority whose duty was to take reasonable care for the plaintiff's wellbeing in the circumstances, within the limits of its resources … In my view, that duty extended to furnishing the plaintiff with appropriate advice when it was intimated that he might leave the hospital. The hospital failed to discharge that duty, and the plaintiff's present condition is attributable to that failure.[39]

The question as to whether Mr Wang and his friends would have accepted the advice to remain at the hospital if spoken to in those terms had to be determined. Mr Wang was unable to say because of his incapacity. The judge did consider the evidence of his friends who were with him on the night in question and came to the view, on that evidence, that he would have.

Considering all of the above and considering the standard expected of a professionally competent registered nurse working in the triage section of an accident and emergency department, ask yourself:

- Would you expect a registered nurse who assessed a patient on arrival with a reported history of traumatic head injury to have made a more detailed note of observations made and taken?
- Given the reported history of traumatic head injury, would you expect a registered nurse to notify the medical officer on duty of the need to assess the patient as a matter of priority?
- Do you agree that a registered nurse should counsel and advise a patient with a reported history of traumatic head injury to wait to be seen before leaving the hospital?

Once again, in relation to the care of Mr Wang, the nursing observation records were clearly deficient. If Mr Wang was assessed as thoroughly as the registered nurse stated in court, then all those observations should have been fully recorded in the patient's observation chart. They are, after all, clinical observations that are directly relevant to a patient's neurological status *and*, given Mr Wang's history of traumatic head injury, were clearly very relevant. Also, the history of traumatic head injury raised a real possibility that Mr Wang's condition may deteriorate, so the need to ensure he was clinically assessed by a medical officer before he left the hospital was obviously the expected standard of care he should have received.

Finally, it is difficult to argue with the proposition as stated by the judge that the registered nurse should have strongly advised and counselled Mr Wang against leaving the hospital before being examined. A competent registered nurse working in the triage area of accident and emergency is there specifically to prioritise patient care based on a scale of seriousness. A patient with a history of traumatic head injury should have been high on the nurse's priority list to be seen as quickly as possible.

CASE EXAMPLE 7.5

McCabe v Auburn District Hospital[40]

Highlights issues for nurses in the recording and reporting of observations following surgery as well as the problem of reliance on verbal handover to the exclusion of the written reports and observations, including a failure to notify a medical officer of abnormal pathology results.

FACTS

Mr McCabe was a 21-year-old man admitted to hospital for an emergency appendicectomy. Postoperatively he did not make the expected uneventful recovery. He could not keep food or fluids down, he developed diarrhoea and a spiking temperature pattern, and he complained of excessive abdominal pain. A chest X-ray and a microurine were ordered and proved negative.

On the morning of the fifth postoperative day, which was a Saturday, the registrar was doing his rounds prior to going off duty but remaining on call at home over the weekend. The patient was still

McCabe v Auburn District Hospital (Continued)

exhibiting the same symptoms. The registrar ordered a full blood count to be done that morning. The blood was taken and the result returned to the ward that afternoon after the registrar had left the hospital. The result disclosed a significantly raised white cell count and other abnormal readings indicative of some form of severe infection. The registered nurse on duty filed the pathology result in the appropriate place in the patient's record and did not attempt to contact the registrar. Likewise, at no time during the weekend did the registrar ring the ward to ascertain Mr McCabe's results. None of the other registered nurses who came on duty that weekend noticed the pathology result.

Not only were the nursing reports written separately from the medical officers, but also the nursing staff members who came and went over the weekend relied on the verbal handover report received at the commencement of each shift.

The result did not come to light until Monday afternoon when the patient's condition was considerably worse. The patient was immediately placed on IV antibiotics and was subsequently returned to theatre for an exploratory operation and found to have widespread peritonitis. He died a few days later after succumbing to renal failure.

Comment and Relevant Considerations Relating to McCabe v Auburn District Hospital

The young man's mother sued the hospital and its staff for negligence in the care of her son and sought compensation for loss of income dependence as well as nervous shock. Based on the facts as outlined above, and the evidence presented, the judge upheld Mrs McCabe's claim against the hospital and its staff. The hospital acknowledged their vicarious liability for the actions of its medical and nursing staff at the outset of the case.

In arriving at his conclusion of negligence by the hospital and its staff, the judge saw fit to criticise the accuracy and reliability of the medical and nursing notes particularly regarding evidence given by other patients and Mr McCabe's friends and relatives as to

his deteriorating condition. The following extracts on this issue appear in his Honour's judgment:

I am of the view that the hospital notes are not, in the current case, reliable. In particular there is unreliability in recording the manifest and observable continuing deterioration of the deceased's condition. I am satisfied that the routine temperature checks even if accurate as to scale were accompanied by failure to note what was there to be seen, namely that the deceased was perspirant and 'hot'. This was evident even to non-medical appreciation … I do conclude … that there were things significant in assessing the patient's deterioration which were overlooked and the written record simply does not truly reflect the currency of events.[41]

And further:

It follows that the ability of the (medical staff) to perceive the deterioration in the patient's condition was inhibited by the inadequacy of the clinical and nursing notes.[42]

And again:

It would be apparent from my earlier findings and remarks that I conclude that the clinical and nursing notes were deficient. Their inadequacy must have been a major factor in bringing about a situation which allowed the patient's condition to deteriorate fatally without timely remedial treatment.[43] [emphasis added]

The comments and findings by the judge are sobering and emphasise the standard the law would expect of nursing staff in the accurate and timely recording of a patient's observations and overall clinical condition as well as notifying the relevant medical officer when a patient's observations are abnormal. It also demonstrates the catastrophic outcome that can result when such observations are simply recorded by nursing staff and not escalated when the patient's clinical condition clearly warrants it. Given the circumstances in this particular matter, a rise in temperature and pulse rate would clearly be of clinical significance and warrant reporting to the medical officer concerned as well as recording the action taken.

Also, in our view, the sequence of events that arose in the care of Mr McCabe raises the important question of whether the standard of care expected of the competent registered nurse in the performance of his or her duties would extend to notifying the medical officer of abnormal pathology results, or indeed of any pathology results. The answer, as always in such a situation, would depend on the facts and circumstances, supported or otherwise by expert opinion from professional nursing peers as well as any relevant policy or procedural directives in place in the hospital or health service.

There is no doubt that registered nursing staff in particular, as part of their study of normal and abnormal pathology, are familiar with a wide range of commonly used clinical and biochemical indicators of the abnormal. In the more highly complex and technical areas of medicine that would not necessarily be so. However, in this incident, it would, we suggest, be readily conceded that a competent registered nurse would recognise an abnormal white cell count and appreciate its significance, to the extent that it was probably indicative of some type of severe infection and, in the circumstances, would have contacted the relevant medical officer immediately.

The fact that a pathology result is abnormal does not of itself signify the necessity for somebody to be contacted immediately, as many patients in hospital will routinely show abnormal pathology results as part of their disease process.

What is significant in considering this issue is the reason why, and the circumstances in which, a particular pathology test is ordered. In the normal situation, pathology tests are ordered as deemed necessary by the patient's medical practitioner, and the results of such tests are returned to the medical practitioner. In hospitals, pathology results are routinely screened on a Monday-to-Friday basis by the medical officers concerned, as they are returned. On weekends or night duty, when medical officers are rostered on call for emergencies only, it is not uncommon for them to be contacted by nursing staff to relay abnormal pathology results following tests that have been ordered to be done during the night or on weekends for a variety of reasons. As a consequence of the pathology result, it may be necessary for the medical officer to initiate treatment and/or medication or make a change to the patient's treatment and/or medication. In such a situation it would be difficult for a competent registered nurse to argue that the standard of care expected of them did not extend to notifying the medical officer concerned of pathology results that the nurse knew to be abnormal, when they knew the medical officer would otherwise not receive them for some time, and when the tests had been ordered to be taken at a time when the medical officer would not normally be present to receive the result.

As indicated earlier, each situation would be determined on its own particular facts and circumstances, but if a nurse is faced with such a situation, any doubts should be resolved by notifying the result to the relevant medical officer. Obviously, notifying the result should be accompanied by an entry to that effect in the patient's record.

In hospitals, procedural guidelines may assist in resolving the majority of problems that arise in this type of situation.

CASE EXAMPLE 7.6

Norton v Argonaut Insurance Company[44]

Highlights issues arising in the administration of medication generally and paediatrics in particular.

FACTS

A 3-month-old infant was admitted to the paediatric ward of a hospital for investigation and treatment for congenital heart disease. On admission his medical practitioner wrote the following medication order on the patient's medication sheet:

Elixir Paediatric Lanoxin 2.5 cc

[0.125 mg] 6qh × 3 then once daily.

The child remained an inpatient for a couple of weeks and received the medication of Paediatric Lanoxin elixir as ordered.

Norton v Argonaut Insurance Company (Continued)

One day, the medical practitioner examined the child and changed the medication order for the Lanoxin to one dose only and he wrote the change of order in the patient's record as follows:

Give 3.0 cc Lanoxin today for 1 dose only.

On the day on which the order was changed, the paediatric ward was particularly busy, with only one registered nurse and one enrolled nurse on duty. Another registered nurse, Mrs Evans, was available and part of her responsibilities required her to provide assistance to ward staff when necessary. On this particular day, she went to the paediatric ward to assist and while checking the patient's records she noticed the change of order for 3 cc of Lanoxin, in which the form of medication or route of administration had not been specified. The medication had not been given, so she decided to administer it herself. Although a registered nurse for many years, she had been out of clinical nursing for some time and she was unaware that Lanoxin was manufactured in elixir form as well as injectable form. Recognising that 3 cc was a large dose to be given intramuscularly, Mrs Evans did consult two other doctors who were present in the ward at the time about the medical practitioner's order. They were unable to assist and they advised that she should follow the written instructions. At no time did she contact the child's doctor. She then made a decision to give the child 3 cc of intramuscular Lanoxin, which was five times the strength of the paediatric elixir. A little over 1 hour after receiving the injection the child died.

The child's parents brought an action against the hospital and the doctor for negligence. The court determined that the doctor was negligent for writing an unclear medication order. The court also found that Mrs Evans failed to meet the standard of care required of a registered nurse and said:

As laudable as her instructions are conceded to have been on the occasion in question, her unfamiliarity with the drug was a contributing factor in the child's death. In this regard we are of the opinion that she was negligent in attempting to administer a drug with which she was not familiar … Not only was Mrs Evans unfamiliar with the medicine in question but she also violated what has been shown to be the rule generally practised by the members of the nursing profession in the community … namely, the practice of calling the prescribing physician when in doubt about an order for medication.[45]

Comment and Relevant Considerations Relating to Norton v Argonaut Insurance Company

The lesson to be learned from this case is that any nurse or midwife who is uncertain about a medication order must take all reasonable steps to contact the prescribing doctor for clarification. If a reasonable effort fails to locate the prescribing doctor, the nurse or midwife should seek the assistance of a person able to assist or give appropriate directions; for example, a clinical manager, supervisor, another doctor familiar with the patient or an administrator able to obtain the assistance of another doctor.

In hospitals with pharmacies, the pharmacist may be able to help a nurse or midwife resolve conflicts over drug dosages. However, such an avenue should be pursued only when all efforts to locate the patient's medical practitioner have failed.

Under no circumstances should a registered nurse or midwife administer a medication to a patient if:

- they are unsure about the drug to be given, its dosage and mode of administration;
- it is unclear whether the patient is allergic to the drug about to be administered;
- based on their own knowledge about the drug and the patient's condition, they may consider the medication is contraindicated.

If in doubt, question and clarify.

To overcome difficulties of this kind, hospitals and health services should have very clear guidelines as to what steps staff should take to clarify a medication order if the patient's prescribing practitioner cannot be contacted within a reasonable time.

The professional and legal responsibilities of a nurse or midwife in dealing with the administration of medications are dealt with in more detail in **Chapter 8**.

Ison v Northern Rivers Area Health Service[46]

Highlights issues relating to advising and informing patients of test results when engaged as a community-based clinical nurse consultant.

FACTS

A registered nurse was employed as a clinical nurse consultant in women's health.

Her major responsibility was to take Pap smears from patients who attended the clinics she conducted, forward those smears to the pathology department in Sydney, receive the results back and notify the clients of those results. It was also her responsibility to maintain various medical records in relation to those activities including the Pap Smear Register.

As a result of a complaint made by a client an investigation revealed that there were 18 different cases where the registered nurse had failed to notify clients of Pap smear results where that notification should have been made. There were a further five cases where there was a failure to notify particular clients of the need to attend for a re-smear because of some uncertainty in the original Pap smear result, and there were additionally 20 files that had been randomly extracted by the employer that demonstrated poor documentation of clients' medical records kept by the registered nurse which was part of her responsibilities.

As a result of all of those matters and a general dissatisfaction her performance as a clinical nurse consultant in women's health, she was dismissed from her employment. She disputed that decision and sought her reinstatement before the Industrial Relations Court of Australia. She was unsuccessful in that application on the basis that she had been treated fairly in the way in which her employer had gone about investigating the complaints made about her work and then procedurally dealing with those matters as well as giving her the opportunity to respond to the allegations.

At the outset it should be said that the registered nurse did not, by and large, dispute the nature of the complaints made against her as detailed above. Instead she raised in her defence the fact that she found herself, as she perceived it, operating in circumstances where she needed additional assistance to help her do her job and that she was doing the best she could in all the circumstances. The court did not support that view and made a number of findings relevant to the question of the standard of care that would have and should have been expected of her in her position.

It was conceded on behalf of the registered nurse that the status of clinical nurse consultant is the highest rank a nurse practitioner could achieve in clinical nursing at that time, requiring as it did an advanced level of nursing practice involving a senior level of knowledge, initiative, responsibility and accountability. There was evidence that as a women's health clinical nurse consultant, the nurse operated in an autonomous fashion as a sole practitioner in the field of women's health in her geographical area.

It was stated by her that when she first commenced in the position, in relation to the taking of Pap smears between 1987 until 1994, she advised her clients in the following terms:

If you don't hear from me regarding your Pap smear result, everything is okay. If I need to contact you about your Pap smear for reassessing it to be unsatisfactory, I will do so by telephone or letter. The results will take 3 or 4 weeks to return to me.[47]

It would seem that from 1994 onwards, as a result of some procedural changes concerning both the categorisation of Pap smear results and the steps to be taken in notifying those results, the nurse advised her clients in words to the effect of:

I will contact you by letter if your Pap smear is fine. If not I will be contacting you by phone.[48]

While that may well have been the intention, she did not observe that procedural standard and also failed to properly maintain her clinical records. For example, one of the clients who attended at her clinic told the court that she first attended the Women's Health Clinic in April 1994 when the nurse had performed a Pap smear. At that time the client had taken with her a letter from her gynaecologist outlining her previous history that stated, relevantly, that she had been treated in 1993 for a CIN lesion of the cervix using radical diathermy and advising that any recurrence of abnormal smears would need to be investigated by colposcopy.

Ison v Northern Rivers Area Health Service (Continued)

This client told the court that, at the time she attended the clinic, the nurse had told her that she would be notified 'either way' of her Pap smear results if there was something abnormal or that she would get a letter in the mail. The client heard nothing despite making both verbal and telephone inquiries in 1994 and 1995. Indeed the client attended the clinic in June 1995 for a further Pap smear consultation and when she inquired as to her last Pap smear results she was told by the nurse that 'it was fine'. Again the client was told that the same procedure would apply — that is, if there was a problem, the nurse would contact her personally and that otherwise notification would be by letter.

The client heard nothing until she was contacted by another nurse in July 1996 advising her that her Pap smear result had come back showing inflammation and suggesting that she should see a gynaecologist. Further inquiries by the client at that time via her GP alerted her to the fact that there had been a problem with the result of her 1994 smear. As the court heard:

> ... [the client] was horrified at what she had learned and promptly visited her own gynaecologist and had treatment ... she was extremely emotional and was of the opinion that 'she was going to die'.[49]

That particular client's experiences and the failure to notify her of her Pap smear results became the initial complaint against the nurse. Evidence was given that the client had commenced civil litigation against the Area Health Service relying on the negligence of the nurse as their employee; it was disclosed during the course of the hearing that the civil litigation had been settled in favour of the client.

When the extent and scale of the nurse's failure to record and properly advise clients of Pap smear results became evident, and when proper investigations had been undertaken by her employer, her services were terminated and she was not reinstated by the court.

Comment and Relevant Considerations Relating to Ison v Northern Rivers Area Health Service

In the hearing to consider her application for reinstatement, and considering all the evidence as to the actions of the nurse in her position as a clinical nurse consultant in women's health, the court had this to say:

> *Having considered the protocols in place at the time ... it is a finding of this court that the applicant would have been more than aware of her direct and personal responsibility to both maintain correct and current medical records, and to notify women clients of health threatening pap smear results. Further, that obligation fell directly to her. The evidence shows that in addition to not following the set protocols, on occasion, the applicant failed to follow her own methodology regarding notification procedures. Mr Schofield described a sole practitioner as one who works unaided, without the assistance of another medical officer along side. It is my view that implicit in that definition is the understanding that the sole practitioner would be capable of applying all relevant regulations and requirements pertaining to that particular profession,*

> *and in that regard the applicant should have been capable of maintaining a correct filing system, with due attention paid to the correct recording of pathology results. The evidence did not bear that out. The court heard evidence of files entitled 'lost files', 'lost reports' and 'to contact', illustrating a less than professional approach to the serious responsibility personal to her.[50]*

On the issue of whether the nurse had sufficient resources and facilities to enable her to do her job according to the standard expected, the court found:

> *Ms Ison had access to sufficient facilities to enable a better standard of client notification be maintained than the one she in fact maintained during the course of her employment. A review was conducted by her employer of a large sample of files. No evidence was produced indicating other women's health nurses failed as Ms Ison did to meet the standards set in the various protocols.[51]*

In short, the court said:

> *... the actions of Ms Ison did not fall solely into the category of 'errors of judgment' but neglect of duty*

on several occasions which potentially could be life threatening to the women patients and accordingly it is the finding of this court that the employer did have a valid reason to terminate Ms Ison.[52]

Once again, it was the nurse's failure to maintain the clinical protocols as documented by her employer that was a critical factor in the court's decision not to reinstate her to her position as clinical nurse consultant. Also, the nurse complained to the court of inadequate resources and facilities as a major reason for her failure to follow the expected clinical protocols to record test results and notify clients of those results. The court found there was no evidence to support this contention. If she had considered she was not sufficiently resourced to enable her to do her job in accordance with her employer's expected protocols, it would be expected that she would have put such concerns in writing and followed through to ensure her employer was properly considering her request for assistance. The clear risk to her clients arising from a failure to notify them of significant test results would demand that she maintain a high standard of record-keeping and prompt notification of test results.

CASE EXAMPLE 7.8

Langley v Glandore Pty Ltd[53]

Highlights issues relating to the standard expected of operating room nurses with specific reference to recognised special interest professional practice standards (Australian Council of Operating Room Nurses).

FACTS

The background to this matter concerns a woman who was operated on for an abdominal hysterectomy. After the operation, it became apparent, as a result of certain symptoms suffered by the woman, that a surgical sponge had been left inside her abdomen. She was required to undergo a further operation some 10 months after the first operation to have that sponge removed. The woman sued the doctor who performed the operation as well as his assistant, and also sued the company Glandore Pty Ltd. That company owned the private hospital where the operation was performed and was also the employer of the nursing staff who assisted at the operation.

When the matter came for hearing in the first instance, it was heard before a judge with a jury. Juries

CASE EXAMPLE 7.8

Langley v Glandore Pty Ltd (Continued)

in civil actions are rare. However, in this case a jury was present, and it was their task after they had heard all the evidence to determine who, of all the parties sued by the woman, had been negligent in leaving the sponge in her abdomen. The jury found that the doctor and his assistant had been negligent and that the nursing staff, as far as their responsibility for checking and counting sponges, had not been negligent.

The two doctors who had been found negligent believed that the decision of the jury was contrary to all the evidence that had been given, particularly in relation to the nurses' responsibility for checking and counting sponges. They argued that the jury verdict was perverse, unreasonable and contrary to all the evidence presented to the court. The two doctors appealed against the decision, arguing that the employer of the nurses, Glandore Pty Ltd, should be made vicariously liable for the negligent actions of the nurses in the matter. While the appeal court agreed that the surgeon had been negligent, they also found that the nurses involved in counting and checking the sponges had been negligent, which meant their employer was vicariously liable for their negligence.

Comment and Relevant Considerations Relating to Langley v Glandore Pty Ltd

In this case, the appeal court found that Dr Langley, as the main surgeon in the case, had been negligent in failing to retrieve the sponge at the conclusion of the operation and failing to identify from the plaintiff's continuing symptoms that a foreign object had been left inside her body. However, the court did not accept that he should bear the full and total responsibility for what was clearly the responsibility of the nurses during the operation — that is, the proper recording of and accounting for the sponges used. Accordingly, the court overturned the decision of the jury because they said that the evidence 'in its totality preponderates so strongly against the conclusion favoured by the jury that it can be said that the verdict is such as reasonable jurors could not reach'.[54] In coming to that decision the court said:

At the trial it was not in contest that it was as a result of negligence on the part of one or

*other of those involved in the operation, that the
sponge had been left inside the patient's body,
and it was not in contest and it could hardly
have been contested that an incorrect count had
been made by the nurses ... the nurses clearly,
under the procedure described, had the primary
responsibility for making an accurate count to
ensure that all of the sponges used had been
recovered from the plaintiff's body ...*

*The relevant established standard for 'counting
of sponges, swabs, instruments and needles' is
called the 'ACORN' standard and it supports the
description of the duties that has been outlined
above ... At the trial, Nurse Kirvisneimi accepted
that she and her fellow nurse had made a counting
error and she was unable to suggest how it had
occurred. None of the witnesses had a recollection
of anything untoward occurring in the course of
the operation.*[55]

A suggestion made in the course of the initial hearing
before the judge and jury was that an emergency may
have arisen that could have justifiably distracted the
nurses from their counting duties. But as the court found,
there was no support for this in the evidence. As the
court stated:

*... if some emergency, of which there was no
evidence, had called for an urgent supply of
sponges, the nurses were not relieved of the duty
of maintaining an accurate count. It was accepted
that if their count was interrupted, they were to
recommence it at the point where they had left it.*[56]

The appeal court found that the nurses had been
negligent in that they:

*... failed to identify the fact that an abdominal pack
had been left inside the plaintiff at the conclusion of
the surgery.*[57]

As a result of that finding, the appeal court allocated
a proportion of the damages awarded to the patient to
be paid by the nurses' employer.

Another matter involving a similar scenario was
dealt with by the courts in the case of *Elliott v Bickerstaff.*[58] The case involved a sponge left inside a patient
following a hysterectomy and colo-suspension. At the

initial trial of the matter, the judge said that while the
surgeon, Dr Elliott, had not been personally negligent,
he should be held liable for the negligent act of leaving
the sponge in the patient because he was responsible
for the overall care of the patient and he could not delegate that responsibility to the nursing staff. Dr Elliott
appealed that outcome arguing he was not liable for
the negligent actions of the nursing staff in the checking and counting of sponges and was entitled to rely
on them when they told him the count was correct. He
gave evidence as to his usual routine practices during
surgery including where he required confirmation
from the theatre nurse that all instruments, swabs and
sponges were accounted for.

The court accepted Dr Elliott's evidence as to
his usual practice as being correct and upheld his
appeal. In doing say, the appeal court said that
Dr Elliott:

*... did not undertake the provision of nursing
services before or after the operation; they were to be
provided by the hospital.*[59]

Accordingly, the appeal court found:

*... [Dr Elliott] was entitled to rely on the theatre
staff in the customary way, and on the evidence
in this case I do not think that his duty of care
relevantly extended beyond feeling for sponges in the
abdominal cavity and asking whether the sponge
count was satisfactory. It follows that in my opinion,
Dr Elliott was not in breach of a non-delegable duty
of care by reason of the negligence of the theatre
staff ... He should be able to concentrate on his own
skilled task without shouldering the responsibilities
of other members of the team.*[60]

Both cases highlight the independent professional
responsibility of nurses and midwives to maintain
their clinical standards notwithstanding they may
be working in a team environment. It cannot be
expected, as a general proposition, that a medical officer be professionally and therefore legally responsible for ensuring that the clinical standards of the
nurse or midwife working alongside him or her are
in accordance with accepted professional nursing or
midwifery practice standards. As always it would depend on the facts and circumstances of the situation
under review.

Coroner's Inquest into the Death of Samara Lea Hoy[61]

Highlights issues relating to the role of a midwife caring for a patient in labour, including monitoring and recording of the fetal heart rate and the accuracy of clinical observations recorded.

FACTS

The child, Samara Lea Hoy, was delivered by Ventouse extraction after a prolonged second-stage labour and died shortly after birth. Because of the circumstances surrounding the death of the child, it was a 'reportable death' and a coroner's inquest was necessary.

During her pregnancy, Mrs Hoy had been managed by her obstetrician, Dr Trueman. Her pregnancy was largely uneventful and, according to the evidence given at the inquest, 'Mrs Hoy did not discuss with Dr Trueman the question of assisted birth or intervention'. She did attend antenatal classes facilitated by one of the midwives where natural birth was emphasised as the preferred method of delivery.

Mrs Hoy presented at the hospital at 6.15 pm in established labour. It was a weekend. Dr Trueman was not on call and his patients were being cared for that weekend by Dr Doolabh. Prior to that day Dr Doolabh had never met Mrs Hoy. He did see Mrs Hoy at about 7.00 pm shortly after her admission to the hospital and then left to go home and be on call as required.

On admission, Midwife Fennell undertook a baseline CTG for 'less than five minutes'. This was in breach of the hospital's policy dealing with 'Assessment and management of first stage of labour', which required the admitting midwife to obtain a baseline CTG observation for a minimum of 10 minutes. Also, during the inquest, Midwife Fennell and the midwife in charge at the time, agreed that a period of 20 minutes or more was required to obtain a good 'reassuring' CTG trace. There was some evidence that Mrs Hoy was not comfortable with the CTG monitor and it was removed shortly after her admission. On that point, according to the coroner:

> Mrs Hoy said in her evidence that she was not encouraged to continue with the CTG. I am prepared to accept Mrs Hoy's evidence that she was not told

the CTG was necessary for the welfare of the baby. Midwife Fennell failed to record Mrs Hoy's refusal to continue with the CTG.

> I find that if it had been explained to Mrs Hoy that a CTG was necessary to assess the ongoing welfare of her baby, she would have had no hesitation of [sic] accepting any discomfort of the CTG and adopted the procedure.[62]

The clinical guidelines adopted by the hospital required CTG monitoring to be undertaken in the presence of certain risk factors.

The partogram completed by Midwife Peller during the evening indicated a rising baseline in the baby's fetal heart rate from the time of Mrs Hoy's admission from 125 bpm at 6.30 pm to 140 bpm at 9.30 pm and 150 bpm at 10.00 pm. Despite that, no steps were taken by the midwives to undertake continuous CTG monitoring although the monitor was readily available in the labour ward and despite the midwives attending to Mrs Hoy that evening agreeing, at the inquest, that fetal tachycardia was one of the indicators that triggered the need for continuous CTG monitoring.

At 10.30 pm, Midwife Fankhauser took over the care of Mrs Hoy. No fetal heart rate monitoring had been undertaken between 10.00 pm and 10.30 pm. At 10.30 pm Midwife Fankhauser was aware that Mrs Hoy was fully dilated and in the second stage of labour. The fetal heart rate was noted to be 170 bpm. Midwife Fankhauser noted that recording on the second-stage document but charted the fetal heart rate at less than 145 bpm on the partogram. No other fetal heart rate recordings were charted after that time despite the hospital's policy requiring this to be done. In considering Midwife Fankhauser's actions at this point, the coroner said:

> The foetal heart rate, as recorded by Midwife Fankhauser at 10.30 pm, when noted against the rising base line on the partogram graph, indicated a clear need to undertake continuous CTG monitoring and inform the obstetrician. This was not done. The assessment and management of second-stage labour policy required a continuous CTG to be undertaken in cases of foetal heart recordings above 160 bpm.

Coroner's Inquest into the Death of Samara Lea Hoy (Continued)

Midwife Fankhauser failed to do this ... [and] failed to follow the normal labour/use of partogram policy. She failed to accurately record the foetal heart rate recordings taken at 10.30 pm or thereafter record the foetal heart rate measurements as required.[63]

The coroner further commented on Midwife Fankhauser's actions that evening as follows:

Another cause for concern was Mrs Hoy's slow progress. This gave another reason for continuous CTG. Given ... that Mrs Hoy had no sign of progress after one hour in the second stage, and the policy of the hospital dictated that the obstetrician should be called in such cases; given the rising foetal heart rate trend as recorded on the partogram and witnessed by Fankhauser, there could be no other conclusion that a continuous CTG monitoring should have been undertaken at 11.30 pm or prior. The above facts cause me to conclude Midwife Fankhauser was derelict in her duty as a midwife. At about midnight, Midwife Fankhauser noted the presence of meconium. This is a sign of foetal distress and again warranted the use of a continuous CTG in accordance with the hospital policy ... There was a systemic break

down in the managing of Mrs Hoy's labour ... Failure to adequately monitor the foetal heart rate was more than likely a cause of death for baby Samara. Had CTG monitoring been utilised and the partogram completed, as required, in all probability intervention may have resulted in the safe delivery of Samara.[64]

The professional failures of Midwife Fankhauser in particular were compounded by the actions of Dr Doolabh when he was finally called at midnight. He attended the hospital at approximately 12.15 am. He did not undertake any vaginal examination of Mrs Hoy, who by this time had been in second-stage labour for 2 hours without progress. According to the evidence, Dr Doolabh adopted a 'wait and see' approach with no CTG monitoring and did not attempt to deliver the baby until 1.40 am. He did so with some difficulty by Ventouse extraction at 1.45 am. At birth, the umbilical cord was wrapped tightly around the baby's neck and she was covered with thick meconium. She was pale and hypotonic, her fetal heart rate had dropped to 40 bpm and she had no spontaneous respiration. Resuscitation was attempted but was unsuccessful.

Comment and Relevant Considerations Relating to the Death of Samara Lea Hoy

The coroner determined the manner and cause of the baby's death as being birth asphyxia due to a tight umbilical cord around the baby's neck. In making that finding, the coroner was scathing in his criticism of the midwifery staff, and Midwife Fankhauser in particular, as well as Dr Doolabh. He found as follows:

- Mrs Hoy was not adequately monitored during labour; in particular, there was a failure to commence continuous CTG monitoring much earlier than was done.
- The maintenance of medical records was 'woefully inadequate'. Information which was required to be recorded was not, and recordings of the fetal heart rate were not made as required and in accordance with hospital policy.

- There was a delay in calling Dr Doolabh. He should have been called at 10.30 pm.
- The delay in calling Dr Doolabh when signs of fetal distress were evident and when a delivery would have been made much earlier 'did contribute to the death of baby Samara'.
- Dr Doolabh's response when he was called was inadequate and, as said by his own peers, substandard.

With particular reference to Midwife Fankhauser, the coroner said:

Midwife Fankhauser's management of Mrs Foy's labour was inadequate ... there is a sufficient body of evidence to warrant her conduct be reviewed ... [and] which might cause a disciplinary body to conclude that she failed to provide Mrs Hoy with an adequate standard of care. The disciplinary board could also conclude that any attempt by Midwife Fankhauser to deliberately alter the records and in turn mislead the Court indicates that she is not a fit and proper person to be registered. Accordingly, I direct the material gathered during these proceedings be referred to the Nursing and Midwifery Board of Australia for its consideration.[65]

In addition to referring Midwife Fankhauser's actions to the registration authority, the coroner further considered the actions of Midwife Fankhauser in deliberately altering the patient's labour progress notes. During the inquest, Midwife Fankhauser admitted that a record of observations initially recorded by her as being taken at 10.30 pm were altered by her some 6 hours after the child's death to make it appear that the observations were taken at 11.30 pm. On that issue, the coroner referred Midwife Fankhauser's actions to the Director of Public Prosecutions (DPP) in Queensland for consideration as to whether she should be charged with the criminal offence of perverting the course of justice.

The actions of Dr Doolabh in the care of Mrs Hoy were also referred to his professional registration body, the Medical Board of Australia.

This case demonstrates very clearly how hospital or health service policies in relation to the delivery of care are not documents that can, or should, be ignored by staff. For example, you will have read in the facts of the case that the hospital's written policy for the Assessment and management of first stage of labour required the admitting midwife to obtain a baseline CTG observation for a minimum of 10 minutes. In Mrs Hoy's case, the admitting midwife undertook the baseline observation 'for less than 5 minutes'. Also, the midwife caring for Mrs Hoy during her labour did not observe the hospital's policy regarding the need to maintain continuous CTG monitoring.

The written policies and clinical protocols of a health service will always be considered by a court as setting the minimum standard of care expected of their employees. In that sense they are not aspirational documents. They are there for a good reason and invariably, when the care of a patient is being carefully scrutinised by a court, the policy and procedural documents

relevant to the patient's care as well as relevant professional standards documents will be subpoenaed. Those documents will then be compared against the patient's records, including observation records, to determine whether the care actually delivered to the patient was in accordance with them. Any omission, without a reasonable explanation, will be relied upon by the plaintiff's lawyers as evidence of an inadequate standard of care and therefore a breach of the duty of care owed to the patient.

CASE EXAMPLE 7.10

Coroner's Inquest into the Death of Bodhi Eastlake-McClure[66]

Highlights issues relating to standards expected of independent homebirth midwives with reference to professional practice standards (Australian College of Midwives).

FACTS

This inquest followed the death of a newborn infant shortly after delivery by caesarean section. The mother, Ms McClure, had been under the care of Ms Sheldrick, an independent midwife. She went into labour early when she notified Midwife Sheldrick that her membranes had ruptured and advised there had also been 'some meconium'.

When Midwife Sheldrick first examined Ms McClure later that day at about 9.30 am, the baby was in the breech position. Midwife Sheldrick remained with Ms McClure all that day and into the night and regularly monitored her blood pressure and the fetal heart rate. Both were within normal limits.

By 9.00 am the next day Ms McClure was still in labour, some 5–6 cm dilated, and the baby was still in the breech position. The decision was made to transfer Ms McClure to the local Base Hospital. Midwife Sheldrick drove Ms McClure to the hospital and, because she could not sit comfortably, she lay down in the back seat of Midwife Sheldrick's car.

Following Ms McClure's admission to hospital she was examined by the consultant obstetrician. The baby remained in the breech position but there was no evidence of meconium at that time. After discussions with Ms McClure and her partner Mr Eastlake, a decision was made for continuous CTG monitoring and an epidural.

Coroner's Inquest into the Death of Bodhi Eastlake-McClure (Continued)

Ms McClure continued to be monitored throughout the day of her admission. At about 3.40 pm the CTG showed that the fetal heart rate may be of concern but the rate settled.

At 5.15 pm that day Ms McClure was making little progress in labour and she was 7 cm dilated. A decision was made to deliver the baby by caesarean section.

Shortly after 6.02 pm the CTG showed a rapid fetal heart rate deceleration and a stat dose of ephedrine was administered and the fetal heart rate returned to normal.

The child Bodhi was delivered by caesarean section at 7.50 pm covered in a thick layer of meconium. Resuscitation was commenced but Bodhi's oxygen saturation and heart rate gradually declined despite cardiac compression and two doses of IV adrenaline. He died at around 9.00 pm.

Comment and Relevant Considerations Relating to the Coroner's Inquest into the Death of Bodhi Eastlake-McClure

In determining the manner and cause of death of the child, the coroner examined a number of questions[67] specifically directed at the actions of Midwife Sheldrick in the care and treatment she gave to Ms McClure. Those questions were:

- Did Ms McClure receive appropriate antenatal care from Midwife Sheldrick?
- Once the baby was found to be in the breech position, should Midwife Sheldrick have encouraged alternative arrangements for the care and delivery of the baby?
- Did Ms McClure receive appropriate advice and treatment from Midwife Sheldrick, including with respect to her transfer to the Base Hospital?

Expert opinion evidence was received from an experienced midwife in relation to the care given to Ms McClure by Midwife Sheldrick. That evidence pointed to a number of actions that Midwife Sheldrick had failed to do during Ms McClure's antenatal period:

- There was no evidence Midwife Sheldrick had advised Ms McClure to have an ultrasound after

20 weeks and in particular once the baby had been discovered to be in the breech position at 33 weeks.
- There was no evidence that Midwife Sheldrick discussed with Ms McClure about consulting an obstetrician in relation to the breech presentation and the possibility of external cephalic version (ECV).
- There was no evidence that Midwife Sheldrick had consulted the Australian College of Midwives *Guidelines for consultation and referral* (ACM Guidelines) to assist her in her clinical decision-making in relation to the care of Ms McClure.

The coroner was extremely critical of Midwife Sheldrick's evidence as to her knowledge of the above-mentioned ACM Guidelines. He stated as follows:

The most disturbing aspect of Ms Sheldrick's evidence was that she frankly admitted not only that she had not followed the guidelines but that, at the time she was caring for Ms McClure and her baby, she was unaware of the existence of the guidelines. Given that the guidelines constitute the midwifery profession's latest thinking on best practice and are the foundational document for practice as a midwife in Australia, this was an astonishing oversight by Ms Sheldrick. The guidelines were first published in 2004. It is difficult to understand how a professional person can remain ignorant of the best practice guidelines published by his or her peak professional body for 8 years if she or he is undertaking appropriate continuing professional development and generally paying attention to the evolution of best practice in that profession.[68] *[emphasis added]*

The above comments emphasise the evidentiary weight that a court will attach to professional standards documents when determining the appropriate standard of care in a given clinical situation.

The coroner was also very clear as to what Midwife Sheldrick should have done, which was to make alternative arrangements for the baby's care and delivery once the breech presentation was confirmed. Again, he referred to the ACM Guidelines, where it states that 'a breech presentation indicates that a midwife should advise a woman that her care should be transferred to an obstetrician for more specialised care' and that 'the midwife may remain involved in providing midwifery services in collaboration with the obstetrician and other clinicians'. Also, the coroner emphasised, the ACM Guidelines provide, with a breech presentation, 'the mother be referred to an obstetrician for ECV at 35 weeks … an obstetrician would have been able to advise the parents concerning the possibility of attempting external cephalic version'.

Given Ms McClure's breech presentation, the coroner stated what Midwife Sheldrick should have done in the following terms:

> It follows that rather than leaving Ms McClure without the advice she needed to make appropriate decisions, Ms Sheldrick ought to have given her a strong recommendation that Ms McClure should see an obstetrician and she should have arranged that referral herself or advised Ms McClure to get her GP to do so.
>
> Once the breech birth had been diagnosed, Ms Sheldrick was obliged as a professional midwife to advise Ms McClure and Mr Eastlake that a birth of a breech baby should be carried out only in a hospital setting with appropriate obstetric care. She should have warned them in strong terms of the serious risk to the baby if they did not accept this advice. She should have made it her very strong recommendation that a breech birth not proceed at home.[69]

Relying on the ACM Guidelines, the coroner found Midwife Sheldrick had failed to provide Ms McClure with proper advice and treatment before her labour began and then 'compounded her error at the onset of labour by failing to advise and, indeed, insisting Ms McClure go to hospital without delay'.

The coroner found that Midwife Sheldrick was deficient in her management of Ms McClure's labour by:

- failing to prepare properly for a breech homebirth;
- allowing the delivery to drag on for a very long time, causing Ms McClure to become exhausted;
- driving Ms McClure to hospital — a journey of about half an hour — in her own car with

Ms McClure lying on the back seat without a seatbelt on;
- failing to ensure that an ambulance was organised to come if necessary;
- failing to warn the hospital of the homebirth and the possible need for urgent intervention in the event of complications arising;
- giving the hospital minimal time to prepare for the arrival of a breech delivery.

Midwife Sheldrick gave evidence that she had assisted in two successful breech births in a home setting and had undertaken some training with an American midwife. The coroner found that 'these experiences gave Midwife Sheldrick a false sense of confidence in her ability to manage Bodhi's delivery skilfully and safely'. He concluded:

> The reality was that she had not the expertise, the support nor the instruments to ensure a safe breech birth at home. As well meaning as Midwife Sheldrick's approach may have been, it was naïve and imprudent as well as unprofessional.[70]

The coroner found that the child had died as a result of meconium aspiration syndrome resulting from undiagnosed fetal distress that had occurred during the unsuccessful homebirth. He concluded that the baby's best chance of survival, given the breech presentation and the presence of meconium in the early stage of labour, was in hospital 'where it may have been detected and timely surgical intervention could have been initiated'. He again cited the ACM Guidelines that, he said, laid such emphasis on cases such as Ms McClure 'being referred to specialist obstetricians for advice and management and why the failure to refer to and comply with the guidelines was such poor midwifery practice on Midwife Sheldrick's part'.

The coroner further concluded that it was not possible to attribute the child's death 'directly or even indirectly' to Midwife Sheldrick's omissions, 'but neither can that possibility be discounted'. He referred his findings to the NSW Health Care Complaints Commission 'for its consideration of a formal complaint against Midwife Sheldrick'.

Coroner's Inquest into the Death of MA[71]

Highlights the responsibilities of nursing staff in mental health units to monitor and observe the patient in accordance with standard clinical protocols.

FACTS

MA had been admitted to the Mental Health Inpatient Unit (MHIPU) of the local Base Hospital some 4 weeks before his death. He had a long history of mental illness involving severe depression, persistent suicidal ideation and previous attempts at self-harm and suicide. He was admitted as an involuntary patient and assessed as 'potentially suicidal' with a sufficiently high level of risk to himself. As a consequence, he was admitted to the high-dependency unit (HDU) and placed on level 1 close observations — that is, 1:1 patient care level observations.

MA was reviewed by the Mental Health Review Tribunal 14 days after his admission. An involuntary patient order was made for a period of 4 weeks noting that MA 'represented a significant risk to himself and that confinement in a closed ward, in this instance the MHIPU, represented the least restrictive environment for his safe and effective care'.

MA remained significantly depressed, distressed and suicidal throughout the period of his admission and his treating psychiatrists were concerned about his suicide risk throughout his admission. A combination of pharmacotherapy was prescribed that the coroner found was frequently and appropriately reviewed.

While MA spent some time in the HDU (High Dependency Unit) of the mental health unit following his admission, he was transferred to the sub-acute unit (SAU) because of his expressed desire not to remain in the HDU. The evidence from the treating psychiatrist and the expert opinion evidence of a psychiatrist was to the effect that MA's mental state would indicate '... that 15 minute observations (performed properly) would have been a sufficient level of clinical vigilance'.[72]

After hearing evidence from MA's treating psychiatrists, the coroner concluded that '... in light of the recognition ... of MA's distress concerning the heightened level of restriction associated with placement in the HDU, the decision not to return MA to the HDU on either the 27 and/or 28 February is a decision which was within the range of appropriate or reasonable care options/decisions'.[73]

On the day of his death, MA was assessed as requiring level 2 observations (every 15 minutes) in accordance with the employer's area standard of practice (SOP) in place at the time, titled 'Patient care levels, specialling and risk assessment for mental health inpatients'.

In relation to the overall management of MA, the coroner accepted the expert opinion evidence from a psychiatrist to the effect that '... no matter how well prepared individual nurses are with post graduate qualifications and experience this will not circumvent let alone prevent all adverse events such as self-harm or suicide' and that '... medication and hospitalisation do not magically mend mental health problems and that complete safety is never guaranteed'.[74]

In acknowledging the above, the coroner noted the following extract from NSW Health MHIPU suicide risk assessment and management protocols:

> *In theory, from a psychiatric nursing point of view, in the MHIPU the risk was to be managed through a combination of therapeutic nursing engagement and patient observations.*[75]

The SOP protocol in place in relation to MA on the day of his death required nursing staff to perform level 2/15-minute observations. On the evidence given at the inquest, that was not done.

Critically, the evidence disclosed that, at approximately 2.40 pm, MA was observed on the CCTV footage to enter his room. Apart from another patient who briefly opened the door to MA's room at approximately 3.05 pm and said MA was 'sitting on the floor', no other person entered MA's room until approximately 5.20 pm when he was found in his room deceased. He was cold to touch and unresponsive, hanging by a bedsheet tied to a mechanical bed raised to the maximum height.

After hearing all the evidence, the coroner was satisfied that MA had already taken steps to end his life by the time the other patient had opened the door of his room at approximately 3.05 pm.

The clear and unequivocal failure on the part of nursing staff to maintain the requisite 15-minute

Continued

Coroner's Inquest into the Death of MA (Continued)

observations of MA were compounded by the fact that entries made in his MHIPU observation sheet by three different nurses on duty at the time stating observations had been undertaken simply did not occur. Based on the evidence given by nursing staff, the coroner found that 'phantom' entries were routinely made on MHIPU observation sheets where no observations or even mere patient sightings had been made. Also, on the day of his death MA was being cared for by a trainee enrolled nurse (TEN) who had four other patients to care for. Her evidence was that it was her understanding that, on the day of his death, MA was on level 4 observations, which was a level assigned when there was 'no foreseeable risk of harm' and that all that was required was that MA was 'sighted' by any member of staff every 2 hours.

The NSW Health guidelines in place at the time relevant to the role of the TEN were to the effect that she was considered a 'cadet' and as such 'must be rostered in a supernumerary position', 'must not be rostered to replace vacancies' and that cadets 'are in a learning role and must not be seen as an additional staff member'. Clearly the TEN's allocation to care for MA and four other patients on the day of his death was said by the coroner to be 'particularly inappropriate' and:

> ... the circumstances do suggest that, as a consequence of the fact that (the TEN) was assigned the care of MA and the TEN was required to undertake that task without an appropriate level of supervision and control by an appropriately qualified and experienced RN, opportunities for effective therapeutic engagement and/ or intervention were lost.[76]

Comment and Relevant Considerations Relating to the Coroner's Inquest into the Death of MA

By the time the inquest into MA's death took place, the Professional Standards Committee under the auspices of the Nursing and Midwifery Board of Australia had conducted an inquiry following complaints received in relation to the actions of the registered nurses on duty on the day of MA's death. Following that inquiry the Committee stated at the commencement of its findings:[77]

> It must be said at the outset that this case is laced with utter tragedy. It concerns the conduct of nursing staff ... when a young man tragically took his own life while an involuntary patient ... By extension it reveals endemic failures of clinical practice, procedure and culture in the hospital at the time.[78]

Given the findings of the Professional Standards Committee, the coroner stated that the focus of the inquest would be to 'search for the causes' of the systemic failures that led to MA's death. Specifically, the coroner identified the 'clinical practice, procedure and culture in the MHIPU at the time of MA's admission, particularly in relation to inpatient observations were governed by the employer's Area Standard of Practice, Safe Operating Procedures titled "Patient Care Levels,

Specialling and Risk Assessment for Mental Health Inpatients" that was in place at the time'.

As stated above, the coroner was satisfied, on the expert opinion evidence presented, that the prescribed pharmacotherapy regimen for MA was appropriate and regularly reviewed. Likewise the decision taken to have MA placed in the SCU rather than return him to the HDU. Given those findings, what became critical in the circumstances leading to MA's death was the level of direct observation of MA required to be made by the nursing staff, which was set at level 2/15-minute intervals. This was clearly not done. As the coroner stated relevantly:

> The SOP is clear, patient care level observations were to be determined by the patient's treating psychiatrist, in consultation with the NUM/the In Charge of Shift Nurse or a delegate.

> It follows that the entries in the Progress/Clinical Notes make plain that on the day in question, the observation level assigned by Dr Bardon to MA, in accordance with the SOP, required nursing staff to perform Level 2/15 minute observations.

> This is a clear and simple directive with the safety and well-being of the patient at its core.

...

Nonetheless, the MHIPU Observation Sheets indicate that the patient care level observations recorded on the relevant dates did not comply with the observation Level set by MA's treating psychiatrist and recorded in the Progress/Clinical Record.

...

Having regard to the evidence as a whole, the Court is satisfied on the balance of probabilities that prior to and as at the day in question nursing staff within the MHIPU were routinely conducting patient care level observations in a manner which was non-compliant with the SOP; and that there was routine non-compliance in relation to both the making and recording of Patient Care Level Observations.

In practice, it appears to have been a procedure which was either routinely misapplied, or routinely ignored.

The fact that the record remained uncorrected over an extended period of time is consistent with a widespread acceptance within the MHIPU of a mode of nursing which neither satisfies applicable professional nursing standards, nor the record-keeping standards of NSW Health.[79]

Overall, having heard evidence from the nursing staff concerned, the coroner found that as at the date of MA's death 'non-compliance with the SOP' was routine practice within the MHIPU.[80] In total contravention of the SOP, patient care level observations were routinely conducted 'en bloc' and retrospectively later in the shift; patients were reportedly left unobserved for extended periods of time and 'phantom entries' were routinely made on MHIPU observation sheets.[81]

What this case illustrates is the importance of nurses and midwives being fully conversant with the employer-sanctioned clinical practice policies in place in relation to the care of their patients. In a mental health setting and against the background of MA's known severe depression and suicidal ideation, close observation was clearly clinically essential. That much was confirmed by the requirement that he be individually observed every 15 minutes.

What became apparent on the evidence was that the significant failure of nursing staff to observe the requisite observations in relation to MA was found by the Professional Standards Committee to be evidence of a 'uniformly cavalier attitude to making and recording patient observations in the MHIPU'.[82] That finding demonstrates a failure of nursing and hospital management to ensure that the clinical policies in place were being routinely followed and maintained. There was evidence to the effect that although nursing management in the MHIPU 'were aware that nurses within the unit were not performing patient care level observations in a manner that complied with the SOP, no corrective action was taken'.[83]

When assessing the failure of the nursing staff in relation to the death of MA, the coroner found that, having regard to all the evidence in relation to the nursing staff, she was satisfied that, 'both prior to and during the period of MA's admission ... there was routine, systemic non-compliance within the MHIPU with the SOP which governed the making and recording of patient observations'.[84]

In addition to the formal findings as to MA's manner and cause of death, the coroner made a number of recommendations directed at the employer and nursing staff in relation to the taking and recording of requisite nursing observations throughout a patient's engagement in psychiatric inpatient care.[85]

SHOULD A NURSE OR MIDWIFE QUESTION TREATMENT OR MEDICATION ORDERS AS PART OF THE DUTY AND STANDARD OF CARE?

A nurse or midwife does have a right and, in many circumstances, a professional and legal obligation to question the orders of a medical practitioner or another health professional; for example, where a nurse or midwife believes, based on his or her knowledge, that:

- given the circumstances, the dose of a medication ordered is excessive; or
- the patient is allergic to the medication; or
- for sound clinical reasons the nurse or midwife believed that the medication or treatment prescribed is contraindicated.

Also, if a nurse or midwife became aware that a patient has not been adequately informed about a proposed treatment and its consequences, he or she should advise the treating medical practitioner and request they discuss the proposed procedure more fully with the patient.

There are also circumstances that arise where a nurse or midwife is of the opinion, based on a patient's observations and clinical condition, that further attention and action by the treating practitioner is warranted. For example, standard observation charts predominantly for pulse rate and temperature recordings are used throughout public hospitals in Australia, and those charts are designed with colour-coded parameters indicated.[86] When a patient's observations fall within those parameters, the nurse or midwife is required to notify the relevant practitioner and discuss those concerns. This is particularly important where close monitoring of the patient is vital and any critical change to the patient's condition manifested by observation and monitoring may well be an indication of problems that require early intervention. The sooner the problem is identified and acted upon the better.

It might be that the treating practitioner may not consider the matters raised by the nurse or midwife to be of any great clinical significance and he or she may choose to ignore the concerns expressed. However, it is far better to err on the side of caution when considering whether to contact a patient's treating practitioner about any change to a patient's condition which the nurse or midwife believes is relevant. A failure to advise the treating practitioner of critical observations and/or changes to the patient's condition may well be a direct cause of the patient's condition deteriorating to the point where it is too late to reverse the damage caused. In such circumstances the nurse or midwife may be deemed to be negligent for failing to notify the patient's treating practitioner in a timely manner and, as a consequence, to have contributed to the damage caused to the patient. Also, when a decision is taken to ring the treating practitioner, it is essential to make an entry to that effect in the patient's record noting the date, time and nature of the concern raised.

There have been cases where the courts, in one form or another, have been critical of the failure of nurses to express their views on appropriate patient management. One such situation is set out in **Case example 7.12**.

CASE EXAMPLE 7.12

Coroner's Inquest into the Death of Timothy John Bice[87]

FACTS

The deceased was a 21-month-old boy who died in a private hospital from circulatory collapse due to dehydration caused by gastroenteritis.

The child was taken to the medical centre of the hospital early on the Wednesday afternoon with diarrhoea, vomiting and general lethargy and was seen by Dr H, who advised the mother that the child was suffering from gastroenteritis and was slightly dehydrated.

The mother was advised to administer regular oral fluids and Panadol for the high temperature and told to bring the child back if she continued to be concerned. The child seemed to improve during the day but suffered a large bout of diarrhoea at about 6.00 pm and was finally taken back to the hospital by his mother at about 9.30 pm. He was seen by another doctor who noted that he was somewhat dehydrated and also had an inflamed throat. The doctor decided to admit the child for review by the paediatrician on admission. The paediatrician, Dr B, saw the child that evening, made a diagnosis of viral gastroenteritis and ordered regular oral foods and observation by the nursing staff.

During Thursday the child suffered frequent bouts of diarrhoea and, after 6.00 pm on the Thursday, frequent vomiting episodes. On the Thursday evening the child became very thirsty, consumed large quantities of fluid, but continued to vomit and was given Maxolon orally at 9.30 pm and, later, another dose intravenously to attempt to alleviate the vomiting. Dr B saw the child at about 10.00 to 10.30 pm but did not examine the child physically at this stage because he testified that he had done so earlier. He testified that there was evidence of dehydration at this stage and that he considered an intravenous drip.

Between 11.00 pm and 2.00 am the condition of the child appeared to stabilise and, when reviewed by Dr B at 2.00 am, he determined that stabilisation had occurred because the child had ceased to vomit. However, at 4.00 am and 5.15 am changes were noted in the child's pulse and respiratory rates which were not reported to the doctor. Between 5.40 and 5.45 am the child had a cardiac arrest. The doctor was notified on two occasions of this event and stated twice that he could not attend. However, he reversed this decision and arrived at the hospital at 6.45 am, by which time the child had died.

Comment and Relevant Considerations Relating to the Coroner's Inquest into the Death of Timothy John Bice

In handing down his findings as to the manner and cause of the child's death, the coroner was quite critical of, among other issues, the failure of the nursing staff, on the Thursday evening, to communicate adequately with the paediatrician, Dr B, about their concern for the child's condition. He expressed that criticism thus:

> *The evidence establishes to my satisfaction that at various times the nursing personnel were concerned with T's condition. An approach was made to the then Director of Nursing, the Witness Sister A. She deposed to this in evidence and as a result apparently sought an interview with the Chief Executive Officer of the Hospital … It is perhaps unfortunate, although understandable, in some respects, that not one of the staff expressed their concern directly to Dr B and I also gathered the distinct impression that most, if not all, of the nursing staff nurtured the hope that intravenous therapy would be commenced some time during the Thursday evening. This appears to me to be a reasonable inference from the evidence given by the staff concerned. One staff member no doubt did approach Dr B. I accept the reluctance of staff members to approach a medical practitioner expressing his/her concern about a patient, but there are times when this protocol should be set aside. It is no doubt true that some practitioners may well resent being approached by a trained sister [sic] in such circumstances … There is no evidence to suggest that Dr B falls in this category. Nevertheless, I consider the trained nursing sisters have the requisite experience to express an opinion concerning a particular patient's condition.[88]*

The coroner in this matter went on to recommend that, as a matter of practice, the nursing staff should communicate their concerns directly with the doctor in future. He expressed that recommendation as follows:

> *There is no doubt on the evidence of Dr D (an expert witness) that he strongly supports the view that experienced nursing staff should have*

> *no compunction or hesitation in approaching a medical practitioner in charge of the case if they (the staff) are or become concerned about the child's condition.[89]*

And later:

> *It is quite clear from the evidence, particularly of Dr D, that trained nursing staff employed at the Adelaide Children's Hospital are encouraged to approach a medical person if they have a concern about a particular patient's condition. This is a commonsense approach to the situation and can really only have beneficial results. I am confident that most, if not all, medical practitioners would not oppose this practice by trained nursing staff in hospitals generally.[90]*

Two Canadian cases are also of interest in the area of the duty and standard of care. In one, nurses were found not to be negligent in failing to further contact the treating practitioner with their concerns about the condition of a patient's leg.[91] The patient subsequently required an amputation of his foot. In delivering his judgment on appeal, the judge said that the reason why the nurses were held *not* to be negligent was that he accepted the evidence of the treating medical practitioner that he would have taken no notice of the nurses even if they had informed him again in relation to their concerns about the patient.

In similar circumstances in another case, the nurses were held to be negligent for not calling the doctors, again despite the fact that the nurses had been expressing and documenting their concerns for 3 days.[92] The reason why they *were* held to be negligent on this occasion was because the doctors gave evidence to the effect that, if they had been informed of the patient's most recent deterioration, they would have acted.

Considerations When Questioning a Medical Practitioner's Orders

The lesson to be learned from the above cases is that, on balance, and if in any doubt, a nurse or midwife should take steps to notify the treating medical practitioner and express his or her concerns *and* at the same time make a written entry in the patient's record of the action taken.

What has to be addressed is the most appropriate and sensible way for a nurse or midwife to deal with such matters, given the possibility that such a situation may get out of hand. In the first instance, as a matter of courtesy and commonsense, the nurse or midwife should discuss her or his concerns directly and discreetly with the medical practitioner involved. Whether such an approach would influence the practitioner to alter the proposed course of treatment would depend very much on the facts and circumstances, but nevertheless a nurse or midwife is clearly entitled to raise his or her professional concerns.

Indeed, in any situation where a nurse or midwife is involved with a medical practitioner in patient or client care, and where a genuine concern is held, a nurse or midwife is not only entitled to discuss the appropriateness or otherwise of the treatment proposed but is also professionally and legally obligated to do so.

Consider the following hypothetical example: If a doctor prescribed a schedule of medications that a nurse or midwife knew or ought to have known or believed to be excessive or harmful to the patient's wellbeing, then the standard of care expected of the professionally competent nurse or midwife would be that he or she express those concerns to the doctor. Further, if the doctor disagreed or refused to alter the medication order following those discussions, and if the nurse or midwife still believed that the particular course of medication proposed was incorrect or inappropriate, then the nurse or midwife would be entitled and, depending on the circumstances, obliged to escalate those concerns formally to the appropriate nurse manager and request assistance. Equally, the nurse or midwife may refuse to administer the medication, as long as he or she does so on reasonable and proper grounds.

The mechanisms by which a nurse or midwife would formalise his or her concerns would vary depending on the circumstances. In a hospital or nursing home, it would be done using the administrative channels available. Outside of a hospital or nursing home, it may be necessary to raise such concerns with the relevant state or territory health authority or medical registration board.

If a nurse or midwife formally raises a complaint concerning the professional competence of a medical practitioner (or any fellow health professional for that matter) the complaint should always be in writing, setting out objectively the details of the complaint and the reasons in support of it.

THIRD AND FOURTH PRINCIPLE IN CIVIL ACTION ALLEGING PROFESSIONAL NEGLIGENCE: DAMAGE SUFFERED AND THE PRINCIPLE OF CAUSATION AND THE SCOPE OF LIABILITY FOR NEGLIGENT ACTS

If the evidence establishes, on the balance of probabilities, that the requisite standard of care expected in relation to the delivery of professional services was not followed, the next step in the process in order to receive compensation requires the following elements to be established on the balance of probabilities:

- that the plaintiff suffered damage — if the plaintiff suffered no damage, no compensation can be awarded; and
- there must be established a causal relationship between the damage and the negligent act relied on and the scope of the negligent person's liability must extend to the harm being complained of.

Both issues are now considered in more detail.

Element 1: Damage

What Type of Damage Does the Law Recognise?

In the context of civil negligence, there are three particular types of damage the courts will recognise and, if proved on the balance of probabilities to exist, award compensation for.

The civil liability legislation of the states and territories refers to 'harm' or 'injury' and, relevantly, defines both; for example, in section 5 of the *Civil Liability Act 2002* (NSW):

> **harm** *means harm of any kind, including the following:*
> *a. personal injury or death,*
> *b. damage to property,*
> *c. economic loss.*
>
> **personal injury** *includes:*
> *a. prenatal injury, and*
> *b. impairment of a person's physical or mental condition, and*
> *c. disease.*

Further definitions are provided for 'mental harm' — for example, in section 27 of the *Civil Liability Act 2002* (NSW):

> **consequential mental harm** *means mental harm that is a consequence of a personal injury of any other kind.*

> **mental harm** *means impairment of a person's mental condition.*

> **pure mental harm** *means mental harm other than consequential mental harm.*

All the other states and territories have adopted similar definitions except that the Northern Territory and Queensland do not define 'mental harm'. For definitions relevant to 'harm' or 'injury' see: *Civil Law (Wrongs) Act 2002* (ACT) sections 32 and 40, *Personal Injury (Liabilities and Damages) Act 2003* (NT) section 3, *Civil Liability Act 2003* (Qld) Sch 2 (Dictionary) and section 51, *Civil Liability Act 1936* (SA) section 3, *Civil Liability Act 2002* (Tas) sections 3 and 29, *Wrongs Act 1958* (Vic) sections 28B and 67, and *Civil Liability Act 2002* (WA) sections 3 and 5Q.

As has already been stated, it is necessary to establish all of the requisite legal principles for a negligence action to succeed. Therefore, the absence of any damage to the plaintiff, even in the presence of a clear breach of the duty of care, will preclude any action from being commenced.

Element 2: The Damage Being Complained of Occurred as a Result of the Negligent Act and the Scope of the Negligent Person's Liability Extends to the Damage Caused

At the outset consider **Case study 7.1**, which explains in a hypothetical example the need to establish a causal relationship between the negligent act and any damage caused to the plaintiff.

To satisfy this element the plaintiff is required to prove, on the balance of probabilities, that there is a direct or causal relationship between the negligent act complained of and the damage suffered by the plaintiff and that the scope of the negligent person's liability extends to the harm suffered by the plaintiff. This is often referred to as the elements of the *principle of causation and the scope of the negligent person's liability.*

For example, section 5D(1) of the NSW *Civil Liability Act* provides that a determination that negligence

---

CASE STUDY 7.1

As a hypothetical example, assume that a nurse in accident and emergency had been directed to put particular drops into a patient's left ear before he was sent home. The nurse got the correct drops, but instead of putting them in the patient's left ear as instructed she misread the instructions and put them into the patient's right ear. What would be the legal consequences for the nurse, if any?

COMMENT AND RELEVANT CONSIDERATIONS

The legal consequences would depend on a number of factors. In the first instance, the medication error as described is a breach of the duty of care a nurse or midwife owes to that patient — the reason being that, if acting in accordance with generally accepted professional standards in the administration of medications, a registered nurse or midwife would not make the medication error described. As a consequence, what the nurse did is in breach of her duty of care to the patient. However, it is highly unlikely that the nature of the drops she put in the wrong ear were such as to cause any physical damage to the patient's right ear. Obviously, if they did, it would be a different matter, but for the purposes of this example we will assume they did not. Accordingly, while it would be hoped the registered nurse would be professionally counselled in relation to the medication error (which should be reported), there would be no legal consequences because the patient did not suffer any damage.

If the drops had caused damage to the patient's right ear, the legal outcome would be different as the patient could establish damage caused by the incorrect administration of the ear drop medication, for which he or she would be entitled to claim compensation.

Remember, if there is no damage, there can be no claim for compensation because it is for the damage caused that the plaintiff is compensated in a civil negligence action.

caused particular harm comprises the following elements:

(a) *that the negligence was a necessary condition of the occurrence of the harm ('factual causation'), and*

(b) *that it is appropriate for the scope of the negligent person's liability to extend to the harm so caused ('scope of liability').*

Provision is made in similar terms in the civil liability legislation of the states and territories (except the Northern Territory) as to the scope and application of these elements in determining liability. See: *Civil Law (Wrongs) Act 2002* (ACT) section 45, *Civil Liability Act 2003* (Qld) section 11, *Civil Liability Act 1936* (SA) section 34, *Civil Liability Act 2002* (Tas) section 13, *Wrongs Act 1958* (Vic) section 51, and *Civil Liability Act 2002* (WA) section 5C.

The common law principle of causation in negligence is often referred to as the 'but for' test; that is, 'but for' the breach of the duty of care alleged, the plaintiff would not have suffered the harm and damage complained of.

Case examples 7.13 and **7.14** illustrate the principle of causation in the examination of cases from the UK and Australia respectively, and **Case study 7.2** presents a hypothetical example.

CASE STUDY 7.2
THE PRINCIPLE OF CAUSATION

Consider this hypothetical example highlighting the principle of causation of a midwife administering medications in a postnatal ward. The midwife mistakenly gives a patient 500 mg of ampicillin. Some 20 minutes after taking the antibiotic, the patient has a massive postpartum haemorrhage and nearly bleeds to death. She suffers all of the attendant medical problems that acute and sudden blood loss can cause and gradually recovers over a period of months.

Knowing that she was given the ampicillin in error, the patient considers bringing a claim alleging negligence on the part of the midwife and claims that the error in administering the ampicillin was the cause of her sudden and precipitate postpartum haemorrhage. Would she succeed in making such a claim?

In considering your answer, it is clear the midwife was in breach of his or her duty of care to the patient by

---

CASE STUDY 7.2
THE PRINCIPLE OF CAUSATION *(Continued)*

administering a medication not meant for her. To succeed in her claim, however, the patient would have to establish, on the balance of probabilities, that 'but for' the midwife's error in administering the wrong medication, the postpartum haemorrhage would not have occurred.

In our view, it would be most improbable that giving 500 mg of ampicillin to the patient 20 minutes before had caused her postpartum haemorrhage. However, if by calling expert medical evidence the patient could establish, on the balance of probabilities, a causal relationship between the two events, then the patient would be entitled to rely on the medication error as the basis for a claim of compensation for the harm she had suffered.

CASE EXAMPLE 7.13
Barnett v Chelsea and Kensington Hospital[93]

FACTS

Mr Barnett went to the accident and emergency department of a hospital in the United Kingdom complaining of nausea and vomiting following the drinking of tea some hours before. The nurse in casualty notified the doctor on duty, who was also not feeling well and not overly inclined to want to see patients. He advised the nurse to send Mr Barnett home with instructions to go to bed and see his own doctor later in the day. Mr Barnett left the hospital but his condition worsened. He returned to the hospital and a few hours afterwards he died from what was later discovered to be arsenic poisoning. Mr Barnett's widow brought an action against the hospital and the doctor alleging negligence on the part of both.

Comment and Relevant Considerations Relating to Barnett v Chelsea and Kensington Hospital

The decision of the court stated that the hospital had a general duty of care to all users to provide a safe and competent service, with safe, competent employees. The standard expected of that duty of care would be that people who present to accident and emergency should have a proper history taken and be examined.

The court stated that this had not been done and accordingly the hospital was liable for allowing such an unsafe situation to occur through the actions of its employees. It was also stated that the doctor was in breach of his duty of care to the patient because he failed to examine him, which is what the ordinary, reasonable doctor in his position would have done.

In this case, Mrs Barnett had established that:

- the duty of care clearly existed;
- the standard of care that would have been expected of the hospital's employees was that they would have taken a history and that he would be examined by the doctor on duty;
- the hospital's employees had been in breach of their duty of care to Mr Barnett;
- the damage suffered by Mrs Barnett was self-evident (Mr Barnett's death).

However, Mrs Barnett failed in her claim against the hospital and its employees because she could not establish that the breach of the duty of care had caused her husband's death. In coming to that decision, the court concluded, on the evidence, that even if Mr Barnett had been properly examined and a history taken, and if he had been admitted the first time he came to accident and emergency, he would still have died.

Expert evidence supported the view that the likelihood of the doctor in accident and emergency diagnosing Mr Barnett's illness as arsenic poisoning was highly improbable. This conclusion was supported by the evidence that, at that time, of the nearly 4 million people who were admitted to the thousands of hospitals in the United Kingdom each year, fewer than 60 had arsenic poisoning. Thus, it was said, the ordinary, reasonable doctor could hardly be expected to have diagnosed arsenic poisoning particularly given the history Mr Barnett had recounted to the nurse in accident and emergency. Remember that Mr Barnett was not able to state that he had taken arsenic because he did not know that fact. He could only recount that he had been drinking tea. In addition, expert medical witnesses stated that it would have taken some hours after admission for sufficient investigations to be completed to permit the correct diagnosis to be made. By then any treatment would have had no effect, and Mr Barnett would have died.

The outcome of the case, as decided by the court on the evidence before it, was that even though the hospital and the doctor were in breach of their duty of care to Mr Barnett and even though the damage was clear, Mrs Barnett could not succeed, because the court found that the arsenic, and not the breach of the duty of care of the hospital's employees, had caused Mr Barnett's death.

By way of interest, Mr Barnett's ingestion of arsenic had occurred by accident. He was employed as a road worker and used a material with an arsenic compound that had accidentally contaminated the tea he was drinking.

A more recent example of the importance of establishing causation is the decision set out in **Case example 7.14**. In that case the judge addressed the application of the 'but for' test as part of the principle of causation and determined that the scope of the defendant's liability extended to the harm caused.

CASE EXAMPLE 7.14

Finch v Rogers[94]

FACTS

Mr Finch was a musician and music student who was diagnosed with a particularly aggressive form of testicular cancer. Dr Rogers operated to remove the affected testicle. There was a delay of some weeks before Dr Rogers took steps to follow up the surgery with postoperative monitoring including blood tests and scans.

When that was done, there was clinical evidence that the cancer had spread to the abdominal lymph glands and as a result Mr Finch had to undergo an extra cycle of chemotherapy. Following the additional cycle of chemotherapy, he developed tinnitus, hearing loss and peripheral neuropathy. In bringing his claim, Mr Finch argued that Dr Rogers had been negligent by not adequately explaining the need for immediate ongoing postoperative monitoring and not undertaking the necessary investigations to determine whether there had been any spread of the tumour. Mr Finch claimed that, because of the delay in that process, he had been required to have the additional cycle of chemotherapy resulting in the damaging and debilitating side effects that he sustained.

Comment and relevant considerations relating to Finch v Rogers

On behalf of Dr Rogers, the breach of the duty of care was admitted, but it was argued that that breach had not caused the damage Mr Finch complained of. Consequently, to succeed, Mr Finch had to establish that there was a causal relationship between the breach of the duty owed to him by Dr Rogers and the damage he sustained. Mr Finch succeeded in his action, and in addressing the issue of causation, the judge said:

> *The evidence does, to my mind, establish as a probability that the fourth cycle materially contributed to the disabilities from which the plaintiff now suffers. But for the fourth cycle, there may have been damage but it probably would not have been disabling.[95]*

And further the judge said:

> *Addressing the issue of factual causation, but for the breach, and the delay which was the consequence of the breach, the following can be said: First, that Mr Finch would probably have been given Indiana BEP chemotherapy on Monday 30 December 1996 or, at the latest, Monday 6 January 1997. Second, that on either day, he would have been regarded as a good prognosis patient. Third, that given his response to chemotherapy (which was good), he would have needed three cycles, not four. Fourth, that he would not have suffered the disabling consequences of ototoxicity and neurotoxicity which were evident after the fourth cycle.*

> *In short, I consider that the defendant's negligence was a necessary condition of the harm that ensued … I further believe that it is appropriate that the scope of the defendant's liability extends to the harm so caused … The consequences were, in each case, a foreseeable result of the breach.[96]*

Applying the principle of causation, that is, 'but for' the fourth cycle of chemotherapy, the judge was satisfied Mr Finch would, on the balance of probabilities, not have suffered the damage he was complaining of. Also, the scope of Dr Rogers' liability extended to the harm suffered by Mr Finch.

Case example 7.15 examines a decision of the High Court that also addressed the issue of having to establish causation.

CASE EXAMPLE 7.15

Tabet v Gett[97]

In addressing the issue of causation, this 2010 decision of the High Court emphasised the point that, for a plaintiff to succeed in an action alleging negligence, he or she must establish each element of the claim in accordance with the requisite standard in civil cases — that being on the balance of probabilities.

FACTS

Reema Tabet, a 6-year-old girl, was admitted to hospital on 11 January 1991. She had recently suffered from chicken pox that had resolved, but both before and after that illness she suffered headaches, nausea and vomiting. She was under the care of Dr Gett, who made a provisional diagnosis of chicken pox, varicella meningitis or encephalitis.

On 14 January 1991, the young child had a seizure. As a consequence a CT scan was undertaken. It disclosed a brain tumour that had apparently been present for the better part of 2 years. The tumour was surgically removed but by that time the child had sustained irreversible brain damage because of the raised intracranial pressure from the build-up of cerebrospinal fluid.

Comment and Relevant Considerations Relating to Tabet v Gett

On behalf of the child a claim was commenced alleging Dr Gett had been negligent in failing to order a CT scan on 11 January or 13 January at the latest. The latter date was identified because on that date the nursing staff observed that the child's pupils were unequal and her right pupil was non-reactive.

In the evidence before the judge who heard the case initially, it could not be established on the balance of probabilities that the taking of a CT scan and the administration of steroids or the insertion of a drain earlier than was done would have averted the child's brain damage. Despite that, the judge determined that 'but for' the delay in diagnosis and treatment by not undertaking the CT scan and associated treatment on 13 January rather than on 14 January after the child's seizure, the child would have had a 40% 'chance' of a better outcome and awarded her compensation.

Dr Gett appealed to the New South Wales Court of Appeal to have the decision overturned and was successful. On behalf of the young girl, an appeal was lodged with the High Court. That appeal was unsuccessful. In dismissing the appeal and specifically on the need for causation to be established on the balance of probabilities, the High Court said:

> *The common law requires proof, by the person seeking compensation, that the negligent act or omission caused the loss or injury constituting the damage. All that is necessary is that, according to the course of common experience, the more probable inference appearing from the evidence is that a defendant's negligence caused the injury or harm. 'More probable' means no more than that, upon a balance of probabilities, such an inference might reasonably be considered to have some greater degree of likelihood; it does not require certainty.*[98]

In dismissing the appeal on behalf of the child, the High Court emphasised that, for the action to succeed, it had to be established, on the balance of probabilities, not only that the doctor's alleged failure had caused the child to suffer harm but also that, by undertaking the treatment a day earlier than was done, the child would have recovered. In other words, the court determined, losing a 'chance' is not establishing the issue in dispute on the balance of probabilities.

THE AWARDING OF COMPENSATION BY THE COURTS

Based on evidence presented, if the plaintiff has established on the balance of probabilities and in accordance with the legal principles the allegation of professional negligence, the court must then determine the amount of financial compensation, otherwise known as damages, to be awarded to the plaintiff.

As a general rule, the common law made provision for ordinary compensatory damages that were classified as specific damages and general damages.

Specific damages were those that can be specifically quantified in monetary amounts. For example, compensation claimed for 2 months' loss of salary can be precisely calculated or medical expenses can be accurately stated.

Very often, one of the largest components of specific damages as part of ordinary compensatory damages is the amount claimed for future economic loss as a result of the loss of the plaintiff's earning capacity arising from the defendant's negligence. Also, the economic cost of providing attendant care needs to the plaintiff on an ongoing basis can be significant, particularly if the plaintiff is young, severely injured with quadriplegia or brain damaged, and will require care for the rest of his or her life.

General damages were those that, as described, were general in nature and were amounts awarded for 'pain and suffering' and 'loss of enjoyment of life'.

One of the factors driving the legislative changes made to civil liability law was the widely held belief that the amounts awarded by the courts as compensation were excessive and driving up insurance costs.

As a consequence, there are now significant legislative constraints limiting the amounts that may be awarded as compensation both for specific damages based on economic loss and for general damages based on non-economic loss. These constraints apply in all states and territories and there is now a threshold test to be met for entitlement to, and a cap on the amount that may be awarded for, non-economic loss.

There is also a cap placed on the damages a court may award for future economic loss based on a plaintiff's earning capacity. Also, there is now a limit that may be recovered for what is termed 'gratuitous attendant care services'. Such services are the care services that a family member, for example a mother or father, wife or husband, will need to provide in order to ensure continuing care for the plaintiff, generally in the family home.

Overall, the legislative changes have made it very difficult for a plaintiff and have significantly reduced the amounts able to be awarded by the courts. Such changes will, we believe, have harsh consequences for many plaintiffs. It remains to be seen whether governments are ultimately persuaded to amend some of the more restrictive provisions in future.

The following are important factors to bear in mind when considering the question of **compensatory damages** generally:

1. In the absence of establishing negligence no damages can be awarded. As has been made clear, to qualify for an award of compensatory damages the plaintiff must establish that somebody was negligent in accordance with the established principles. There are situations where the plaintiff is unable to do that and is therefore unable to bring a negligence action against anybody. Consider this example: A person driving a motor vehicle along a highway comes to a bend in the road. In negotiating that bend he drives too fast, the car goes out of control, runs off the highway and hits a tree. The driver suffers serious injuries, including paraplegia.

   In this situation, the driver of the motor vehicle would not be able to bring an action in negligence against anyone because he would not be able to find fault with anyone, apart from himself perhaps, and he cannot sue himself. At best he would become entitled to an invalid pension or maybe assistance from the National Disability Insurance Scheme.

   The outcome would be different, however, if instead of running off the road out of control, the driver of the car sustained his injuries when the driver of another vehicle failed to give way at an intersection. In that type of accident the injured driver would be able to find somebody who had been negligent — that is, the driver of the other motor vehicle. More importantly, the driver's insurance company would be liable to pay the amount of compensation awarded if negligence is established.

2. If the plaintiff should succeed in proving negligence, he or she must also ensure that the person or party made liable has adequate financial resources to pay the amount awarded, either directly or by access to an insurance policy. The task of the courts is not to provide the money awarded to the plaintiff, but rather to assess and state the amount of damages the plaintiff is entitled to once negligence has been established or admitted. The plaintiff must then recover that amount from the defendant or the defendant's insurer.

3. Common law principles have long determined that, if a person dies as a result of the negligent act of another, the person's right to bring an action in negligence 'dies' with them. Clearly, such a principle has harsh consequences when a person dies as a result of another person's negligent act leaving behind a family who had been financially dependent on that person's income and could have reasonably looked forward to that income for many years to come. To overcome the harshness of that common law principle, parliaments have intervened and passed legislation that permits the relatives of a person killed in such circumstances to bring an action claiming compensation for the loss of income they could foreseeably have been able to rely on. In New South Wales this legislation is known as the *Compensation to Relatives Act 1897*, but in the other states and territories it has somewhat different titles.[99]

Generally speaking, the category of relatives who can bring such an action is clearly defined in the Act and generally includes de facto spouses/partners.

DEFENCES TO AN ACTION ALLEGING PROFESSIONAL NEGLIGENCE

When a plaintiff brings an action alleging negligence, the plaintiff must establish his or her allegation on the balance of probabilities. Equally it is possible for the defendant to refute the allegation of negligence made by the plaintiff by raising certain defences.

In raising a defence, the defendant must establish that defence on the balance of probabilities by calling the appropriate evidence. The general defences available to a defendant are:

■ a general denial and rebuttal of the allegation;
■ contributory negligence;
■ voluntary assumption of risk.

A General Denial and Rebuttal of the Allegation

This is the most common form of defence raised and arises where the defendant can establish that:

- no duty of care was owed to the plaintiff; or
- whatever the defendant did was reasonable in all the circumstances in that it was shown to be 'widely accepted' by 'peer opinion' to be 'competent professional practice'; or
- the plaintiff suffered no damage; or
- there was no causal relationship between the breach of the duty of care alleged and the damage to the plaintiff; or
- the damage being complained of was not within the scope of the defendant's liability.

If the defendant can establish one or more of the above principles, he or she will be able to successfully resist any claim for compensation made by the plaintiff.

Contributory Negligence

This is often referred to as a 'partial defence' to an action in negligence. The essence of contributory negligence as a defence is to apportion a determined percentage of blame to the plaintiff for the damage caused and penalise the plaintiff by reducing the damages awarded accordingly.[100] The determination of apportionment of blame, if any, is done by the judge, but the defendant must establish it on the balance of probabilities.

A good example of a case in which contributory negligence is often raised as a partial defence is that of personal injury involving the failure of a passenger in a motor vehicle accident to wear a seatbelt. For example, a front seat passenger in a motor vehicle fails to secure the seatbelt and, as a result of the driver's negligence, an accident occurs. On impact, the passenger is thrown through the windscreen onto the bonnet, suffering severe facial lacerations and head injuries. The passenger sues the driver for negligence and, as part of the damages complained of, seeks compensation for the consequences of the facial and head injuries suffered.

In his or her partial defence of contributory negligence, the driver will allege that if the passenger had secured the seatbelt, the facial and head injuries he or she is now complaining about would not have been sustained and that this is a fact readily known or which ought to have been known by the passenger. Therefore, the failure or negligence on the part of the passenger to wear a seatbelt has contributed to the damage he or she is now complaining of.

If the driver, as the defendant, can successfully establish the partial defence of contributory negligence, the court is entitled to reduce, by a percentage, the damages awarded to the plaintiff. This percentage represents the plaintiff's share or portion of the fault in causing the damage being complained of. Damages are reduced in percentage terms so that the court may determine that the plaintiff was 10% (or 50% or 85%, and so on) to blame for the damage and reduce the amount awarded accordingly.

Voluntary Assumption of Risk

This defence is commonly known as the defence of *volenti non fit injuria* ('no injury is done to one who voluntarily consents'). Its basis is that no action in negligence can arise if the plaintiff knowingly and willingly consents to run the risk of injury. A person who participates in a dangerous sport cannot complain if he or she is injured, as the defence of *volenti* would claim that, in agreeing to participate in such dangerous activities, the person had voluntarily assumed the risk of injury.

For a defendant to raise *volenti* as a defence, he or she must establish, on the balance of probabilities, that the plaintiff knew of and understood the risk of injury arising from the activity undertaken and, knowing and understanding that, freely and voluntarily consented to run the risk of injury by participating in that activity.

Not surprisingly, this defence arises most often in relation to sporting activities. However, such a defence will not succeed if a person in the course of a game goes beyond the normal 'rough and tumble' of a particular sporting activity and recklessly or negligently injures a fellow player. In such a situation the defence of *volenti* will fail. Damages have been awarded to people injured in sporting activities where they have established that they were exposed to an unreasonable risk of harm or where a fellow player has acted recklessly and beyond what would be considered reasonable in all the circumstances and which has resulted in injury.

As a result of the changes made by the civil liability legislation of the states and territories (see **Table 7.1**), a defendant is not liable in negligence for harm suffered by a plaintiff where the injury was as a result of an 'obvious risk' of a dangerous recreational activity (such as any sport) engaged in by the plaintiff. Accordingly, the plaintiff would bear the onus of proving that he or she was not aware of the 'obvious risk' raised as a defence by the defendant.

VICARIOUS LIABILITY

In determining liability in certain situations, it is necessary for the courts to consider whether the liability and therefore the financial consequences for an individual's negligent act can be transferred to another person. In determining this issue, the courts will consider the principles encompassed within the doctrine of vicarious liability.

The doctrine of vicarious liability provides that, where an employee has been negligent in the course and scope of employment and a person suffers damage as a result, the employer will be made liable. That does not mean that the personal liability of the individual is transferred to the employer, but rather that the responsibility for the negligent act is directed at the employer. In simple terms, it means the employer has to pay the plaintiff the sum of money awarded by the court as a result of the employee's negligent act.

Historically the doctrine has its origins in the old master–servant relationship, which made the master liable for all the wrongs of his servants. Over the years, with social, industrial and technological change, this has been replaced by the employer–employee relationship. Despite the change of terminology, the doctrine of vicarious liability has been retained insofar as imputing liability within the employer–employee relationship.

It can be very difficult for employers to avoid liability under this doctrine, primarily for practical economic reasons. If the individual employee were to remain financially liable to compensate the innocent plaintiff who has been badly damaged by the employee's negligent act, many such plaintiffs would go without, for the simple reason that most employees do not have sufficient financial resources to meet any financial damages awarded to an injured plaintiff. Obviously the employer is in a better financial position, better able to plan and insure for such losses and better able to distribute such losses through its financial system. Also, an employer is under a legal obligation to provide a safe system of work for employees and to ensure employees comply with safe work standards.

In pursuing an attitude of almost strict liability against the employer in this area, the law has also provided the employer with the power to recover such money paid out, either wholly or in part, from the negligent employee. The right to seek total recovery of monies paid is known as seeking an indemnity from the employee concerned; the right to seek partial recovery is known as seeking a contribution.

When considering whether the employer is vicariously liable for the negligent acts of an employee, the following principles have to be determined:

- that the person was an employee;
- that the negligent act arose in the course and scope of employment.

Who is an Employee for the Purposes of the Doctrine of Vicarious Liability?

In the first instance, an employee has to be distinguished from what is generally referred to as an independent contractor. The closest analogy to an independent contractor is the self-employed person, although as far as the law is concerned that may not necessarily be the case.

The common law principles developed by the courts to distinguish between an employee and an independent contractor is to apply one of two tests: the **control test** or the **organisation test**.

The Control Test

Relying on the control test, a person is an employee if the employer exercises authority over that person in the performance of the person's work and is able to give the person instructions in relation to such work. In most situations other indicators of control can be determined by the answers to these questions:

- Is the person paid a weekly or regular wage that has tax deducted?

◼ Is the person entitled to the benefits of an industrial award — for example, annual leave, sick leave?

◼ Does the employer provide the necessary plant and equipment to enable a person to carry out the duties that person is engaged to perform?

If the answers to the above questions are in the affirmative, there is probably no doubt that the person concerned is an employee. The great majority of people working in differing types of employment are employees, and nurses and midwives are no exception.

The question as to whether a person is an employee or an independent contractor may not always be readily apparent, even when using the control test, as particular circumstances may exist which make it difficult to determine. Ultimately each case must be determined on its own facts and circumstances. Nevertheless, past decisions by the courts have expanded the application of the control test to include work as diverse as that undertaken by a trapeze artist[101] and bicycle couriers.[102]

More recently, the High Court has further considered the distinction between employees and independent contractors in two cases. The first involved a young person working for a labour hire company who sent him to work on a building site of a construction company.[103] When he left the job he claimed accrued leave entitlements and superannuation and was told he was not entitled to them as he was an independent contractor. The High Court determined he was an employee of the labour hire company and in doing so, emphasised the importance of examining questions of control of how, where and when work is performed. The second case involved two truck owner-drivers who provided transport services to a company over many years.[104] Both truck drivers had entered into independent contractor agreements between the company and each driver's respective partnership arrangements. In that case, the High Court determined the two owner-drivers were independent contractors emphasising the contractual terms entered into between the parties. Notwithstanding the importance of considering the terms of any written agreement, ultimately it is important to consider the character of the relationship established by the rights and obligations in the contract between the parties which is where the issue of control becomes important.

The Organisation Test

The application of the control test in relation to claims of negligence by the medical staff of hospitals ran into considerable legal difficulties for many years.

The courts took the view that, although hospitals were required to exercise due care in the selection of staff, they could not be made liable for the professional negligence of medical and nursing staff in carrying out their professional duties because they were unable to control them in the exercise of their professional judgment. Accordingly, the courts determined that hospital management could not be made vicariously liable for the negligent acts of such staff.

To overcome the limitations of the control test, the courts ultimately devised an alternative known as the organisation test. For that test to apply, the question to be asked is: Is the person part of the employer's organisation? Such a test has also been applied in the context of the following question: Is the person's work subject to coordinational control as to the *where* and *when* rather than the *how*?[105]

The attitude taken by the courts now is that hospitals are liable for the negligence of all staff, including nurses, midwives, resident medical officers, part-time anaesthetists and consultants, on the basis that they are part of the hospital organisation.

Using the organisation test, the full extent of the liability of hospital and health authorities for such staff was determined in a decision of the English appeal courts in 1954[106] where it was stated:

In the first place I think the hospital authorities are responsible for the whole of their staff, not only for the nurses and doctors but also for the anaesthetists and the surgeons. It does not matter whether they are permanent or temporary, resident or visiting, whole time or part time. The hospital authorities are responsible for all of them. The reason is because, even if they are not servants, they are the agents of the hospital to give the treatment. The only exception is the case of consultants or anaesthetists selected and employed by the patient himself.[107]

The organisation test has general application in Australian courts.[108]

There are occasions, however, when a court has considered the application of the organisation test and found it not applicable to the facts and circumstances of the particular case before it. For example, when a patient is a private patient and engages the doctor directly in his or her consulting rooms. Following the private consultation, the patient agrees to a particular treatment and is subsequently admitted to a particular hospital for that treatment. In those circumstances the hospital may not be liable for the negligence of the doctor when treating the patient in the hospital. Ultimately it would depend very much on the facts and circumstances of each case. Obviously, if the damage caused to the patient came about as the result of faulty hospital equipment being used by the doctor, or the negligence of the hospital staff, the hospital would be liable.

The Nurse or Midwife as an Independent Contractor as Distinct from an Employee

As stated earlier, the doctrine of vicarious liability revolves around the employer–employee relationship. While the great majority of nurses and midwives working in Australia are employees, as legally understood, some are not. Some are what the law refers to as independent contractors, or, as is more commonly understood, self-employed people. Where that situation exists, the need for professional indemnity insurance clearly arises.

The most obvious category of nurses or midwives working as independent contractors would be independent homebirth midwives or private duty nurses.

Despite the belief of many nurses and midwives, a nursing agency is generally not an employer. Although it would be necessary to consider the contractual terms as well as the particular facts and circumstances before a conclusive view could be expressed, in most circumstances the agency's purpose is to find work for the nurse or midwife, for which it charges the patient or client a commission.

If engaged in such a way, a nurse or midwife should maintain his or her own professional indemnity insurance policy, particularly if engaged to work in the patient's own home. In such a work situation, liability for a negligent act causing damage to the patient or client would rest squarely with the nurse or midwife, who would then rely on his or her professional indemnity insurance to pay any damages for which he or she may be found personally liable.

The position may not be so clear when an agency nurse or midwife is employed to work in a public or private hospital, as frequently happens in times of staffing shortages. If an agency nurse or midwife were negligent while employed in such a manner, the hospital would generally be considered directly liable, particularly if it could be shown that it engaged the services of an agency nurse or midwife and then required that nurse or midwife to work unsupervised in an area in which it knew, or ought to have known, he or she was not competent to work — for example, an intensive care unit. Alternatively, on the basis of the organisation test within the doctrine of vicarious liability, the hospital would be vicariously liable. However, it would still be open to the plaintiff to bring an action against the nurse or midwife on the basis of their personal liability but generally the personal financial circumstances of the nurse or midwife would deter such an action.

Apart from agency nurses, some nurses and midwives are employed directly by the patient — for example, homebirth midwives. In such a situation, the midwife is clearly an independent contractor and is required to have professional indemnity insurance.

A very good example of the professional and legal consequences that can follow a failure by an independent midwife to have professional indemnity insurance occurred in New South Wales in 2013.[109] In that case, the court found the homebirth midwife had been negligent in both recommending and carrying out the homebirth in 2006. The child was born following a protracted and difficult labour and was left with severe physical and intellectual disabilities. The court awarded the child and his mother $6.6 million in damages. Unfortunately the midwife had no professional indemnity insurance and little in the way of assets. The likelihood is that the mother and child will never receive the money awarded by the court.

As a general rule, because of the variable nature of the work undertaken, agency nurses as well as homebirth midwives should have professional indemnity insurance.

What Constitutes the Course and Scope of Employment?

The doctrine of vicarious liability clearly envisages that the employer's liability is confined to those negligent acts that arise within the course and scope of an employee's work.

The attitude of the courts as to what constitutes the 'course and scope of employment' is not subject to precise definition and has generally tended to be given the widest possible application, probably largely as a result of the courts' eagerness to ensure that a plaintiff will not go uncompensated because of an individual employee's negligent act and an inability to pay any monetary compensation awarded by the courts.

Generally speaking, the course and scope of employment will embrace all the authorised acts of an employee, even if such authorised acts are performed in an incorrect and unauthorised way.

If a nurse or midwife administered medications contrary to authorised hospital procedure and protocol and, in doing so, negligently gave the wrong drug, and the patient suffered damage, would the hospital be vicariously liable?

The answer is yes, because the giving of medications is well recognised as being part of the course and scope of the work of a nurse or midwife, and the fact that she or he gave them out in an unauthorised way contrary to the employer's policy does not allow the hospital to escape its liability.

The result of that example might well be different if the nurse prescribed the medication. As a general rule, nurses and midwives are not authorised to prescribe medications (nurse practitioner provisions and emergency circumstances aside). Should a nurse or midwife routinely take it upon herself or himself to prescribe medication, and a patient suffered damage as a result, then it could be argued that she or he had gone outside the course and scope of their work, and the hospital would not be vicariously liable for the damage caused and, more significantly, the payment of any compensation awarded.

Alternatively, an emergency situation might well be different. For example, in areas such as intensive care, registered nurses are sometimes authorised to administer, in the absence of a medical practitioner, a medication regimen that may be given in certain life-threatening situations. The authority for such emergency treatment would generally be found in the appropriate hospital policy document or clinical protocol, drawn up and approved by the medical officers concerned.

Where initiation of the administration of medications by registered nurses or midwives in emergency situations is sanctioned in appropriate circumstances, such actions will clearly come within the course and scope of employment. The same situation may arise in the labour ward where a midwife is authorised by a clinical protocol to administer certain medications in an obstetric emergency. As always, it is necessary to look at each case in the light of its own particular facts and circumstances.

To take the actions of a nurse or midwife outside the course and scope of employment, the actions of the nurse or midwife must consist of more than doing an act in a way or at a time that is prohibited by the employer. The employee's actions must also be so totally unrelated and removed from his or her normal course of employment that the employee is considered, on the occasion in question, to be 'in the position of stranger' vis-a-vis his or her employer.[110]

When an employee goes outside the course and scope of employment, it is often said that he or she is out on a 'frolic of his/her own'.

Where nurses or midwives are concerned, the temptation to embark on such a 'frolic' more often than not involves the use of motor vehicles and, in so doing, nurses or midwives working in the community are the most likely to be affected.

Problems Arising from the Use of Motor Vehicles Provided by the Employer for Use in the Course and Scope of Employment

When an employer provides an employee with a motor vehicle for the purposes of carrying out his or her work, the general intention is that the vehicle will be used only in the course of employment. A motor vehicle is often the cause of an employee going outside the course and scope of employment and embarking on a 'frolic of his/her own' because its use is relatively easy and temptingly convenient.

The question to be considered is to what extent, if at all, can an employee driving the employer's motor vehicle diverge from his or her normal work journey and still remain within the course and scope of employment. The attitude taken by the courts in such matters is to consider the extent and purpose of such divergence, bearing in mind that practical considerations do not often permit the most direct route to be used.

The following are examples of different views expressed by the courts.

1. A long-distance truck driver who turned off the highway to go to a hotel to get a drink negligently collided with a motor cycle. The court determined that the driver was acting in the course of employment, because it was reasonable to diverge from the highway for the purpose of obtaining refreshment. Accordingly the employer was vicariously liable.[111]

2. A courier was sent to deliver wine and collect empty bottles. On the return journey he agreed to give a friend a lift in a different direction from his usual route. An accident occurred caused by the courier's negligence. The court determined that the courier had diverged from the course of his employment and had undertaken a completely different journey. Accordingly the employer was held not to be vicariously liable.[112]

The above examples illustrate that an employee is not required to take the most direct route, and that a reasonable divergence from that route will not necessarily take the employee outside the course and scope of employment. Once again, it would be necessary to consider the facts and circumstances of each case, having regard to the views expressed by the courts.

A further problem arises when an employee gives a lift to a person while engaged in the course of employment and does not diverge from it.

Consider this example: A nurse working in the community is driving her employer's motor vehicle back to the community health centre after completing her visits for the day. It is mid-afternoon in summer and extremely hot. On the way back she notices an elderly woman walking slowly along the footpath and recognises her as a former client of the health centre. Concerned for her because of the heat, the nurse pulls over and asks the woman where she is going and if she can help. As it happens, the elderly lady is on her way to the outpatients' department at the local hospital. Coincidentally, the community health centre is situated in the grounds of the hospital and the nurse offers to drop her off. The elderly lady agrees and gets into the car. On the journey to the hospital the nurse negligently collides with another vehicle and the elderly lady is injured. The nurse's employer has consistently made it clear that staff members are not to give lifts to people, other than clients on authorised journeys.

Given the above facts, the nurse was clearly doing what she was not authorised to do, and yet her actions could not be said to be so totally unrelated or removed from her normal course of employment as to place her in the position of a stranger vis-a-vis her employer. In addition, at no time did the community nurse diverge from her usual route as part of the course and scope of her employment.

Is the nurse's employer vicariously liable for the injuries occasioned to the elderly woman as a result of the nurse's negligent driving?

Although no situation precisely resembling the above example has been dealt with by the courts on a reported basis, the courts have considered the position where an employee engaged in the course of employment gives a lift to a stranger contrary to the employer's instructions. In such situations, the courts have generally come to the view that the employer was not vicariously liable, on grounds that the employee was on a frolic of his or her own. The courts would consider all the facts and circumstances but, on balance, the fact that the nurse was acting outside the clear instructions of her employer in relation to giving lifts to strangers or even former patients, except in clearly authorised circumstances, would most likely render her actions as being outside the course and scope of her work as a nurse.

Consider another example: A community midwife was given permission to drive the employer's car to and from work but was instructed not to use it for personal errands. During days off the midwife used the car to go and visit friends some distance away. On the return journey an accident occurred as a result of the midwife's negligent driving. Although no one was injured, extensive property damage was done to two other vehicles. The owners of the two vehicles claimed compensation for the cost of repairing their vehicles from the owner of the vehicle that 'caused' the accident, that is, the midwife's employer. Would the employer have to pay?

In the circumstances outlined, the employer would be able to defend such a claim. The midwife was clearly not acting in the course and scope of her employment, having embarked on a frolic of her own, contrary to the employer's express instructions. Accordingly, the employer would not be vicariously liable, and the vehicle owners would have to recover their damages from the midwife.

It should be apparent, where a nurse or midwife is driving a motor vehicle owned by their employer and using it in the course and scope of employment, that there be clear written guidelines from the employer as to who may be transported in the motor vehicle and whether the motor vehicle may be used for private as well as business use.

Do not confuse the provision of a motor vehicle owned by the employer and used in the course and scope of employment with the provision of a motor vehicle as part of one's salary package. In the latter situation, the vehicle is clearly owned by the employee and the doctrine of vicarious liability has no application.

An Employer's Right to Seek a Financial Contribution or Total Financial Indemnity from a Negligent Employee

Where the employer is found to be vicariously liable and has to financially compensate the plaintiff for the negligent acts of one or more of its employees, the common law provided the employer with the right to recover the money paid out, either wholly or in part, from the negligent employee.

At first glance such a right would seem somewhat harsh and punitive. Indeed it has been all but abrogated in Australia.

Reality reveals that, in Australia, as a matter of common policy, employers do not pursue their common law right to recover a contribution or indemnity from negligent employees and that damage caused by such accidents is covered by insurance taken out by employers. The Commonwealth Parliament and the parliaments of New South Wales, the Northern Territory and South Australia have passed legislation to prevent employers from recovering monies from employees which the employers have been required to pay out as a result of being found vicariously liable.[113] However, no such protection exists for the employee if the negligent act arises from the employee's serious and wilful misconduct. What would be deemed to be serious and wilful misconduct is not defined.

In those states and territories with no legislative protection, the common law principles of contribution and indemnity could still be used, although, as a matter of

policy, it would be surprising if such a right were ever pursued in the courts.

Notwithstanding the doctrine of vicarious liability, it is still open to a plaintiff to bring his or her action against the negligent employee directly if he or she so chooses, thereby effectively bypassing the employer as a source of financial compensation. This decision would, for all practical purposes, be significantly constrained by the plaintiff's need to ensure that, if he or she is successful, the employee has sufficient personal financial resources to make such a task worthwhile. More often than not the plaintiff will pursue the employer as the better financial risk.

Under the South Australian legislation referred to earlier, provision is made that, should the plaintiff bring the action against the employee directly and succeed, the employee can recover the money he or she has to pay from the employer as long as the employee has no other form of indemnity insurance. The New South Wales legislation does not make such provision and certainly there is no such right in common law as far as the other states or territories are concerned.

The common law right of contribution or indemnity has led to the need for professionals generally, including health professionals, to consider professional indemnity insurance.

PROFESSIONAL INDEMNITY INSURANCE REQUIREMENTS FOR HEALTH PROFESSIONALS, INCLUDING NURSES AND MIDWIVES

In 1995, when the Commonwealth Government released its final report on compensation and professional indemnity in healthcare,[114] it found, among other matters, that there were 'strong public policy reasons to support government legislation requiring all health professionals to have adequate professional indemnity cover as a condition of practice'.

That recommendation was acted on by the states and territories in the context of moving to a system of national registration for health professionals. For nurses and midwives, that took effect in July 2010 by the passing of the uniform *National Law* by each of the states and territories. For example, in New South Wales it is known as the *Health Practitioner Regulation*

National Law (NSW). The provisions of the *National Law* in place in each of the states and territories since 2009 are in identical terms.

Section 129 of the *National Law* covers professional indemnity insurance arrangements and requires that a registered health practitioner must not practise in his or her field of registration unless 'appropriate professional indemnity insurance arrangements' are in force in relation to that practitioner's professional practice. In relation to the majority of nurses and midwives who are employed in the public or private sector by a hospital or designated health service (as distinct from independent contractors), the employer would have public liability and indemnity insurance in place and the individual nurse or midwife would not need to have her or his own professional indemnity insurance.

In those states where recovery from a negligent employee, whether on a total indemnity or contribution basis, is prohibited (New South Wales, the Northern Territory, South Australia and Commonwealth employees) the issue does not arise. In the other states and the Australian Capital Territory, it can be assumed that appropriate professional indemnity insurance arrangements are in place for all healthcare practitioners employed by the public sector and major private sector hospital and healthcare providers.

In some areas of the private sector, the situation may not be so clear-cut, and nurses and midwives employed in the private sector in the Australian Capital Territory, Queensland, Tasmania, Victoria and Western Australia should inquire about their employer's professional indemnity insurance arrangements.

Those nurses and midwives who are practising as independent contractors must ensure they secure appropriate professional indemnity insurance cover. Under the *National Law* provisions, independent midwives in the course of attending homebirths had a 2-year exemption from the mandatory requirement for professional indemnity insurance. That exemption initially expired in June 2012 but was later extended subject to certain conditions. (See **Chapter 4**, specifically Professional Indemnity Insurance Requirements for Privately Practising Midwives.)

In New South Wales, in addition to the requirement for mandatory professional indemnity insurance under the *Health Practitioner Regulation National Law*

(NSW), section 19 of the *Health Care Liability Act 2001* reaffirms the mandatory requirement that medical practitioners must have professional indemnity insurance as a condition of registration and practice. Further, for medical practitioners, section 19 also states that a failure to have professional indemnity insurance as required is deemed to be unsatisfactory professional conduct. Similar provisions exist in the other states and territories.

In addition to nurses, midwives and medical practitioners, other health professional groups covered by the provisions of the *National Law* in relation to the regulation of their profession include dental and medical practitioners, physiotherapists, pharmacists, optometrists, podiatrists, osteopaths, occupational therapists, psychologists and chiropractors.

The system of national registration and the professional obligations arising in relation to it are covered in detail in **Chapter 4**.

THE EMPLOYER'S DIRECT LIABILITY FOR NEGLIGENT EMPLOYEES

In addition to the application of the doctrine of vicarious liability, the law has also imposed a direct personal liability on the employer. That duty cannot be delegated and is known as a non-delegable duty of care.

What that means is that the law imposes on hospital and healthcare employers a general duty of care that is owed to the users of their health services. That duty of care requires that they provide a safe and competent health service and generally do all that is reasonable and proper in the delivery of that service to ensure that patients are not exposed to an unreasonable risk of harm. Clearly, it is reasonably foreseeable that a failure to do that may result in harm and damage to users of the service.

Inherent in such a general duty of care is the duty to employ safe and competent employees and to provide such employees with appropriate education as well as clear standards, policies and procedures and the necessary assistance to ensure employees are able to carry out their tasks safely and competently. When a patient or client suffers damage as a result of the negligence of a nurse or midwife in carrying out his or her professional services, the fault can often be directly attributed to the employer as a breach of the employer's direct duty to the patient that includes a duty to hire safe competent employees who are expected to work within safe clinical standards mandated by the employer.

THE NURSE OR MIDWIFE AS A GOOD SAMARITAN

One of the concerns frequently expressed by nurses and midwives is the liability they believe may arise if they stop and render first aid at a motor vehicle accident or other emergency. As a result of misinformation, nurses and other health professionals have often been actively discouraged for many years from rendering such assistance. Whatever the origins of such a belief, a number of issues require clarification and certain fears need to be put to rest in relation to this matter.

At the outset it must be said that there is no Australian case in which a 'good samaritan' has been sued by a person claiming that the actions of the good samaritan were negligent and as a result caused them harm.

As far as common law principles are concerned, there is no legal duty to stop and render assistance in any type of emergency, and that includes a motor vehicle accident. There are some exceptions to that rule:

- There is a legal duty to help where the person requiring assistance is directly related. For example, if the family home caught fire, the law would expect that, as far as was reasonably possible, the parents would attempt to rescue their children from the blaze.
- There is a legal duty to help when the person requiring assistance is under the control of another person where a duty is involved. For example, if a physical education teacher were involved in conducting a swimming class and one of the students got into difficulties, he or she would be under a duty to do all that was reasonably possible to assist the student.
- Specific legislation sometimes requires that a person must render assistance. For example, the most common legislative provisions apply to motor vehicle accidents where the requirement to stop and render assistance applies to the drivers of the motor vehicles involved in the accident.

No such legal requirement applies where a person comes across the scene of the accident while driving.

The legislative changes to civil liability law introduced by the states and territories (**Table 7.1**) incorporated provisions in relation to a person acting as a good samaritan. For example, section 56 of the *Civil Liability Act 2002* (NSW) defines a 'good samaritan' as:

… a person who, in good faith and without expectation of payment or other reward, comes to the assistance of a person who is apparently injured or at risk of being injured.

As provided by section 57 of that Act, a person acting as a good samaritan does not incur any personal civil liability in relation to any act or omission when assisting a person who is injured or at risk of being injured in an emergency.

The protection from civil liability for a person acting as a good samaritan does *not* apply if it is the good samaritan's intentional or negligent act or omission that caused the injury or risk of injury in respect of which the good samaritan first comes to the assistance of the person.

Under section 58, the protection from civil liability for a good samaritan also does not apply if:

2. a. *the ability of the good samaritan to exercise reasonable care and skill was significantly impaired by reason of the good samaritan being under the influence of alcohol or a drug voluntarily consumed (whether or not it was consumed for medication), and*
   b. *the good samaritan failed to exercise reasonable care and skill in connection with the act or omission.*
3. *This Part does not confer protection from personal liability on a person in respect of any act or omission done or made while the person is impersonating a health care or emergency services worker or a police officer or is otherwise falsely representing that the person has skills or expertise in connection with the rendering of emergency assistance.*

The provisions applying to good samaritans in the respective legislation of the other states and territories are set out below.

Australian Capital Territory: see *Civil Law (Wrongs) Act 2002* section 5. The 'good samaritan' is defined in similar terms to the New South Wales definition. No civil liability will attach to a good samaritan who acts in good faith and without recklessness. That exemption from liability will not attach if the good samaritan is significantly impaired by alcohol or drugs.

Northern Territory: see *Personal Injuries (Liabilities and Damages) Act 2003* section 8. The 'good samaritan' is defined in similar terms to the New South Wales definition. No civil liability will attach to a good samaritan who acts in good faith and without recklessness.

Queensland: see *Civil Liability Act 2003* section 26, which provides that no civil liability will attach where a person is rendering first aid or other assistance in an emergency and who does so in good faith and without reckless disregard for the safety of the person requiring assistance. Also, see *Law Reform Act 1995* section 16, which states that liability does not attach to a medical practitioner, nurse or 'other person' in rendering care, aid or assistance in an emergency if the act was done in good faith and without gross negligence and without expectation of fee or reward.

South Australia: see *Civil Liability Act 1936* section 74, which provides that no civil liability will attach to a 'good samaritan' acting without expectation of reward, and in good faith and without recklessness who comes to the aid of a person in an emergency. That immunity will not operate if the good samaritan's capacity was significantly impaired by alcohol or recreational drugs.

Tasmania: see *Civil Liability Act 2002* sections 35B and 35C, where the provisions closely resemble the New South Wales provisions, except the Tasmanian Act provides that the 'good samaritan' exemption is expressed as relating to the provision of assistance, advice or care at the scene of the emergency or accident (s 35B(2)(a)) or in providing advice by telephone or another means of communication to a person at the scene of the emergency or accident (s 35B(2)(b)).

Victoria: see *Wrongs Act 1958* section 31B. The definition of a 'good samaritan' is in relatively similar terms to that applying in New South Wales. Also, a good samaritan is not liable in any civil proceedings for anything done or not done in good faith.

Western Australia: see *Civil Liability Act 2002* sections 5AB and 5AD. The 'good samaritan' is defined in similar terms to the New South Wales definition. No civil liability will attach to a good samaritan who acts in good faith and without recklessness.

It is puzzling to know why good samaritan provisions were considered necessary in the civil liability legislation, particularly given there are no reported cases in Australia where such an action has been brought.

TIME LIMITS OR LIMITATION PERIODS FOR BRINGING A CIVIL NEGLIGENCE CLAIM

As in most civil litigation, the law imposes time limits or limitation periods for bringing a claim in negligence. Such limits will vary depending on the type of damage or injury that is being alleged. For example, in relation to a claim for damages for 'dust diseases' such as mesothelioma alleged to have been caused by exposure to asbestos particles, no limitation period is set in New South Wales, the Northern Territory or Victoria.[115]

Changes have been made by the states and territories to the relevant legislation setting limitation periods with respect to claims for personal injury or death. As a general rule, there is now a period of 3 years in which plaintiffs can commence such claims.[116] What is critical is determining when the limitation period begins to run. As a general rule, it is when the plaintiff suffers the damage complained of, although there are different approaches as to how that is determined between the states and territories. For example, in the Australian Capital Territory, Northern Territory, Queensland and South Australia the limitation period starts to run from the time the injury occurred. In New

South Wales and Tasmania the time begins to run from the date when the personal injury is 'discoverable', and in Victoria and Western Australia it runs from the date on which the action 'accrues'.

As a general rule, the prescribed limitation period for children does not begin to run until the child reaches the age of 18 years. Accordingly, depending on the limitation period applying in the particular state or territory, the young person would have until the age of 21 where the limitation period is 3 years and until the age of 24 where the limitation period is 6 years.

PROVISIONS FOR AN APOLOGY WITHIN THE CONTEXT OF POTENTIAL CIVIL LIABILITY FOR NEGLIGENCE

Very often, persons who commence negligence litigation against health professionals are reported as being motivated by the failure or refusal of the health professionals and health authorities to tell them 'how and why' things went wrong and never receiving an expression of regret or apology for the negligent actions.

The main reason given by health professionals and authorities for not admitting errors and apologising is because such statements are seen as an admission of liability with professional, financial and insurance implications.

This phenomenon has been addressed in the civil liability legislation enacted by the states and territories, although there are differences as to how the issue is dealt with.

For example, in New South Wales, section 69 of the *Civil Liability Act 2002* gives protection from liability for an apology in the following terms:

1. *An apology made by or on behalf of a person in connection with any matter alleged to have been caused by the person:*
    a. *does not constitute an express or implied admission of fault or liability by the person in connection with that matter, and*
    b. *is not relevant to the determination of fault or liability in connection with that matter.*
2. *Evidence of an apology made by or on behalf of a person in connection with any matter alleged to have been caused by the person is not admissible in any civil proceedings as evidence of the fault or liability of the person in connection with that matter.*

Section 68 of that Act defines an apology as follows:

apology means an expression of sympathy or regret, or of a general sense of benevolence or compassion, in connection with any matter whether or not the apology admits or implies an admission of fault in connection with the matter.

All other states and territories make provision for an 'apology' or 'expression of regret'. The respective provisions are: *Civil Law (Wrongs) Act 2002* (ACT) sections 12–14, *Personal Injuries (Liabilities and Damages) Act 2003* (NT) sections 12 and 13, *Civil Liability Act 2003* (Qld) sections 71 and 72, *Civil Liability Act 1936* (SA) section 75, *Civil Liability Act 2002* (Tas) section 7, *Wrongs Act 1958* (Vic) sections 14I and 14J, and *Civil Liability Act 2002* (WA) section 5AH.

There is considerable similarity between the respective legislative provisions of the states and territories. The extent to which such provisions are used by health authorities and health professionals is unknown but can only be encouraged where appropriate.

CONCLUSION

Knowledge of the law and the application of the legal principles relating to the determination of professional negligence are of utmost importance to all nurses and midwives. They reinforce the legal and professional obligation of nurses and midwives to ensure they incorporate and maintain professional practice standards into all aspects of their care and treatment.

CHAPTER 7 REVIEW QUESTIONS

Following your reading of **Chapter 7**, consider these questions in reaching the objectives of this chapter. Guidance on which part of the chapter will assist you in answering the questions can be found at http://evolve. elsevier.com/AU/Staunton/law/. You may, of course, consider other sources as part of your considerations.

1. What is the legal test used to determine the standard of care expected in the delivery of your professional services as a nurse of midwife? In considering your response, refer as necessary to the civil liability legislation of your state or territory.

2. What do you understand to be 'peer professional opinion'? How would that be established by a court?

3. In addition to 'peer professional opinion', what are other sources of evidence that courts would consider in determining the appropriate standard of care expected of a nurse or midwife in a particular clinical situation?

4. As a nurse or midwife, is it professionally appropriate for you to question the treatment or medication orders of a medical practitioner or other health professional? If so, give an example where you might do so and what steps you would take to deal with such a situation.

5. Should a registered midwife working as a home-birth midwife have professional indemnity insurance? If so, why is it necessary?

6. While driving on your day off, you come across a motor vehicle accident. The people in the vehicles are clearly injured. Are you under a legal obligation to stop and render assistance? If so, what are those obligations?

7. Select one of the case examples numbered **Case example 7.3** to **Case example 7.11**. Read the case details and commentary and identify the specific clinical failures identified by the respective court in relation to the actions of the nurse/s or midwife/midwives in question.

ENDNOTES

1. *Donoghue v Stevenson* [1932] AC 562, at 619.
2. Ibid.
3. *BT (as administratrix of the estate of the late AT) v Oei* [1999] NSWSC 1082.
4. Now the *Public Health Act 2010* (NSW).
5. *Rogers v Whitaker* [1992] HCA 58; (1992) 175 CLR 479.
6. Ibid, at [12].
7. Ibid, at [14].
8. Ibid, at [16].
9. *Chappel v Hart* (1998) 195 CLR 232; *Rosenberg v Percival* (2001) 205 CLR 434.
10. *Chappel v Hart* (1998) 195 CLR 232 at 276–7.
11. Ibid.
12. National Health and Medical Research Council: *Making decisions about tests and treatments: principles for better communication between healthcare consumers and healthcare professionals: endorsed*, 2006 and current. Always check NHMRC website for updates.
13. Nursing and Midwifery Board of Australia: Enrolled Nurse Standards for practice: Reviewed 1/2/2017: Endorsed Ahpra 2023.
14. *Langley v Glandore Pty Ltd (in liquidation)* [1997] QCA 342 (30 October 1997); (1997) Aust Tort Reports 81-448 at 64, 560.
15. Ibid, at 64, 567.
16. Coroner's inquest into the death of Bodhi Eastlake-McClure, Deputy State Coroner Dillon, NSW Coroner's Court, 7 August 2014.
17. *Lahey Estate v Craig* (1992) 123 NBR (2d) 91.
18. *Thompson Estate v Byrne* (1992) 104 Nfld and PEIR 9.
19. *Versteegh v The Nurses Board of South Australia* (1992) 60 SASR 128.
20. Now *Public Health Act 2010* (NSW).
21. Now *Public Health Regulation 2012* (NSW).
22. Now *Public Health Act 2010* (NSW) s 78.
23. Now *Public Health Regulation 2012* (NSW) reg 40.
24. Now *Public Health Act 2010* (NSW) s 52.
25. Now *Public Health Act 2010* (NSW) s 79.
26. Ibid.
27. *BT (as administratrix of the estate of the late AT) v Oei* [1999] NSWSC 1082 at [92]–[94].
28. Coroner's inquest into the death of Paul Lau, Coroner's Court of NSW: No 2015/181507, 29 March 2018.
29. Ibid, at [46].
30. Ibid, at [154].
31. Ibid, at [153].
32. Ibid, at [170].
33. *Sha Cheng Wang v Central Sydney Area Health Service* [2000] NSWSC 515; (SC (NSW), Hidden J, No. 17083/90, 9 June 2000, unreported).
34. Ibid, at [39].

35. Ibid, at [21].
36. Ibid, at [48].
37. Ibid, at [64]–[65].
38. Ibid, at [69].
39. Ibid, at [70]–[71], [76]–[77].
40. *McCabe v Auburn District Hospital* (SC (NSW), Grove J, No. 11551 of 1982, 31 May 1989, unreported).
41. Ibid, p 17.
42. Ibid, p 18.
43. Ibid, p 31.
44. *Norton v Argonaut Insurance Company* (1962) 144 So 2d 249 (Ct App La).
45. Ibid.
46. *Ison v Northern Rivers Area Health Service* (Industrial Relations Court of Australia, Tomlinson J, No. 44/97, 3 March 1997, unreported).
47. Ibid, at 3.
48. Ibid.
49. Ibid, at 15.
50. Ibid, at 22.
51. Ibid, at 24.
52. Ibid, at 27.
53. *Langley v Glandore Pty Ltd (in liquidation)* [1997] QCA 342 (30 October 1997); (1997) Aust Tort Reports 81-448.
54. Ibid, at 64, 569.
55. Ibid, at 64, 567.
56. Ibid, at 64, 567–8.
57. Ibid, at 64, 569.
58. *Elliott v Bickerstaff* [1999] NSWCA 453 (16 December 1999).
59. Ibid, at [101].
60. Ibid, at [102]–[103].
61. Coroner's inquest into the death of Samara Lea Hoy, Southport Coroner's Court, Feb–Jun 2010.
62. Ibid, at 4.
63. Ibid, at 6.
64. Ibid, at 6.
65. Ibid, at 23.
66. Coroner's inquest into the death of Bodhi Eastlake-McClure, NSW Coroner's Court, Deputy State Coroner Dillon, 7 August 2014.
67. Ibid, at [30].
68. Ibid, at [35]–[36].
69. Ibid, at [39]–[40].
70. Ibid, at [49].
71. Coroner's inquest into the death of MA, NSW Coroner's Court: No. 2014/65501: 2 February 2018.
72. Ibid, at [66].
73. Ibid, at [30].
74. Ibid, at [54].
75. Ibid, at [56].
76. Ibid, at [169].
77. Ibid, at [14] where reference is made to the Findings of the Professional Standards Committee Inquiry constituted under Part 8 of the *Health Practitioner Regulation National Law* (NSW) in the inquiry into a complaint in relation to Mr Abraham Thomas Registration No. NMW 0001711533; Ms Donna Hayden Registration No. NMW0001406174, presently unregistered; and Ms Julie Rumble Registration No. NMW0001010046, presently unregistered [Ref: 4603/17] dated 28 April 2017.
78. Ibid, at [15].
79. Ibid, at [100]–[109].
80. Ibid, at [113].
81. Ibid, at [113].
82. Ibid, at [14].
83. Ibid, at [120].
84. Ibid, at [131].
85. Ibid, at [249].
86. The colour-coded parameters that appear on standard observation charts are known as 'Between the Flags' and are coloured red and yellow. When a patient's baseline observations fall within either of those colour-coded parameters, clinical policy standards require the relevant treating practitioner to be notified.
87. Coroner's inquest into the death of Timothy John Bice, Adelaide Coroner's Court, Jul–Aug 1989.
88. Ibid.
89. Ibid.
90. Ibid.
91. *McDonald v York County Hospital* (1973) 41 DLR (3d) 321.
92. *Bergen v Sturgeon General Hospital* (1984) 28 CCLT 155.
93. *Barnett v Chelsea and Kensington Hospital* [1969] 1 QB 428.
94. *Finch v Rogers* [2004] NSWSC 39.
95. Ibid, at [134].
96. Ibid, at [147] and [148].
97. *Tabet v Gett* [2010] HCA 12.
98. Ibid, at [111].
99. *Civil Law (Wrongs) Act 2002* (ACT); *Compensation (Fatal Injuries) Act 1974* (NT); *Supreme Court Act 1995* (Qld); *Civil Liability Act 1936* (SA); *Fatal Accidents Act 1934* (Tas); *Wrongs Act 1958* (Vic); *Fatal Accidents Act 1959* (WA).
100. *Civil Law (Wrongs) Act 2002* (ACT) s 102; *Law Reform (Miscellaneous Provisions) Act 1965* (NSW) s 9(1) and *Civil Liability Act 2002* (NSW) ss 5R and 5S; *Law Reform (Miscellaneous Provisions) Act 1956* (NT) s 16(1); *Law Reform Act 1995* (Qld) s 10(1) and *Civil Liability Act 2003* (Qld) ss 23 and 24; *Law Reform (Contributory Negligence and Apportionment of Liability) Act 2001* (SA) s 7 and *Civil Liability Act 1936* (SA) s 44; *Wrongs Act 1954* (Tas) s 4(1) and *Civil Liability Act 2002* (Tas) s 23; *Wrongs Act 1958* (Vic) ss 26(1) and 44; *Law Reform (Contributory Negligence and Tortfeasors' Contribution) Act 1947* (WA) s 4(1) and *Civil Liability Act 2002* (WA) s 5K.
101. *Zuijs v Wirth Bros Pty Ltd* (1955) 93 CLR 561.
102. *Hollis v Vabu Pty Ltd* (2001) 207 CLR 21.
103. *CFMEU & Anor v Personnel Contracting Pty Ltd* (2022) HCA 1.
104. *ZG Operations Australia Pty Ltd & Anor v Jamesek & Ors* (2022) HCA 2.
105. Fleming J G, *The law of torts*, 9th ed, Law Book Company, Sydney, 1998, p 416.
106. *Roe v Minister for Health* [1954] 2 QB 66.

107. Ibid, p 82.
108. *Albrighton v Royal Prince Alfred Hospital* (1980) 2 NSWLR 542; *Ellis v Wallsend District Hospital* (1989) 17 NSWLR 553.
109. *Patterson v Khalsa* (No 3) [2013] NSWSC 1331.
110. Fleming, op. cit., p 421.
111. *Chaplin v Dunstan* (1938) SASR 245.
112. *Storey v Ashton* (1986) IR 4 QB 476.
113. *Insurance Contracts Act 1984* (Cth) s 66; *Employees Liability Act 1991* (NSW) ss 3, 5 and 6; *Law Reform (Miscellaneous Provisions) Act 1984* (NT) s 22A; *Civil Liability Act 1936* (SA) s 59.

114. *Compensation and professional indemnity in healthcare: final report*, Australian Government Publishing Service, Canberra, November 1995.
115. *Dust Diseases Tribunal Act 1989* (NSW) s 12A; *Limitation Act 1981* (NT) s 12(2)(a).
116. *Limitation of Actions Act 1958* (Vic) s 27B(2)(d); *Limitation Act 1985* (ACT) s 16B(2); *Limitation Act 1969* (NSW) ss 18A and 50C; *Limitation Act 1981* (NT) s 12(1); *Limitation of Actions Act 1974* (Qld) s 11; *Limitation of Actions Act 1936* (SA) s 36; *Limitation Act 1974* (Tas) s 5(1); *Limitations of Actions Act 1958* (Vic) s 5(1AA); *Limitation Act 2005* (WA) s 13(1).

Section 4   NURSING PRACTICE

8

THE ADMINISTRATION OF DRUGS

LEARNING OBJECTIVES

In this chapter, you will:

- examine the state, territory and Commonwealth legislation relating to the management and control of medicines in Australia
- consider mechanisms for identifying those nurses, nurse practitioners and midwives who are authorised to administer or endorsed to prescribe medicines
- identify strategies for the safe management and administration of drugs
- explore common problems relating to the management and administration of drugs that might result in an adverse event.

INTRODUCTION

This chapter sets out in detail the legislative and policy requirements for nurses, nurse practitioners (NPs) and midwives in relation to the management, administration and, more recently, the prescription of drugs. It considers not only the correct way to manage these matters, but also the reasons why adverse medication events occur and what can be done to avoid them.

The Australian Institute of Health and Welfare reported that the Australian Government spent $13.9 billion on all PBS and RPBS medicines in 2020–21, with PBS accounting for 98% of the spend. That averaged out to $541 per person. Spending increased by 8.4% compared to 2019–20.[1]

In addition, many medicines are purchased over the counter without a prescription, including analgesics (painkillers), cough medicines and vitamins, and complementary and alternative medicine (CAM) use has become an established part of healthcare for many Australians. CAM is estimated to be used by up to two out of three Australians, and in 2017 was estimated to account for a further $3.5 billion in expenditure every year.[2]

The Pharmaceutical Society of Australia notes that 250 000 hospital admissions annually are a result of medication-related problems, at an annual cost of $1.4 billion, and a further 400 000 additional presentations to emergency departments are likely to be due to medication-related problems. Up to 50% of the harm caused is considered to be preventable.[3]

The great majority of medications that nurses and midwives administer on a day-to-day basis are considered to be, and are defined by legislation as, poisons. That is, generally speaking, they are substances that, by their very nature, are inherently dangerous to one's health if not used appropriately.[4] Accordingly, it is considered necessary to identify them and lay down clear provisions as to how such substances may be obtained, the basis on which a person may have possession of them, who may prescribe them, how they must be stored and other specific provisions for certain substances.

The Commonwealth and each state and territory has legislation that covers the control and supply of poisons and therapeutic goods (see Box 8.1). Among other things, these pieces of legislation set out the specific responsibilities of nurses, NPs and midwives in

BOX 8.1

LIST OF STATUTES AND REGULATIONS GOVERNING MEDICATIONS IN AUSTRALIA

Cth	*Narcotic Drugs Act 1967*
	Narcotic Drugs (Licence Charges) Act 2016
	Therapeutic Goods Act 1989
	Therapeutic Goods (Charges) Act 1989
	Therapeutic Goods Regulations 1990
	Therapeutic Goods (Charges) Regulations 2018
ACT	*Dangerous Substances Act 2004*
	Drugs of Dependence Act 1989
	Drugs of Dependence (Personal Use) Amendment Act 2022
	Medicines, Poisons and Therapeutic Goods Act 2008
	Medicines, Poisons and Therapeutic Goods Regulation 2008
NSW	*Drug and Alcohol Treatment Act 2007*
	Drug Court Act 1998
	Drug Misuse and Trafficking Act 1985
	Drug Supply Prohibition Order Pilot Scheme Act 2020
	Poisons and Therapeutic Goods Act 1966
	Poisons and Therapeutic Goods Regulation 2008
	Poisons and Therapeutic Goods (Poisons List) Proclamation 2016
NT	*Misuse of Drugs Act 1990*
	Misuse of Drugs Regulations 1990
	Medicines, Poisons and Therapeutic Goods Act 2012
	Medicines, Poisons and Therapeutic Goods Regulation 2014
Qld	*Drugs Misuse Act 1986*
	Drugs Misuse Regulation 1987
	Health (Drugs and Poisons) Regulation 1996
	Medicines and Poisons Act 2019
	Therapeutic Goods Act 2019
	Therapeutic Goods Regulation 2021
SA	*Controlled Substances Act 1984*
	Controlled Substances (Controlled Drugs, Precursors and Plants) Regulations 2014
	Dangerous Substances Act 1979
	Dangerous Substances (Dangerous Goods Transport) Regulations 2008
	Dangerous Substances (General) Regulations 2017
	Health Care Act 2008
	Health Care Regulations 2008

Tas	*Misuse of Drugs Act 2001*
	Poisons Act 1971 (Note: under section 14(1) and (2), the Minister may adopt Part 4 of the Uniform Standard (SUSMP) as the Poisons List, and may amend its application to Tasmania.)
	Poisons (Adoption of Uniform Standard) Order 2012
	Poisons (Application of Uniform Standard) Order 2021
	Poisons (Declared Restricted Substances) Order 2017
	Poisons (Drugs Of Dependence) Order 2009
	Poisons (Exempted Public Institutions) Order 2020
	Poisons (Midwifery Substances) Order 2011
	Poisons (Notifiable Restricted Substances) Order 2009
	Poisons (Prescribed Periods) Order 2009
	Poisons (Public Institutions) Order 2000
	Poisons Regulations 2018
	Poisons (Specified Substances) Revocation Order 2023
Vic	*Drugs, Poisons and Controlled Substances Act 1981*
	Therapeutic Goods (Victoria) Act 2010
	Drugs, Poisons and Controlled Substances (Commonwealth Standard) Revocation Regulations 2014
	Drugs, Poisons and Controlled Substances (Confiscation) Regulations 2014
	Drugs, Poisons and Controlled Substances (Industrial Hemp) Regulations 2018
	Drugs, Poisons and Controlled Substances (Poppy Cultivation and Processing) Regulations 2014
	Drugs, Poisons and Controlled Substances (Precursor Chemicals) Regulations 2017
	Drugs, Poisons and Controlled Substances (Precursor Supply) Regulations 2021
	Drugs, Poisons and Controlled Substances (Volatile Substances) Regulations 2014
	Drugs, Poisons and Controlled Substances Regulations 2017
WA	*Medicines and Poisons Act 2014*
	Medicines and Poisons (Validation) Act 2022
	Medicines and Poisons Regulations 2016

relation to the various types of drugs that they have to deal with and administer in their work. The possibility of making drug-related errors, and the legal consequences that can flow from this, are such that nurses and midwives need to be aware, not only of specific legislative requirements that apply to them, but also how to minimise the possibility of errors occurring.

The information contained in this chapter will be of value to registered nurses and midwives and also to enrolled nurses. In the past, only registered nurses and midwives were allowed to administer medications against a prescription. However, education programs now enable enrolled nurses across Australia to administer medications. At the time of writing, all enrolled nurses are presumed to be able to administer medications under the new national registration scheme. Enrolled nurses who are not educated to administer medications are expected to advise the Nursing and Midwifery Board of Australia (NMBA), so that a notation can be put against their registration to advise employers and the general public that they are not educated or able to administer medications. When an enrolled nurse who is not educated to administer medications completes the relevant required program of study, they are then able to apply to the NMBA to have the notation lifted from their registration.[5]

The legislation that governs the management of medication has different titles in the different jurisdictions (see Box 8.1). Not only are there statutes that govern the control of drugs, there are also very specific regulations and orders that set out exactly how medications must be managed and the degree of control to which specific medications and drugs are subject. The legislation embraces all conceivable types of poisons available, ranging from agricultural poisons and domestic pesticides to drugs of addiction. The relevant legislation in each state and territory is relatively similar in how it classifies and identifies poisons and therapeutic goods, but there are differences in the detailed provisions that apply in some areas. In addition, as part of these various statutes, certain criminal offences are indicated where a person deals with certain poisons in a manner contrary to the provisions, particularly drugs of addiction. Criminal charges in relation to well-publicised drug offences, such as the possession or supply of heroin or cocaine, arise under other legislation.

For the sake of clarity and because of varying legal requirements, the types of poisons or drugs available are divided into various sections, called schedules, which are determined by the Poisons Standard, currently Poisons Standard June 2023 (Cth), established under paragraph 52D(2)(b) of the *Therapeutic Goods Act 1989* (Cth). Such provisions are then incorporated into the various statutes in each jurisdiction. For legal definitions, it is still necessary to check with each relevant state or territory authority, but the Standard for the Uniform Scheduling of Medicines and Poisons (SUSMP), contained in the various schedules of the Poisons Standard, provides the template for each jurisdiction.[6]

Each of the 10 schedules of the SUSMP 24 provides a comprehensive list of poisons that are classified according to the degree of control recommended to be exercised over their availability to the public. The SUSMP points out, in the Principles of Scheduling, that poisons are not scheduled on the basis of a universal scale of toxicity, stating:

Poisons are not scheduled on the basis of a universal scale of toxicity. Although toxicity is one of the factors considered, and is itself a complex of factors, the decision to include a substance in a particular Schedule also takes into account many other criteria such as the purpose of use, potential for abuse, safety in use and the need for the substance.

This instrument lists poisons in 10 Schedules according to the degree of control recommended to be exercised over their availability to the public.

Poisons for therapeutic use (medicines) are mostly included in Schedules 2, 3, 4 and 8 with progression through these Schedules signifying increasingly restrictive regulatory controls.[7]

The classification of the 10 schedules is reproduced in Table 8.1.

The specific schedules that are most relevant to nursing staff are those generally identified as Schedule 4 substances and Schedule 8 substances.

Schedule 4 substances are commonly referred to as 'prescription only' or restricted substances and cover all drugs that are able and required to be provided on the prescription of a medical practitioner, nurse practitioner, endorsed midwife, dentist or veterinary surgeon.

Schedule 8 substances are called 'controlled drugs' and sometimes 'drugs of addiction'. Apart from the Schedule 8 drugs, there are few drugs that nurses or midwives administer on a day-to-day basis that do not come within Schedule 4. For example, such drugs as antibiotics, anti-hypertensives and anticoagulants clearly fall into Schedule 4, as they can be obtained only on prescription.

In some jurisdictions, certain drugs are declared to be Schedule 4 substances but in terms of storage and security are required to be dealt with in the same manner as Schedule 8 substances. Although Schedule 8 substances are commonly referred to as controlled

	TABLE 8.1	
	Classification of Poisons Under the Schedules of the SUSMP (Poisons Standard)	
Schedule	**Title**	**Description**
Schedule 1	Blank	This Schedule is intentionally blank.
Schedule 2	Pharmacy medicines	Substances, the safe use of which may require advice from a pharmacist and which should be available from a pharmacy or, where a pharmacy service is not available, from a licensed person.
Schedule 3	Pharmacist only medicines	Substances, the safe use of which requires professional advice but which should be available to the public from a pharmacist without a prescription.
Schedule 4	Prescription only medicines and prescription animal remedies	Substances, the use or supply of which should be by or on the order of persons permitted by State or Territory legislation to prescribe and should be available from a pharmacist on prescription.
Schedule 5	Caution	Substances with a low potential for causing harm, the extent of which can be reduced through the use of appropriate packaging with simple warnings and safety directions on the label.
Schedule 6	Poisons	Substances with a moderate potential for causing harm, the extent of which can be reduced through the use of distinctive packaging with strong warnings and safety directions on the label.
Schedule 7	Dangerous poisons	Substances with a high potential for causing harm at low exposure and which require special precautions during manufacture, handling or use. These poisons should be available only to specialised or authorised users who have the skills necessary to handle them safely. Special regulations restricting their availability, possession, storage or use may apply.
Schedule 8	Controlled drugs	Substances which should be available for use but require restriction of manufacture, supply, distribution, possession and use to reduce abuse, misuse and physical or psychological dependence.
Schedule 9	Prohibited substances	Substances which may be abused or misused, the manufacture, possession, supply or use of which should be prohibited by law except when required for medical or scientific research, or for analytical, teaching or training purposes with approval of Commonwealth and/or State or Territory Health Authorities.
Schedule 10 (previously Appendix C)	Substances of such danger to health as to warrant prohibition of supply and use	Substances which are prohibited for the purpose or purposes listed for each poison.

drugs, in New South Wales they are known as drugs of addiction, (sometimes) in Tasmania as narcotic substances and in Western Australia as drugs of dependence. Whatever the minor variation in titles, the type of drugs that come within this schedule are usually the narcotic analgesics such as opium, opium derivatives (such as morphine) and synthetic opium derivatives (such as pethidine).

Some substances that nurses and midwives administer from time to time are not required to be provided on prescription. They are often referred to as 'nurse- or midwife-initiated medications' and can be administered by nursing or midwifery staff without a medical officer's authority or prescription. These medications usually include substances such as antacids, aperients and paracetamol. Nurses and midwives should not automatically assume their right to administer such substances without reference and should do so only in accordance with clearly written guidelines drawn up by the hospital or health authority.[8]

The specific list of drugs under the various schedules changes fairly frequently as new drugs are developed and introduced. It is therefore essential that nurses and midwives maintain their awareness of this aspect and that any relevant addition or change to the list of drugs in Schedule 4 or Schedule 8 be communicated to them. Hospitals are automatically notified of relevant changes to the poisons legislation by the state or territory health departments, generally by way of departmental circulars. To the extent that they are relevant, such circulars should be acted upon where necessary and distributed to all staff concerned.

EXAMINING THE RELEVANT REGULATIONS

As already indicated, the various state and territory Acts and the division of the schedules are essentially similar in fundamental layout and content, and it is not intended to incorporate the precise details of each state or territory's legislative provisions in this text. The Regulations that accompany each of the Acts, and that are extremely important to nurses and midwives, vary in the precise words used concerning requirements as to the authority to prescribe, possess, control, supply, store and so on, but not to any significant degree. Some Regulations are more precise and detailed than others, and nurses and midwives in each state and territory should read their relevant Regulations carefully. When doing so, it is important to note the distinction between the words 'prescribe', 'dispense' and 'administer'. In general terms, medical and nurse practitioners and endorsed midwives (and others) prescribe, pharmacists dispense, and nurses and midwives (and others) administer. The degree of commonality in the various state and territory Regulations can best be summarised as follows:

- Schedule 4: restricted substances;
- Schedule 8: controlled substances.

Schedule 4: Restricted Substances

As a general rule, only medical and nurse practitioners, endorsed midwives, dentists and veterinary surgeons can issue a prescription for a restricted substance. Prescriptions are required to contain specific details, such as the name and address of the patient, date, drug and dosage. Some states and territories require that the prescriber writes 'legibly' although this may be overcome with electronic prescribing. In an emergency, a medical practitioner can direct the dispensing of a restricted substance orally, including by telephone, subject to certain requirements.

Except in hospitals, no person other than a pharmacist or a pharmacist's assistant can dispense a prescription for a restricted substance. In hospitals where a pharmacist is employed, he or she is responsible for storing and recording restricted substances. In hospitals where no pharmacist is employed, the director of nursing or, in his or her absence, the person acting in the position, or the medical superintendent, has this responsibility. More often than not, in remote areas such a task falls to the registered nurse in charge because there is no medical practitioner on the premises. In remote areas, the rule is that access to the drug storage room must be restricted to Ahpra registered staff who are able to possess and supply medicines.[9] Whoever is responsible for storing and supplying restricted substances must not issue such a substance from hospital stocks unless he or she has a proper prescription or the appropriate ward requisition slip from the nurse in charge of the ward.

Restricted substances can be administered in hospitals only on the written authority of a medical or nurse practitioner or an endorsed midwife, except in the case of an 'emergency' when the medical or nurse practitioner or endorsed midwife may verbally authorise the administration of a restricted substance. If the medical or nurse practitioner or endorsed midwife verbally authorises the administration of such a substance, he or she must confirm that verbal authority generally within 24–48 hours by writing in the patient's notes.[10]

Schedule 8: Controlled Substances

Certain persons are authorised to be in possession of and to supply certain drugs of addiction for the purposes of their profession or employment. This list can vary between jurisdictions and also depending on the location. However such persons generally include:

- a pharmacist;
- a medical practitioner;
- the director of nursing of a public hospital where no pharmacist is employed or, in the pharmacist's absence, the person acting in the position;
- the nurse or midwife in charge of a ward in a public hospital;

- a nurse or midwife employed in a community health centre;
- a nurse employed in air ambulance duties;
- a director of nursing and/or midwifery of a private hospital or nursing home; or
- an Aboriginal or Torres Strait Islander health practitioner.

It is important to remember that where a nurse or midwife, or any other person for that matter, is given authority to be 'in possession and supply' of drugs of addiction then provision is also made for such authority to be withdrawn if it is breached or exceeded.

Only a medical or nurse practitioner, endorsed midwife, dentist or veterinary surgeon can issue a prescription for a drug of addiction. The requirements for such prescriptions are similar to those for restricted substances. In an emergency a medical or nurse practitioner or endorsed midwife can direct the dispensing of a drug of addiction orally, including by telephone, subject to certain requirements. Except in hospitals, no person other than a pharmacist or a pharmacist's assistant can dispense a prescription for a Schedule 8 drug.

The nurse or midwife in charge of a ward or clinic is required to keep all drugs of addiction stored separately from other goods, with the exception of certain other restricted substances, such as Schedule 4 restricted substances. The storage area should be a separate receptacle or cupboard securely fixed to the premises, which should be kept securely locked when not in use. Any person, including a nurse or midwife, authorised to be in possession of and to supply drugs of addiction is to keep the safe or cupboard in which they are stored securely locked and keep the key on his or her person.[11] If the authorised person is absent from the premises, the key to the cupboard or safe must be left in a secure location.

Approval can be given by state or territory health authorities for drugs of addiction to be kept in approved first-aid kits for use in an emergency in isolated localities, in an occupational health centre, in search and rescue operations or in other approved situations. In such approved situations a register must still be kept.

Ward Registers or Drugs Books

The nurse or manager in charge of a facility where Schedule 8 drugs are stored is required to keep a register of controlled drugs in that facility; this is known as a medicine register. For example, under sections 205 and 206 of the *Medicines and Poisons (Medicines) Regulation 2021 (Qld)* a medicine register, for an Schedule 8 safe or approved store, is a document that is required to state when each type of medicine is put in, or taken from, the safe or store for a dealing; and the amount of the type of medicine in the safe or store at any given time. The manager is required to take all reasonable steps to make and keep a medicine register for the safe or store; and to keep the medicine register with, or as close as practicable to, the safe or store. The register may be paper (s 209) or electronic (s 208). If any drug of addiction is lost, destroyed or rendered unusable, a person authorised to possess such drugs must be notified. In the case of a drug of addiction that is unusable and has to be destroyed, the destruction of the drug must be undertaken by the pharmacist, director of nursing or medical superintendent in the presence of another person and a record made in the register of such loss or destruction. Where an ampoule of a drug of addiction is only 'part used' and the remainder discarded, the entry in the register should record that fact. See **Clinical example 8.1**.

CLINICAL EXAMPLE 8.1

A patient is ordered 75 mcg of fentanyl and the only ampoules available are 100 mcg ampoules. Therefore, the register records that the patient received 75 mcg and the remaining 25 mcg was destroyed on the basis that it had been rendered unusable.

The relevant Regulations usually specify what a nurse is required to do if there is a discrepancy or drugs are missing — for example, notify a relevant person or body. The process for such notification should also be spelled out in the employer's policy and procedure manual.

Storage of Drugs for Voluntary Assisted Dying

As was discussed in **Chapter 6**, voluntary assisted dying has been introduced into all jurisdictions in Australia except the ACT and the NT at the time of writing. Clearly the medications associated with voluntary assisted dying are used to end life, rather than for traditional therapeutic purposes, and as such all the statutes make provision for the storage, prescription, administration and disposal of the medications to be used for voluntary assisted dying. Each jurisdiction has slightly different provisions, so the nurse or midwife needs to check their own legislation, but some useful documents have been developed to assist with the processes.[12]

PROBLEM AREAS WITH DRUGS

Although a sound knowledge of the relevant legislation relating to drugs and poisons is essential for all nurses and midwives, what is equally important is an awareness of the problem areas in relation to drugs and how to avoid or deal with them. Mistakes can and do occur, and it is unlikely that any system devised will ever entirely eliminate the probability of drug-related errors occurring. Hospital administrators, medical and nurse practitioners, endorsed midwives, and registered and enrolled nurses and midwives should recognise their respective responsibilities in this area and take steps to minimise the risk of errors occurring and, when they do, to minimise the damage that flows from them — the law would expect such a response to be reasonable, considering the clear duty of care that is owed to the patient.

The Australian Commission on Safety and Quality in Health Care (ACSQHC) has identified medication safety as one of its priorities. In the second version of the ACSQHC National Standards, Medication Safety is a stand-alone standard — Standard 4.

The aim of the Medication Safety Standard is:

> ... to ensure that clinicians safely prescribe, dispense and administer appropriate medicines, and monitor medicine use. It also aims to ensure that consumers are informed about medicines, and understand their own medicine needs and risks.[13]

The environment in which medicines are regulated, prescribed, supplied, administered and monitored in Australia is complex, and the Commission has selected four overarching criteria by which to assess medication safety. These are as follows:

Clinical governance and quality improvement to support medication management

Organisation-wide systems are used to support and promote safety for procuring, supplying, storing, compounding, manufacturing, prescribing, dispensing, administering and monitoring the effects of medicines.

Documentation of patient information

A patient's best possible medication history is recorded when commencing an episode of care. The best possible medication history, and information relating to medicine allergies and adverse drug reactions are available to clinicians.

Continuity of medication management

A patient's medicines are reviewed, and information is provided to them about their medicines needs and risks. A medicines list is provided to the patient and the receiving clinician when handing over care.

Medication management processes

Health service organisations procure medicines for safety. Clinicians are supported to supply, store, compound, manufacture, prescribe, dispense, administer, monitor and safely dispose of medicines.[14]

One of the major changes has been the introduction of a National Standard Medication inpatient chart, in both paper and electronic form, by the ACSQHC. The ACSQHC states that 'the charts support the delivery of appropriate care for hospitalised patients to help communicate information consistently between clinicians on the intended use of medicines for an individual patient'.[15] There are charts available for use in adults, paediatrics, day surgery, general practice and also some specific charts for practices such as subcutaneous insulin, residential medication charts for aged care and a clozapine titration chart.[16]

Importantly there is also a list of national terminology, abbreviations and symbols.[17] All health professionals need to be familiar with these standardised terms, as their use will reduce the risk of error significantly.

Administrative Considerations

In Australia almost all health organisations are required to have a permanent medication management committee made up of relevant personnel to formulate specific policy in relation to drug control and administration.[18] Some hospitals and health centres may be too small to warrant such a committee, but even in these circumstances hospital and health administrators are required to lay down firm and clear policies for employees concerning the administration of drugs.

The policies should:

1. ensure that the relevant legislative provisions are implemented and adhered to;
2. ensure that all staff members concerned are advised of any relevant changes to the legislation that may occur from time to time. This can be easily achieved by bringing such changes to the attention of staff through standard communication strategies;
3. ensure that staff members are informed and instructed about the use, requirements for handling, storage, contraindications and other matters relating to new drugs;
4. ensure that policies exist for contentious issues that arise — for example:
   a. legibility of medication orders;
   b. procedures to be followed by staff when making and taking verbal medication orders, especially in emergencies;
5. specify procedures for checking drugs of addiction and certain restricted substances, such as how often each substance is counted and by whom;
6. identify procedures to be followed if medication orders are to be transcribed;
7. clarify what medications, if any, outside Schedule 4 and Schedule 8 substances can be given by nursing and midwifery staff without a medical officer's authority or prescription — for example, on the basis of what are commonly referred to as 'nurse- or midwife-initiated medications';
8. where appropriate, determine standard medication protocols, commonly referred to as Standing Orders, to be followed by nursing and midwifery staff in emergencies or in areas such as obstetric delivery wards.

Clinical Considerations

In the day-to-day task of administering medications, nurses and midwives should bear the following 12 considerations carefully in mind to help reduce the possibility of errors occurring.

1. The guiding principle behind the administration of medication is: **if in any doubt, question and clarify with the prescribing practitioner concerned**. A useful maxim is often described as 'the five rights' of medication safety: the *right* patient should receive the *right* dose of the *right* drug via the *right* route at the *right* time.[19] However, to these five have now been added a further four — the *right* documentation, action, form and response.[20] Read medication sheets carefully. If the prescription is still handwritten and the handwriting is illegible or there is any other confusion about the prescription, take steps to clarify it and, if need be, have it rewritten before the drug is administered. Computerised medication sheets do alleviate the legibility problem, but there may still be issues about the clarity of the prescription. However, if a nurse or midwife is present at the time the medication sheet is written up, they should ensure that the entry is comprehensible and, if not, have it clarified immediately.
2. Check the labelling of the drug carefully. If it is an ampoule or tablet in a blister pack, check the labelling on the ampoule or blister, not the box or container it is in.
3. Leave medications in the packaging they arrive in from the pharmacy — don't transfer them to another container. Most of the Regulations make provision for such a situation.
4. Do not transcribe a patient's medication orders from his or her medication sheet into any other part of the patient's notes or other documents unless absolutely unavoidable. This eliminates the risk of transcription errors and the possibility that some other person may give a drug to a patient based on the transcribed error. Transcribing medication orders is not against the law as such, but it has become such an important issue for healthcare staff because of the great danger of errors arising in such a practice. Therefore, it is essential that in whatever system

is devised in relation to medication the necessity to transcribe such orders is eliminated or reduced to an absolute minimum.

5. If it is necessary, in an emergency situation, to take a drug order over the telephone, the following six steps should be observed:

   a. Obtain the patient's notes if possible.

   b. Ask the prescribing practitioner to repeat the order at least once — and more if it is unclear.

   c. Repeat the order back to the prescribing practitioner.

   d. If another nurse or midwife is present and available, ask them to listen to the order as a second check.

   e. Make an immediate entry in the patient's notes (not on a scrap of paper) recording the date, time, drug, amount, number of doses and so on, and sign the entry. Ask the second nurse or midwife, if available, to countersign the entry. A problem that sometimes arises here is where to make the entry in the patient's notes — that is, in the medication sheet or in the body of the patient's notes. Unless contraindicated by hospital policy, there is no legal reason why the entry cannot be made on the medication sheet. It would certainly seem the most sensible thing to do, particularly as the prescribing practitioner has to countersign and confirm the order generally within 24–48 hours. Some hospitals take the view that the patient's medication sheet constitutes a hospital prescription form, and as nurses and midwives in general (unless endorsed to prescribe as nurse practitioners or endorsed midwives) cannot prescribe drugs, they cannot write on the medication sheet. Whichever view is taken, it is more important to make the entry directly into the patient's notes and that the hospital administration makes a clear policy on such a matter, which it then communicates to the staff concerned.

   f. Appropriate steps should be taken to ensure that the prescriber confirms the verbal order in writing in the patient's notes within a specified time. In most states and territories, the Regulations specify the time, which usually ranges from 24 to 48 hours.

6. Registered nurses and midwives are presumed to have specific knowledge and expertise in relation to drugs, which they acquire as part of their training and education. That knowledge and expertise should cause them to question medication orders carefully in certain situations rather than blindly follow instructions; for example:

   a. if a dosage seems excessive in all the circumstances;

   b. if the drug seems inappropriate having regard to known contraindications, drug interactions, side effects or allergies;

   c. if the drug is one they have not encountered before.

7. If, after carefully checking the drug and dosage with the patient's medical practitioner, the nurse or midwife is still concerned, he or she should communicate that concern to a person in authority for further checking. That may not be possible in isolated situations, but in most hospitals a system to deal with such concerns should be devised.

8. Whatever procedure for further checking does or does not exist, any query raised by a nurse or midwife with the prescribing practitioner concerning the suitability or dosage of a particular drug ordered for a patient should be documented immediately by the nurse or midwife in the patient's record. In making such an entry, care should be taken that it is factual and objective. See **Clinical example 8.2**.

9. Registered nurses and midwives should not be required to administer complicated drug regimens in specialised or high-dependency areas, unless they are assessed as competent to do so or have undertaken education in the specialty. This is particularly so with children where drug dosages are required to be fractionally precise and the margin for error is extremely small.

10. Where certain drugs are required to be checked prior to administration, they should be checked by two people. In situations where nurses or midwives work alone or in isolation this may not be possible. This problem frequently occurs with community nurses and midwives who are required to administer

CLINICAL EXAMPLE 8.2

Assume that the prescribing practitioner has prescribed an intravenous dose of 0.5 mg of digoxin for a patient. The registered nurse on duty feels that such a dose administered intravenously is excessive in the circumstances and wishes to check it with the prescribing doctor. In doing so, it is suggested that the following entry may appear in the patient's notes:

15.5.15: 14.00 Contacted Dr Brown concerning his order of 0.5 mg of digoxin IV. Dr Brown directed that the order be amended to 0.05 mg of digoxin IV. Medication sheet amended accordingly. P Smith RN.

OR

15.5.15: 14.00 Contacted Dr Brown concerning his order of 0.5 mg of digoxin IV. Dr Brown confirmed order. P Smith RN.

If the second example is the outcome and the nurse is still concerned, contact should be made with a person in authority, if such a system has been devised. If it has, the following entries may then appear:

15.5.15: 14.15 Contacted Dr Jones concerning Dr Brown's order of 0.5 mg of digoxin IV.

14.30 Received a telephone order from Dr Jones to change the order to read 0.05 mg of digoxin IV. Medication sheet amended accordingly. P Smith RN.

In the event that Dr Jones confirms Dr Brown's order, the following entry may appear instead of the last entry above:

14.30 Dr Jones telephoned and stated that he had discussed the order of 0.5 mg of digoxin IV with Dr Brown and he confirmed Dr Brown's order. P Smith RN.

medications in the home — for example, the drawing up of insulin for diabetic patients. In such situations the nurse or midwife concerned has no alternative but to administer the drug after carefully checking it alone. However, the patient is often highly knowledgeable about their own illness and

regimen, and if they are able to check and assist it is always useful and instructive to involve them.

11. Where a community nurse is required to visit a patient in their home on a weekly basis, the nurse may be required to leave prescribed medications in a dosette box for the patient to self-administer at set times during the week. When that situation arises, the nurse should take all reasonable steps to ensure the medications are correctly administered, such as giving careful explanations and, if need be, written instructions to the patient and/or relatives as to the time and method such medications are to be taken, as well as any other relevant instructions. Where there is a language barrier between the nurse and patient, it may be necessary to arrange for an interpreter to be present. There are free online interpreter services in most health services and government organisations that can be organised to assist.[21]

12. There are also situations where an unregistered carer can assist a person to take their own medications. This occurs in residential aged care facilities and in home care. However, the critical difference is that the person knows and manages their own medications but is unable to administer them by themselves and asks for assistance from the carer. This situation is potentially fraught for the carers, especially if the person is perhaps forgetful or unable to express the effectiveness of their medication, as the carer does not have the knowledge and skills to assess the impact of the medications on the individual. A recent review of carer medication errors demonstrated that home medication administration errors made by carers are a potentially serious patient safety issue. Carers made similar errors to those made by professionals in other contexts and a wide variety of contributory factors were identified.[22] The ACSQHC recommends the following:

Patients and carers should be provided with enough information about medicine-related treatment options. This information needs to be in a form that is easy to understand and useful to patients. Appropriate education and provision of written medicine-related information to patients are essential to encourage safe and effective medicine use, and promote adherence to treatment regimens. This may include the supply of a medicines list (or profile), education about the medicines and any changes, and consumer medicine information (CMI) leaflets.[23]

Electronic Medication Management

The ACSQHC identifies the breadth of electronic medication management (EMM) as applying to:

- prescribing systems, such as general practitioner desktop systems or hospital clinical information systems that have electronic ordering;
- decision support systems, such as evidence-based order sets, allergy checking and medicine interactions;
- dispensing systems, such as pharmacy software and automated dispensing systems;
- ordering and supply solutions, such as the electronic transfer of prescriptions (ETP) and inventory solutions;
- electronic medical records in the acute and primary care sectors.[24]

Following the prescription of a medication electronically, a nurse would sign onto the system and select the medications to be given. They may also identify a reason why the medication was not administered, such as the patient being absent, or they would confirm the administration of each dose. An electronic signature would then be stamped against the medication administered, recording the time of administration. Some systems trigger alerts when medications are due or overdue. Documentation of reasons for medication omission are often mandatory using these systems.[25]

The most recent review of the evidence in relation to electronic medication management makes the following findings:

... electronic medication administration record systems in hospitals are associated with reduced medication administration errors

(e.g. dose omissions, timing errors), improved quality indicators and enhanced medication documentation. Studies measuring efficiency of medication administration following electronic medication administration record implementation present mixed results. Electronic medication administration records are rarely implemented in the absence of other integrated health information technology, thus their effects should be considered in tandem with such technologies. Implementing electronic medication administration record systems requires significant workflow changes and ongoing monitoring to maximise system benefits and reduce unintended consequences, such as new medication errors associated with system use.[26]

ENDORSEMENTS FOR ADMINISTERING MEDICATION UNDER THE NEW NATIONAL REGISTRATION SCHEME

Under the national registration scheme, there is provision under section 94(1) of the schedule of the *Health Practitioner Regulation National Law Act 2009* (Qld) for a National Board (in this case the NMBA) to endorse the registration of a registered healthcare practitioner (in this case either a nurse or midwife) 'as being qualified to administer, obtain, possess, prescribe, sell, supply or use a scheduled medicine or class of scheduled medicines' if the registered nurse or midwife:

a. *holds either of the following qualifications relevant to the endorsement —*
   i. *an approved qualification;*
   ii. *another qualification that, in the Board's opinion, is substantially equivalent to, or based on similar competencies to, an approved qualification; and*
b. *complies with any approved registration standard relevant to the endorsement.*[27]

These endorsements are discussed in detail in **Chapter 4** but suffice it to say here that nurse practitioners are specifically endorsed under section 95, and a specified class of midwives are also endorsed to prescribe under section 96.

CRIMINAL AND PROFESSIONAL ISSUES RELATING TO THE ADMINISTRATION OF DRUGS

It is not unknown for a nurse or midwife to have a drug addiction. Health impairment was the third most frequent complaint lodged about nurses and midwives in the *2021/2022 annual report* of the Ahpra and National Boards.[28] Nurses and midwives are often able to maintain such a habit because of their relatively easy access to drugs generally and, as registered nurses and midwives, to drugs of addiction in particular. The provisions of the various *Poisons Acts* and *Regulations* authorise registered nurses and midwives to be 'in possession of and supply certain drugs of addiction'. Such authority is generally symbolised by the possession of keys to the cupboard where these drugs are kept.

If this authority to possess and supply drugs is breached by self-administration, or by supplying or administering to a person other than a patient, the authority can be withdrawn. Apart from anything else, such an action also constitutes a criminal offence under the provisions of the poisons or crimes legislation of each state and territory.

Should a registered nurse or midwife be found guilty (convicted) of such an offence, he or she will invariably be required to appear before the relevant panel or tribunal described in Part 8 of the schedule of the *Health Practitioner Regulation National Law Act 2009* (Qld) in the appropriate state or territory. The powers under that Act include the power to remove a nurse's name from the register, subject to certain provisions, thereby effectively preventing the nurse from pursuing employment in his or her profession or placing conditions on the nurse's right to practise. However, there are also support pathways (sometimes known as impaired registrants pathways) that assist nurses to manage their impairment through regular psychological and physical monitoring.[29] It is not uncommon for registered nurses to have their registration cancelled or suspended for varying periods of time as a result of convictions arising from drug offences related to their employment. In 2017 the NMBA introduced an independent support program for impaired nurses and midwives that includes support for nurses and midwives with a substance abuse problem.[30]

CONCLUSION

The rules governing the administration and management of drugs have changed quite a lot since the last edition of this textbook (published in 2019), and further changes are expected, particularly with developments in electronic prescribing. Nurses and midwives need to follow local policy and national developments closely.

CHAPTER 8 REVIEW QUESTIONS

Following your reading of **Chapter 8**, consider these questions in reaching the objectives of this chapter. Guidance on which part of the chapter will assist you in answering the questions can be found at http://evolve.elsevier.com/AU/Staunton/law/. You may, of course, consider other sources as part of your considerations.

1. Do you think the way medicines are regulated in Australia could be improved? If so, how?

2. Do you believe the mechanisms for identifying those nurses, nurse practitioners and midwives who are authorised to administer or endorsed to prescribe medicines are sufficiently rigorous? Explain your answer.

3. What common problems are you aware of relating to the management and administration of drugs that can result in adverse events?

4. Are you using electronic medication management in your workplace? Do you think it improves medication safety and, if so, how does it achieve this?

ENDNOTES

Note: all links were last accessed on 20 July 2023.

1. Australian Institute of Health and Welfare, *Medicines in the health system*, 2022, https://www.aihw.gov.au/reports/medicines/medicines-in-the-health-system.

2. von Conrady D and Bonney A, 'Patterns of complementary and alternative medicine use and health literacy in general practice patients in urban and regional Australia', (2017) *Australian Family Physician* 40(5), https://www.racgp.org.au/afp/2017/may/patterns-of-complementary-and-alternative-medi-2.

3. Pharmaceutical Society of Australia, *Medicine safety: take care*, 2019, https://www.psa.org.au/wp-content/uploads/2019/01/PSA-Medicine-Safety-Report.pdf.

4. Australian Government, *Guiding principles for medication management in the community*, 2022, https://www.health.gov.au/sites/default/files/2022-11/guiding-principles-for-medication-management-in-the-community.pdf.

5. Nursing and Midwifery Board of Australia (NMBA), *Fact sheet: enrolled nurses and medicine administration*, 2022, https://www.nursingmidwiferyboard.gov.au/Codes-Guidelines-Statements/FAQ/Enrolled-nurses-and-medicine-administration.aspx#.

6. Poisons Standard 2023, https://www.legislation.gov.au/Details/F2023L00864. (Note: amendments are made to the Standard throughout the year. Check the website regularly for currency if you require accurate information about a schedule.)

7. Ibid.

8. Australian Government, *Guiding principles for medication management in the community*, 2022, https://www.health.gov.au/sites/default/files/2022-11/guiding-principles-for-medication-management-in-the-community.pdf, p 43.

9. See for example, the Australian Government initiative of Remote primary health care manuals (2023), *Clinical procedures manual: managing a remote clinic dispensary* https://www.remotephcmanuals.com.au/content/documents/manuals/medicines/Managing_a_remote_clinic_dispensary.html.

10. See, for example, the very detailed advice in NSW Health (2022), Policy Directive PD2022_032 *Medications Handling* at S. 6.3, p 93, https://www1.health.nsw.gov.au/pds/ActivePDS-Documents/PD2022_032.pdf.

11. See, for example, Government of South Australia, Department for Health and Ageing, SA Health, *Code of practice for the storage and transport of drugs of dependence*, 2012, https://www.sahealth.sa.gov.au/wps/wcm/connect/public+content/sa+health+internet/about+us/legislation/controlled+substances+legislation/code+of+practice+for+the+storage+and+transport+of+drugs+of+dependence.

12. See, for example, Queensland Health, *Managing, storing, and disposing of voluntary assisted dying substances— Guidance for health services*, 2022, https://www.health.qld.gov.au/__data/assets/pdf_file/0033/1166568/substance-management-guidance-health-services.pdf.

13. Australian Commission on Safety and Quality in Health Care (ACSQHC), *National Safety and Quality Health Service standards — Medication safety standard*, 2023, https://www.safetyandquality.gov.au/standards/nsqhs-standards/medication-safety-standard.

14. Ibid.

15. Australian Commission on Safety and Quality in Health Care (ACSQHC), *National Standard Medication Charts*, 2019, https://www.safetyandquality.gov.au/our-work/medication-safety/medication-charts/national-standard-medication-charts.

16. Ibid.

17. Australian Commission on Safety and Quality in Health Care (ACSQHC), *Recommendations for terminology, abbreviations and symbols used in medicines documentation*, 2016, https://www.safetyandquality.gov.au/our-work/medication-safety/safer-naming-and-labelling-medicines/recommendations-terminology-abbreviations-and-symbols-used-medicines-documentation.

18. See, for example, NSW Health, *Medication handling policy directive PD2022_032*, 2022, https://www1.health.nsw.gov.au/pds/ActivePDSDocuments/PD2022_032.pdf, p 15.

19. Federico F, 'The five rights of medication administration', (2023) *Institute for Health Care Improvement*, https://www.ihi.org/resources/Pages/ImprovementStories/FiveRightsofMedicationAdministration.aspx.

20. Elliott M and Liu Y, 'The nine rights of medication administration: an overview', (2010) *British Journal of Nursing* 19(5):300–5. https://europepmc.org/article/med/20335899.

21. See, for example, SA Health (undated), *Working with interpreters refugee health fact sheet*, https://www.sahealth.sa.gov.au/wps/wcm/connect/318f8c4d-bd97-4978-9ae2-a53fbfcfc262/Working+with+interpreters_Refugee+Health+Service.pdf?MOD=AJPERES&CACHEID=ROOTWORKSPACE-318f8c4d-bd97-4978-9ae2-a53fbfcfc262-opo8K0; NSW Health, *NSW health care interpreting services*, 2022, https://www.health.nsw.gov.au/multicultural/Pages/health-care-interpreting-and-translating-services.aspx.

22. Parand A, Garfield S, Vincent C, Franklin BD, 'Carers' medication administration errors in the domiciliary setting: a systematic review', (2016) *PLoS One*, 11(12), https://pubmed.ncbi.nlm.nih.gov/27907072/.

23. Australian Commission on Safety and Quality in Health Care (ACSQHC), 'Continuity of medication management. Medication Safety Standard', *NSQHS Standards*, https://www.safetyandquality.gov.au/standards/nsqhs-standards/medication-safety-standard/continuity-medication-management.

24. Australian Commission on Safety and Quality in Health Care (ACSQHC), *Electronic medication management*, 2023, https://www.safetyandquality.gov.au/our-work/medication-safety/electronic-medication-management.

25. Australian Commission on Safety and Quality in Health Care (ACSQHC), 'Evidence briefings on interventions to improve medication safety', *Electronic medication administration records, Volume 2, Issue 3*: https://www.safetyandquality.gov.au/sites/default/files/2021-08/evidence_briefings_on_interventions_to_improve_medication_safety_3_electronic_medication_administration_records_july_2021.pdf.

26. Ibid, p 1.

27. Ahpra and National Boards, *Health Practitioner Regulation National Law Act 2009* (Qld), section 94(1), https://www.ahpra.gov.au/about-ahpra/what-we-do/legislation.aspx.

28. Ahpra and National Boards, *2021/2022 annual report*, 2023, N1 Supplementary Tables, https://www.ahpra.gov.au/Publications/Annual-reports/Annual-Report-2022.aspx.

29. See, for example, the information contained in Nursing and Midwifery Council of NSW, *Do you have an impairment?*, 2019, https://www.nursingandmidwiferycouncil.nsw.gov.au/have-an-impairment.

30. Nurse and Midwife Support, *Your health matters*, 2022, https://www.nmsupport.org.au/.

DOCUMENTATION AND CONFIDENTIALITY OF AND ACCESS TO PATIENT RECORDS (INCLUDING E-RECORDS, INCIDENT REPORTING AND OPEN DISCLOSURE)

LEARNING OBJECTIVES

In this chapter, you will:

- consider the purpose of keeping and making patient records
- examine best practice in report writing and in the proper use of patient records
- explore the implication of and best practice in the use of e-health records
- reflect on the requirement for confidentiality in relation to patient information and patient records
- look at the rights of patients to have access to their own health records
- become aware of how adverse events and clinical incidents are reported, documented and managed, including the need for open disclosure.

INTRODUCTION

This chapter focuses primarily on the use and compilation of healthcare records, including confidentiality. It also considers the principles of adverse event management and incident reporting, including open disclosure.

THE ROLE OF CLINICAL DOCUMENTATION IN HEALTHCARE DELIVERY

Writing in patients' records is an integral part of the work undertaken by nurses and midwives. The patient's record, particularly the reports written by healthcare personnel incorporated within it, should constitute an ongoing account of the patient's healthcare treatment. Accordingly when the patient next presents for care and treatment, their previous health records provide an important history of past treatment given and progress made. In turn, that information provides the background to assist with future care and treatment as required. In addition, a patient's record is used for teaching, quality and research purposes.

From time to time, healthcare records will be required as evidence in court. It is important to stress that this is not the most important reason for writing good healthcare records. However, where the care and treatment of a patient is under critical scrutiny, courts place great reliance on a patient's healthcare record, considering them as a contemporaneous, objective and generally reliable evidence of what occurred at critical times of a patient's care and treatment. As was noted by the coroner investigating the death of a patient in a Sydney hospital:

> *Good record-keeping is a critical element of sound, safe medical practice … The keeping of good records should not be driven by fear of lawyers or a 'tidy town' mentality, but by the recognition of the urgency of patient safety … Taking and recording observations of vital signs is probably the most important of the records that must be kept up to date, but progress notes are almost equally important. Progress notes are slices in time that enable clinicians to monitor patients as they improve, stabilise or deteriorate.*[1]

When a patient's healthcare record is required by a court, the relevant health authority or the individual medical practitioner is served with a subpoena requiring them to produce the relevant records. The records can be used in civil and criminal proceedings and in coronial inquests.

In civil proceedings against a hospital or health service or an individual healthcare professional, a person's healthcare record may often be used as evidence to support an allegation that a certain treatment was wrongly given or that there was a failure to give particular care or treatment. The record can also be used as supporting evidence of other matters that may be in dispute — in civil proceedings, for example, that a particular injury occurred as a result of an accident, and the circumstances in which it was alleged by the patient to have occurred.

In criminal proceedings, records can be used as evidence that a particular incident such as an assault and/or injury actually happened, and to show the nature and extent of the injury. For example, in relation to a charge of sexual assault, it may be that the first place the victim presented for help was the emergency department of a hospital. On arrival the victim would invariably give an account of events leading up to his or her presence at the hospital. In such a situation, the health professional's record of the words used in relation to the complaint made and the injuries sustained may become important evidence in the criminal charge that may well follow.

In coronial inquests, the purpose of the inquiry is to determine the manner and cause of death (see **Chapter 11**). Here the records may be used to track a person's deterioration, to identify whether any errors or adverse events occurred during the patient's stay, or to ascertain the condition of the person when they were first (and possibly subsequently) seen by the health professional.

For whatever purpose patients' records may be required in legal proceedings, such records, including nursing or midwifery records, will be subject to close and careful scrutiny. It is important, therefore, that these records meet the standard expected of them. If the records are an accurate and factual account of good care, they will provide valuable assistance in a court of law.

Relevant Considerations in Documentation

In some jurisdictions there are now strict requirements for the way in which reports must be written. For example, NSW Health now has a policy — *Health care records — documentation and management* — that contains mandatory requirements for documentation.[2] This policy includes specific advice for nurses and midwives and, because it is so comprehensive, these extracts are reproduced in **Appendix A** at the end of this chapter.

There are a number of different techniques or models of documentation including:

- progress notes;
- various types of charting by exception, such as documenting variance and charting clinical incidents;
- problem-oriented medical records; and
- more standardised formats, such as clinical or critical pathways, clinical algorithms and pre-designed clinical care plans, which are becoming more prevalent with electronic records.

Although some organisations still use only handwritten records, computerised systems are now far more commonplace in our healthcare system; some organisations use a combination of both. Electronic health records, or e-health records as they are known, are explored in more detail later in this chapter.

Certain points are common to all forms of records and should always be borne in mind. The Australian Commission on Safety and Quality in Health Care (ACSQHC) identifies that clinical records should be 'clear, legible, concise, contemporaneous, progressive and accurate'. A number of these (and other) points are summarised below with some practical examples:

- Reports should be accurate, concise and complete. Accuracy is obviously essential and it is important to distinguish between what is personally observed and what is related as part of a patient's complaint of illness or injury. For example, in accident and emergency, there is a difference in the record between writing 'patient assaulted by two men' and 'patient reported that he had been assaulted by two men'. Unless the assault was actually witnessed, the patient's complaint of injury is clearly hearsay evidence and must be reported as such. 'Concise and complete' may sound like a contradiction in terms, but primarily it is important to avoid unnecessary verbosity.

■ In particular, as part of ensuring the reports are complete, reference should always be made where a patient refuses any treatment or medication or acts in a manner contrary to healthcare advice. For example, providing they have capacity, it is a patient's right to refuse their medication or indeed any intervention they choose, as was discussed in **Chapter 6**. However, it is important to document the refusal so that any adverse outcomes can be monitored and accounted for should they occur. This would be particularly important for midwives when women can naturally hold strong views about the management of their pregnancy and labour that may sometimes go against the advice of the midwife. If there is no record of such a refusal occurring, the record is incomplete.

■ If reports are still being handwritten, they should be legible. Incorrect interpretation of a person's handwriting can lead to mistakes and has done so in the past. Remember, if unsure about what is written, always check. This problem will hopefully be overcome with the introduction of e-records, although typographical and entry errors can still occur and any concerns or uncertainties still need to be raised with the person who has entered the data.

■ Remember that some computer programs have predictive text and also auto-correct, which can create problems if the language is technical and not easily recognised by the computer program. It is good practice to check the accuracy of wording once it has been entered.

■ When making an entry into a patients e-health record, always ensure the correct patient record is logged on and remember to close it off as soon as the entry is completed. This practice should overcome the error that occurred in prescribing medications as detailed in **Case example 7.3**[3] where the prescribing practitioner forgot to close the patient's e-health record and inadvertently charted medications in the wrong patient's record that ultimately resulted in the patient's death.

■ Reports should be written objectively. This critical distinction can best be summarised as follows: 'Learn to record what you see, not what

---

BOX 9.1
WRITING OBJECTIVE, DEFINITE STATEMENTS OF FACT

1. A statement such as the 'patient appears to be drunk' would be more accurately reported in the following, or similar, terms:
   ■ patient is unsteady on his or her feet;
   ■ patient's speech is slurred;
   ■ patient's breath smells strongly of alcohol.
2. A statement such as the 'patient appears to be shocked' would be more accurately reported in the following, or similar, terms:
   ■ patient is pale and sweating;
   ■ patient's pulse rate and blood pressure are specified;
   ■ patient has peripheral cyanosis, or patient's fingers and toes are blue.
3. A statement such as the 'patient appears to be sleeping' can be contentious. How to report the patient's sleep status, especially in night duty reports, is one area in which nurses and midwives commonly seek guidance. The justification for the use of the word 'appears' in this context has been that some qualification and/or caveat is required in cases where the nurse has written 'patient slept well', but the next morning the patient reports that he or she didn't sleep well at all. This can be difficult for nurses and midwives as, even if the patient had one unobserved period of wakefulness but was sleeping on all occasions when they checked on them, for the patient that interruption to their sleep, coupled with the strange bed and strange sounds of the hospital ward, may well feel like a very poor night's sleep indeed.

---

you think you see'. Three examples are given in **Box 9.1**.

A simple rule to follow is to write only an objective, definite statement of fact; that is, record what you heard, saw or did and provide as much specific clinical information as possible, such as measurements of clinical signs and results.

■ For people who are so unwell they require constant attention throughout the night, the question of sleep becomes almost a side issue. Although it is hoped that a patient will sleep for as much of the night as is possible, it is still good practice to observe patients at regular intervals. Here the most accurate and definite record that the clinician can give is to document the patient's sleep status as at the time of observation — for example: 'Patient observed at regular intervals (if possible mention the time). When so observed, patient was sleeping'. Obviously where the patient does not sleep it should also be appropriately and accurately reported. The use of the word 'appears' as a means of qualification is not appropriate in clinical documentation.

■ Entries in reports should be made at the time a relevant incident occurs. This is known as 'contemporaneous reporting'. Nurses (probably more so than midwives) have traditionally written their reports at the completion of each shift. There is no legal reason for this, and it would be more appropriate to make a relevant entry as soon as possible after an incident or episode of care occurs. Not only will the nurse or midwife better recall the event, in some cases if the nurse waits until the completion of the shift to record an occurrence that episode may have been overtaken by subsequent events — particularly if a patient's condition worsens and various treatments are commenced and tests undertaken. Trying to recreate the accurate sequential order at that stage can prove confusing. Any entry that is made should be prefaced by the date and time and followed by the writer's signature.

■ Always make an entry in a patient's record if you contact a fellow health practitioner of your concerns about a particular patient. For example, a patient's observations may be deteriorating, the patient may have refused medication or you become concerned about a patient's condition for a particular reason and believe the treating doctor or another relevant health practitioner should review the patient. When you contact the relevant treating practitioner, always make an entry in the patient's notes stating the date and time and the reasons why you contacted him or her and sign the entry. This habit will stand you in good stead if the patient's condition deteriorates further and the question may later arise: when was the medical or other health practitioner first contacted about the patient's condition? If you make an entry at the time, you will be able to point to that, instead of trying to rely on your memory as to whether you did make contact, at what time and what was conveyed. Developing that practice will also overcome the problem where you insist you did ring the practitioner, but he/she denies that or does not remember.

■ Abbreviations should not be used in reports unless they are accepted healthcare organisation abbreviations. The diversity of healthcare organisations in which nurses and midwives undertake their clinical placements and later work leads to a diversity of abbreviations used — often with confusing and misleading results. Every healthcare facility, as a matter of administrative policy, should have a list of accepted abbreviations accompanied by the accepted meaning of each abbreviation. No other abbreviations should be used in the patient's records. It is also critical that those abbreviations are accepted by all health professionals, as different professional groups can use the same acronyms or abbreviations to describe different phenomena related to their own area of practice.

■ If medical terminology is used in the records, the nurse or midwife must be sure of the exact meaning, as otherwise it could prove misleading.

■ Any errors made while writing an entry in a patient's record should be dealt with by drawing a line through the incorrect entry and initialling it before continuing. Total obliteration of the incorrect entry may suggest that there is something to hide. Writing over mistakes with emphasis and inserting words left out between lines can also cause confusion and misunderstanding and should definitely be avoided. Liquid correcting fluid should never be used to correct mistakes.

■ With e-health records a correction at the time of entry can be made by deletion. However, any attempt to amend a record at a later date must be made transparently with an addendum to the record, signed and clearly acknowledged as an alteration. Most computer systems can track alterations and amendments to text and it would be unfortunate if an innocent attempt to correct a record appeared to be a clandestine or even a fraudulent cover-up.

■ No entry concerning the patient's treatment should be made in a patient's record on behalf of another

BOX 9.2
REDUCING THE RISK OF MAKING INCORRECT ENTRIES

A number of factors are worth remembering that may reduce the risk of an incorrect entry being made:

- Check the patient's name on the record before making an entry.
- Do not make an entry in a patient's record that refers to an identifying room or bed number only. Patients are often moved while staff are absent (for example, during a meal break), and remembering a patient simply as 'the patient in room 12' can sometimes cause incorrect entries to be made in the chart at the end of room 12 (apart from any other considerations).
- Make sure that the patient's name and identifying number is on every sheet of the patient's record before making an entry on that sheet. Some observation sheets are single sheets which are not immediately incorporated into the body of the patient's record. If these single sheets are not identified before any entry is made, there is the risk that the wrong patient's observations may be recorded on the sheet unwittingly, or the sheet may be wrongly identified after an entry is made and then filed in the wrong patient's record.
- Avoid wherever possible making notes concerning a patient on loose paper for rewriting into the patient's notes. Not only is it common for such scraps of paper to be lost but every time an entry is transcribed in this fashion there exists a margin for error in the transcription itself, as well as the risk that the entry will be made in the wrong patient's notes. It is also a duplication of work and therefore wastes time.

nurse or midwife. Examples of this have unfortunately arisen, particularly in relation to fluid balance charts. This can be understandably problematic if adverse events occur and the particular patient's records are closely and critically scrutinised.

See **Box 9.2** for further guidance on reducing the risk of making incorrect entries.

INTEGRATED RECORD-KEEPING

Integrated documentation in the patient's record is essential. In the past, nurses, midwives and medical officers traditionally wrote separate reports about a patient, and these reports were separately filed. On many occasions neither party read the reports of the other. That such a situation ever arose is odd enough; that it might continue is unsatisfactory and contrary to best practice.

To obtain a comprehensive picture of the patient's condition and progress, it is essential that the reports of all healthcare personnel caring for the patient be part of an ongoing integrated holistic record. It is also much safer, as it requires all personnel involved to read their colleagues' reports. Not only is such an undertaking instructive and illuminating for everybody but it must also help ensure that all personnel are aware of what is happening to the patient — clearly the most important consideration of all. Most hospitals and health services have already introduced such an integrated system and this is perpetuated through e-health records.

READING THE PATIENTS' RECORDS

Nurses and midwives must ensure they read their patients' records thoroughly and regularly. Many hospitals and some health centres rely on a system of verbal reporting at the commencement of each shift as the main way of passing on the history and any relevant information concerning the patient that has arisen during the previous shift. If the nurse or midwife is unfamiliar with the patient, they should read the written record to gain a more extensive overview, even if a verbal report has been delivered.

The verbal handover is generally an efficient way of quickly reporting on all patients to all relevant staff on a shift-by-shift basis. However, the verbal report must be seen as an adjunct to the written report and not a substitute for it. Important information and pathology results that may not have been mentioned in the verbal report may not be known and noted, sometimes until it is too late. It is also possible that a colleague may simply forget to mention an important fact during a verbal handover that can often be ascertained by reading the patient's clinical notes.

THE VALUE OF GOOD RECORDS WHEN USED AS EVIDENCE IN COURT

Sometimes the quality of the patient's record-keeping has been high, and this has been advantageous for nurses and midwives in terms of both their verbal evidence and their written evidence. Conversely the inadequacy of a patient's record has been adversely commented upon. For example, see **Case example 7.5** in Chapter 7, where the court found that the inadequacy of the nurses' notes 'must have been a major factor in bringing about a situation which allowed the patient's condition to deteriorate fatally without timely remedial treatment'.[4] However, **Case example 9.1** illustrates the opposite outcome, where the nursing and other records were considered 'the most reliable evidence' concerning the patient's care and treatment.[5]

The Difficulties for Nurses and Midwives When Records Produced in Court are Poor

Unfortunately, on numerous occasions the poor quality of patients' records has meant that the courts have (understandably) taken them literally and found their depiction of patient care wanting. Perhaps because nursing and midwifery both have such a strong oral tradition, the records have never been the major focus of authenticity.[6] Greater reliance has traditionally been vested in the oral handover.[7] Thus, questions such as 'at what time did you take Mrs Smith's 6 o'clock observations?', however illogical they may sound to listeners, are a consequence of the fact that 4-hourly observation charts are often pre-printed with the times 2, 6, 10, 2, 6, 10.[8] This type of chart should no longer be used as it leads to a number of anomalies. For example, if a nurse or midwife has a caseload of eight people, only one can have their observations recorded exactly on the hour. In addition, the records often take the form of graphs or plans, meaning times are abbreviated or rounded off to save space. However, if an observation is taken and found to be abnormal, and particularly if a person is seriously ill or a patient's condition is deteriorating, the exact time of the observation must be written.

The above example does not excuse poor recording practices, but it goes some way to explaining them. This is problematic for nurses and midwives who would wish their records to be accorded professional authority. When witnesses have poor recollection of events, particularly if considerable time has passed since the relevant incident occurred, judges rely on written evidence made at the time of the event. Accordingly, those who do not produce accurate records will find it difficult to have their account of a particular incident treated as legitimate if it is inconsistent with the written evidence. When charts and times have been tendered in courts and tribunals and have been found to be inaccurate, the witness's credibility has suffered as a consequence. For example, a finding that 'these times were all approximate times, were not accurate times and cannot be relied upon' led to the judge declaring that 'I accept [the anaesthetist's conflicting] evidence in view of the inexactitude of the nurses' times as shown by the contradictions on the charts'.[9]

The extent to which a patient's medical records are considered critical in relation to legal proceedings is illustrated by the following passage from a text for medical practitioners relating to emergency department administration and legal matters:

> *Comprehensive records, written when you saw the patient, are the keystone of your defence if you are sued. The better the records, the better is your chance of a successful defence. It does not matter what you did, if you did not write it down, you did not do it. Conversely, if you did write it down, you did do it.*[10]

The above passage also underscores the importance that nursing and midwifery staff should place on recording their entries in an accurate, objective and timely manner, taking into account the whole of the patient's condition.

CASE EXAMPLE 9.1

Spasovic v Sydney Adventist Hospital[11]

In this case, the patient claimed that the nurses employed at the hospital and the doctors who cared for him failed to exercise reasonable care in assessing and treating complaints he made and symptoms he exhibited, in particular a headache, which were caused by a small cerebral haemorrhage from an arterio-venous malformation (AVM) in his brain. He claimed that, because of their failure to assess and treat him, he was discharged from hospital without the small cerebral haemorrhage or the AVM having been diagnosed. Later on the same day he suffered a major cerebral haemorrhage from the AVM, which caused him to have very serious permanent disabilities.

Comment and Relevant Considerations Arising From *Spasovic v Sydney Adventist Hospital*

The healthcare records of the patient were a central plank of the evidence offered in defence by the hospital and the medical staff. The lawyers representing the hospital made the following representation, as reported by the judge, James J:

> It was submitted by counsel ... that I should accept the Hospital's medical records and particularly the Hospital notes (that is the Integrated Progress Notes), as reliable evidence and indeed the most reliable evidence concerning the plaintiff's headache and events happening during the plaintiff's stay in the Hospital.

> As was submitted ... the Hospital's medical records and particularly the Hospital notes have the virtues, as evidence, of being contemporaneous records; of having been made by or under the supervision of trained observers; of having been made, not for the purposes of litigation or out of self-interest or with hindsight, but for the purpose of disinterestedly recording, progressively, what was happening during the plaintiff's stay in the Hospital; and of being, on the face of them, quite detailed and not merely perfunctory.

> The virtue of having been made without hindsight, that is of having been made without knowledge of the plaintiff's major haemorrhage on 20 January 1996 and its consequences, is a virtue possessed by the entries in the Hospital notes and by very little other evidence, lay or expert, in the case. I have also had the benefit of seeing and hearing many of the nurses who made notes give evidence and I formed a generally favourable impression of them.[12]

The judge concluded that he had decided, in general, to accept the records as being 'an accurate record of the matters purportedly recorded in them'.[13] This case provides a striking example of how good records, made with the sole purpose of providing good nursing care, not only furnished evidence of the existence of good nursing care but also enabled the judge to find both the written and verbal evidence provided by the nurses to be reliable.

DOCUMENTATION AND REPORT WRITING IN AN AGED CARE FACILITY

A relatively small proportion of our elderly population lives in nursing homes, as these individuals are no longer able to care for themselves or be cared for in the community and will require long-term nursing care with progressive deterioration over time. Thus, they are especially vulnerable and require specialised nursing care. Over the years, the need to protect both the environment in which these frail elderly people live and the standard of care they receive has been recognised and enshrined in legislation at state, territory and Commonwealth level. The major piece of legislation is the *Aged Care Act 1997* (Cth), which (*inter alia*) makes reference to Records Principles that must be kept by an aged care provider relating to the environment, care and management of elderly people.[14]

Reference to the Principles provides, among other matters, that an approved aged care provider must keep the following types of records:

- individual care plans;
- medical records, progress notes and other clinical records of care recipients;
- all incidents involving allegations or suspicions or reportable incidents;
- confirmation that a copy of the Charter of Rights has been given to the care recipient;
- vaccination records for care recipients and staff (specifically influenza and COVID-19).

Given that residents are usually in an aged care facility for a longer time than a normal hospital stay, questions about how often to document their care and what to document are commonly raised. There is no hard-and-fast requirement in relation to this and, generally, the operator of an aged care facility should have a clear policy in place in relation to the need for ongoing documented care.

One approach would be to have a record of a resident's condition as of a change of shift as well as in the event of any untoward incident that arises. For example, if the resident had a fall or became unwell for whatever reason and required specific attention and intervention, it would be expected that it would be immediately documented as well as the steps taken to deal with it and which persons were notified.

The reason for nominating the change of shift as one approach for documenting a resident's condition is to better establish a timeline as to when a resident's condition started to deteriorate. For example, if a resident is observed to be unwell and continues to deteriorate, the first question a clinician would ask would be 'When did this problem first arise?' If there is no shift-by-shift record of the resident's condition, there is no definitive way of knowing how long the condition has persisted, which may have significant consequences for ongoing care and treatment decisions.

Another approach of course is to chart by exception. That is, no entry is required to be made if the resident's condition remains stable and it is only when a specific incident arises requiring clinical intervention that an entry is made in the resident's care record.

Whichever approach is taken, it should be the subject of a clear written policy endorsed by the aged care provider.

In some respects, the provisions relating to the determination of funding needs for a resident in the aged care sector requires quite detailed documentation to be undertaken and maintained. The Aged Care Funding Instrument (ACFI)[15] administered by the Commonwealth is a funding instrument that assesses the relative care needs of residents and provides the mechanism for allocating the Federal Government subsidy to aged care providers in order to enable them to deliver the identified care needs to residents. The ACFI consists of 12 questions about care needs covered in three domains. Diagnostic information about mental and behavioural disorders and other medical conditions is also collected. The three ACFI domains are reproduced in **Box 9.3**.

The ACFI assessment pack is extremely detailed. It is recommended that various charts are kept for a number of days to have a full assessment of residents' care needs. Nurses who intend to work in the aged care sector will need to be familiar with these assessment and documentary requirements and to keep abreast of updates on the Department of Health website.[17] Organisations that provide aged care also offer valuable updates and advice in relation to documentation requirements.[18]

BOX 9.3
AGED CARE FUNDING INSTRUMENT DOMAINS[16]

- Activities of Daily Living Domain (ACFI Questions 1–5; Nutrition, Mobility, Personal Hygiene, Toileting and Continence). Ratings calculated from completing checklists in this domain determine the level of the subsidy.
- Behaviour Domain (ACFI Questions 6–10; Cognitive Skills, Wandering, Verbal Behaviour, Physical Behaviour and Depression). Ratings calculated from completing checklists in this domain determine the level of the subsidy.
- Complex Health Care Domain (ACFI Questions 11–12; Medication and Complex Health Care Procedures). Ratings calculated from completing checklists in this domain determine the level of the subsidy.

E-HEALTH RECORDS AND THE AUSTRALIAN DIGITAL HEALTH AGENCY

E-Health Records

More and more, Australian hospitals and healthcare providers are moving to electronic health (e-health) records. Such a development has certain advantages. For example, such records may be readily transferred within established e-health systems and such systems certainly address many of the difficulties encountered relating to the legibility of handwritten records. In addition, many computerised systems for prescribing already have built-in systems for detecting errors, which have been demonstrated to reduce adverse events in prescribing.[19] However, the record can reflect only the care delivered, and not the quality of it. Having said that, the record may well provide standardised formulae for documenting care that may enable more consistent information to be documented and shared. As a consequence, the majority of the considerations discussed in this chapter will continue to be relevant for all records, both handwritten and computerised.

Australian Digital Health Agency

The Commonwealth together with state and territory governments have been working to better coordinate health records and enhance health outcomes for some years utilising digital platforms. The culmination of that coordination was the establishment of the Australian Digital Health Agency (ADHA) in 2016, which is jointly funded by the Commonwealth and state and territory governments and reports to state and territory Health Ministers through the Health Council of COAG (Council of Australian Governments). The ADHA describes its purposes as:

Better health for all Australians enabled by seamless, safe, secure digital health services and technologies that provide a range of innovative, easy to use tools for both patients and providers.[20]

The seven strategic priorities of the ADHA are:

1. *Health information that is available whenever and wherever it is needed*
2. *Health information that can be exchanged securely*
3. *High-quality data with a commonly understood meaning that can be used with confidence*
4. *Better availability and access to prescriptions and medicines information*
5. *Digitally-enabled models of care that improve accessibility, quality, safety and efficiency*
6. *A workforce confidently using digital health technologies to deliver health and care*
7. *A thriving digital health industry delivering world class innovation.*[21]

The establishment of the My Health Record (MHR) system established under the provisions of the *My Health Records Act 2012* (Cth) would be the best-known outcome of the work of the ADHA. The MHR system has been developed over a number of years. In essence, it consists of online summaries of individuals' health information including medicines they are taking, known allergies and treatments received including immunisation records (the latter having become critical during the COVID-19 pandemic). The MHR system is designed to enable an individual's doctors, hospitals and other healthcare providers to access the individual's health information, in accordance with established access controls. Individuals are also able to access their MHR online.

All Australians can register for a personally controlled electronic health record and have access to a summary of their own health information whenever they need it. The document types and information that can be uploaded, entered, downloaded and viewed are listed as: Shared Health Summary, Event Summary, Discharge Summary, Medication Records, e-Referrals and Specialist Letters.[22]

People can include their Medicare data and enter personal information themselves, such as whether they have any allergies or adverse reactions, and any medications they are currently using. Other information that a patient can add includes the contact details of the holder of their advance care directive and a list of emergency contacts.

Parents can create a record for their children with information about scheduled health checks and childhood development milestones.

Records were created for every Australian who wanted one after 31 January 2019. The MHR legislation also provides that a person may choose to opt out of the MHR system at any time by permanently deleting his/her record. The privacy provisions of the MHR Act have also been strengthened to:

- permit every Australian to permanently delete their records, and any backups, at any time;
- explicitly prohibit access to My Health Records by insurers and employers;
- provide greater privacy for teenagers 14 years of age and over;
- strengthen existing protections for people at risk of family and domestic violence;
- clarify that only the MHR Agency, Department of Health and Medicare (and no other government agency) can access the MHR system;
- explicitly require law enforcement and other agencies to produce a court order to access information in My Health Records;
- make clear that the system cannot be privatised or used for commercial purposes.[23]

CONFIDENTIALITY OF HEALTHCARE RECORDS

Given the concerns about internet and computer security that exist in the general population, questions of privacy and confidentiality are specifically relevant to health record administrators, consumers and clinicians.

Privacy and confidentiality in relation to healthcare records are now discussed in more detail.

The requirement for nurses and midwives to observe a duty of confidentiality and privacy is spelled out in the Nursing and Midwifery Board of Australia (NMBA) *Code of conduct for nurses in Australia* and *Code of conduct for midwives in Australia*, specifically at section 3.5 within the Domain of practising safely, effectively and collaboratively and under Principle 3, Cultural practice and respectful relationships. Section 3.5 is set out in **Box 9.4**. Reference is also made in section 3.5(e) to the NMBA policy in managing social media.[24]

It is self-evident that, if nurses are to expect their patients to proffer highly sensitive information so they can care for them appropriately, patients must feel secure that the nurses and midwives will not divulge that information without their consent. If the patient does consent to the sharing of confidential information, the duty of confidentiality is not relevant, but the information can be shared only to the extent that the patient has consented. For example, if the person is happy for the nurse or midwife to share information with the team but not the family, there is still a duty to maintain confidentiality as specified.

There are a number of exceptions to this rule in each state and territory. The first is where it is mandated or permitted by statute or court order to share the information. An example of the former is mandatory reporting of notifiable diseases and suspected child abuse. An example of the latter is a subpoena requiring the production of specific data gathered in research. However, in the latter example, a judge could exercise judicial discretion in deciding whether it should be admitted into evidence if the information produced is not considered helpful in establishing the issue in dispute.

The second major exception is where the information is 'in the public interest'. This common law principle is best described as being an interest that is common to the public at large and that may or may not involve the personal or proprietary rights of individual people. In the healthcare system, the disclosure of an individual's healthcare details would generally be unlikely to pass the public interest test. At the same time, publication of healthcare data relevant to the overall health of the population would undoubtedly

---

BOX 9.4
PRINCIPLE 3: CULTURAL PRACTICE AND RESPECTFUL RELATIONSHIPS

3.5 CONFIDENTIALITY AND PRIVACY

Nurses have ethical and legal obligations to protect the privacy of people. People have a right to expect that nurses will hold information about them in confidence, unless the release of information is needed by law, is legally justifiable under public interest considerations or is required to facilitate emergency care. To protect privacy and confidentiality, nurses must:

  a. respect the confidentiality and privacy of people by seeking informed consent before disclosing information, including formally documenting such consent where possible

  b. provide surroundings to enable private and confidential consultations and discussions, particularly when working with multiple people at the same time, or in a shared space

  c. abide by the NMBA Social media policy and relevant Standards for practice, to ensure use of social media is consistent with the nurse's ethical and legal obligations to protect privacy

  d. access records only when professionally involved in the care of the person and authorised to do so

  e. not transmit, share, reproduce or post any person's information or images, even if the person is not directly named or identified, without having first gained written and informed consent. See also the NMBA Social media policy and Guidelines for advertising regulated health services

  f. recognise people's right to access information contained in their health records, facilitate that access and promptly facilitate the transfer of health information when requested by people, in accordance with local policy, and

  g. when closing or relocating a practice, facilitating arrangements for the transfer or management of all health records in accordance with the legislation governing privacy and health records.

Source: Nursing and Midwifery Board of Australia (NMBA), *Code of conduct for nurses in Australia*, 2018, Section 3.5, Principle 3.

---

meet the public interest test. The public interest test tends to fall into two areas; the first is sometimes described as the 'iniquity rule' — that is, the information discloses the commission of a crime or misdeed; the second is the 'balancing rule' — where the disclosure must be balanced in the public interest against the need for confidentiality. Disclosure of criminal activity or other civil wrong, even if it involves disclosing confidential information, may sometimes be justified on this ground. However, that disclosure must be in the public interest. If the public interest is not advanced by the disclosure, it will not be permissible to breach confidentiality.

Regulations exist to allow epidemiological data to be released under strict conditions for research purposes. Such data are released only to bona fide researchers and on condition that the confidentiality of data is maintained.[25]

Overall, the expectation is that we will take great care to respect the confidences entrusted to us by our patients. Each state and territory has legislation which requires people who deal with healthcare records to maintain confidentiality.

Advice Available to Nurses and Midwives on Documentation and Confidentiality

In addition to advice on what and how to document, there is also valuable advice available from most health departments and some employers on the relationship between documentation and confidentiality.

All of the states and territories have policy directives in relation to privacy and confidentiality that incorporate the basic rights, including the right to privacy, enunciated by the Australian Commission on Safety and Quality in Health Care (ACSQHC) in their policy document *Australian charter of healthcare rights*.[26] For example, the policy document *Confidentiality and privacy in healthcare*[27] prepared by the Victorian Department of Health provides specific advice about the privacy applying to both handwritten and e-records. Also, the policy of NSW Health in relation to the topic is contained in the document titled *NSW Health: your health care rights and responsibilities*.[28] That policy document sets out a guide for NSW Health staff, as well as a guide for patients, carers and families.

In addition to specific legislative provisions or policy directives, healthcare workers and public health organisations can owe a common law duty of confidentiality to their clients/patients. This duty arises from the nature of the relationship between health workers and their clients/patients.

Healthcare providers may be sued in the civil courts by clients/patients for breaches of confidentiality that cause damage or harm to the person or the person's reputation. If successful, monetary compensation may be awarded or the court may issue orders to prevent the breach occurring.

A defence to a common law action for breach of confidentiality would be that the disclosure was lawful where there was a statutory obligation or power to justify disclosure. However, where a confidentiality obligation exists, a client/patient may seek court orders to prevent the breach occurring, in addition to seeking compensation for any damage that has occurred.

The increasing complexity of our society has resulted in the perceived need for a variety of government and private sector agencies to acquire and store information of a personal and often sensitive nature about individuals, which seriously threatens the notion of individual privacy in the conduct of our daily lives. The need to compile a healthcare record about a patient or client is obvious and the use to which such records are formally put has already been stated and cannot be seriously questioned. The very nature of healthcare records is such that highly personal and sensitive material is often contained in them. It is therefore important that hospitals and health centres recognise and respect the right of individual privacy as far as their patients or clients are concerned and that steps be taken to respect that privacy, particularly in relation to healthcare records.

The use and storage of and access to a patient's or client's healthcare record should be (and in most cases is) the subject of a clear written policy by every hospital and health organisation. A policy document does not have the legal and binding force of legislation, but should be recognised for what it is meant to be — a clear statement of policy directives in relation to a particular issue of general importance in an organisation, which quite often embodies legal principles and/or requirements.

As previously discussed, electronic information, mail and communication systems are increasingly used as effective means of maintaining and transferring documentation and information in the healthcare environment. Precautions must be taken to ensure that clinical staff are fully informed of appropriate, safe and secure use of electronic information systems. It should be assumed that any and all clinical documentation will be scrutinised at some point.

Legislative Provisions in Relation to the Right of Access to Healthcare Records and Privacy Considerations Including a Patient's Right of Access to their Own Healthcare Records

A patient's right of access to their own healthcare records was addressed in the High Court decision of *Breen v Williams* (**Case example 9.2**). Following that decision, the Australian Government set out the legislative requirements known as the Information Privacy Principles in the *Privacy Act 1988* (Cth), to inform federal agencies in relation to access to personal information. That task is overseen by the Office of the Australian Information Commissioner (OAIC).

The current Australian Privacy Principles were introduced in 2014 under section 14 of the *Privacy Act 1988* (Cth) and are referenced in Schedule 1 of the Act.[29] They are reproduced in Box 9.5.

Of particular interest is Australian Privacy Principle (APP) 12 — access to personal information —

which states that, 'If an APP entity holds personal information about an individual, the entity must, on request by the individual, give the individual access to the information'.[30] There are a number of exceptions to that requirement, relating to the health, security and the privacy of others, *inter alia*, but it is clear that the intent of the principle is to ensure that individuals can have access to their own records.

The OAIC also regulates the privacy aspects of the e-health record system. Its website contains a substantial amount of information in the personally controlled electronic health record system (PCEHR).[31] The legislative provisions specifically relating to personally controlled e-health records are as follows:

- *Personally Controlled Electronic Health Records Act 2012* (Cth)
- *PCEHR Rules 2012* (Cth) (Note: the name of the Rules is this acronym as opposed to the spelled out words)
- *Personally Controlled Electronic Health Records Regulation 2012* (Cth).

The OAIC also regulates the privacy provisions of the PCEHR Act and has a range of functions, including:

- investigating complaints about the mishandling of personal information in an e-health record;
- providing education and guidance about privacy for individuals, healthcare providers, the system operator and other participants in the system; and
- accepting data breach notifications from the system operator, and repository operators and portal operators.

REPORTING AND DOCUMENTING ADVERSE EVENTS AND CLINICAL INCIDENTS

Since the mid 1990s, studies have been undertaken in most Australian states to examine the most appropriate mechanism for incident reporting in the healthcare system. Since that time, incident reporting has gradually developed and is now an integral part of healthcare practice.

In 2004, the Australian Commission on Safety and Quality in Health Care (ACSQHC) developed and recommended to Health Ministers a national specifica-

---

BOX 9.5
AUSTRALIAN PRIVACY PRINCIPLES[32]

Principle 1 — open and transparent management of personal information
Principle 2 — anonymity and pseudonymity
Principle 3 — collection of solicited personal information
Principle 4 — dealing with unsolicited personal information
Principle 5 — notification of the collection of personal information
Principle 6 — use or disclosure of personal information
Principle 7 — direct marketing
Principle 8 — cross-border disclosure of personal information
Principle 9 — adoption, use or disclosure of government-related identifiers
Principle 10 — quality of personal information
Principle 11 — security of personal information
Principle 12 — access to personal information
Principle 13 — correction of personal information

CASE EXAMPLE 9.2

Breen v Williams[33]

In contrast with health departments' guidelines, which support the patient's right to have access to his or her medical records, this 1995 decision by the High Court discounted such a proposition as a legal right both at common law and as a fiduciary duty owed by the medical practitioner to his or her patient. Ms Breen had commenced action in the Supreme Court of New South Wales seeking an order that her plastic surgeon give her access to her medical records. She had spent 5 years attempting to obtain her medical records to support her participation in a class action in the United States over breast implants. Ms Breen claimed she had a proprietary right and interest in the information contained in her medical records, or was otherwise entitled to the information, and sought orders giving her access to her medical records to examine and copy them. The doctor argued that because his medical notes were:

... prepared by me in the belief that they will remain private to me, they often contain conclusions, commentary and musing which might well be different in form and substance if the notes were prepared by me in the knowledge that the patient was entitled to a copy of my records.[34]

The initial judge hearing the matter refused Ms Breen's application on the grounds that:

The defendant was not made the plaintiff's medical adviser for the purpose of making him a collector or repository of information for the plaintiff to have available to her for whatever purposes she chooses. Collecting and retaining information was ... a subsidiary purpose, to lead only to medical advice and treatment to be administered by him or on his referral.[35]

Ms Breen appealed to the New South Wales Court of Appeal, which dismissed her appeal by a majority.[36] She then appealed to the High Court, where her appeal was also dismissed. Justice Brennan gave the following reasons for doing so:

I would hold that information with respect to a patient's history, condition or treatment obtained by a doctor in the course or for the purpose of giving advice or treatment to the patient must be disclosed by the doctor to the patient or the patient's nominee on request when (1) refusal to make the disclosure requested might prejudice the general health of the patient, (2) the request for disclosure is reasonable having regard to all the circumstances and (3) reasonable reward for the service of disclosure is tendered or assured. A similar duty may be imposed on the doctor by the law of torts but, in particular situations, for example, some emergency treatments, the relationship between doctor and patient may not give rise to a duty that extends so far ... .

An undertaking to provide information is one thing; a duty to give the patient access to and to permit the patient to copy the doctor's records is another. The doctor's duty to provide information not only can be discharged, but in some circumstances ought to be discharged, without allowing the patient to see the doctor's records. Where that duty can be performed without giving the patient access to the doctor's records, there is no foundation for implying any obligation to give that access. There is no evidence in this case to suggest that access to the respondent's records might have been necessary to avoid or diminish the possibility of prejudice to the appellant's health.[37]

tion for incident reporting and management systems to support the reporting and management of incidents at the local level. It was designed to identify better ways to manage hazards and risks and to improve systems of care delivery. As a consequence, the need for incident reporting is now an established part of our safety and quality framework in Australia.

The ACSQHC developed the National Safety and Quality Health Service (NSQHS) Standards, whose aims are to protect the public from harm and improve the quality of health service provision. Those Standards provide a nationally consistent statement about the level of care that consumers can expect from health services. The first edition of the NSQHS Standards was released in 2011, and they have been used to assess health service organisations in relation to safety and quality since January 2013. The second edition was released in November 2017, and they were further reviewed in May 2021.[38]

Under Standard 1, the Clinical Governance Standard, Action 1.11, the health service under review is required to have organisation-wide incident management and investigation systems. The organisation must provide evidence that it:

a. *Supports the workforce to recognise and report incidents;*

b. *Supports patients, carers and families to communicate concerns or incidents;*

c. *Involves the workforce and consumers in the review of incidents;*

d. *Provides timely feedback on the analysis of incidents to the governing body, the workforce and consumers;*

e. *Uses the information from the analysis of incidents to improve safety and quality;*

f. *Incorporates risks identified in the analysis of incidents into the risk management system; and*

g. *Regularly reviews and acts to improve the effectiveness of the incident management and investigation systems.*[39]

Incident-reporting systems have now been developed in each of the states and territories. Queensland and the ACT utilise the Riskman reporting system; New South Wales the Incident Management System; Victoria the Victorian Health Incident Management System; Western Australia the Datix Clinical Incident Management System; South Australia the Safety Learning System; Tasmania the Safety Reporting and Learning System; and Northern Territory the Clinical Senate system.

The procedure followed when adverse incidents are reported is generally similar. For example, in New South Wales each incident is coded by severity and the likelihood of recurrence under the Harm Score and rated numerically from 1, being the most severe, to 4. Victoria has a rating system known as the Incident Severity Rating with six levels of Harm from No Harm to Death.[40]

As follow up, NSW Health requires Harm Score 1 events be subject to a Serious Adverse Event Review such as a root cause analysis (RCA).[41] A RCA is an in depth investigation as to the cause of and circumstances under which the adverse event occurred.

The outcome of an RCA investigation is regarded as confidential and is protected by what is known as statutory privilege,[42] under the *Health Administration Act 1982* (NSW). In effect, the application of statutory privilege is expressed as providing that a person 'is neither competent or compellable to produce any document or disclose any communication to a court, tribunal, board, person or body if the document was prepared, or the communication was made' for the dominant purpose of a Serious Adverse Event Incident report such as a RCA. A similar provision applies in relation to the report of a quality assurance committee. In New South Wales, this right to keep information obtained during the course of an investigation confidential has been confirmed by the Administrative Decisions Tribunal.[43]

In Western Australia the *Health Services (Quality Improvement) Act 1994* extends a similar privilege (referred to as qualified privilege) to the reports of registered Quality Improvement Committees. That is, the Minister for Health is empowered under section 7 of that Act to approve a specified committee to be a Quality Improvement Committee. Similar to provisions in New South Wales, section 10 of the Western Australian statute provides that a person is 'neither competent or compellable' to give evidence or produce any document relevant to registered Quality Improvement Committee activities or functions.

In Western Australia, the Office of Patient Safety and Clinical Quality, the authority responsible for oversight of the work of Quality Improvement Committees, explains that the qualified privilege scheme is designed to encourage hospitals and health professional to:

■ *conduct quality improvement activities*
■ *investigate the causes and contributing factors of clinical incidents by protecting:*
  – *certain information from disclosure*
  – *clinicians involved in the activity from civil liability.*[44]

Guidelines issued by the WA Department of Health about Quality Improvement Committees explain that it is important to review what went wrong to improve safety and quality, and to find ways to prevent the event from happening again. It is generally believed that people will be more likely to talk about the mistakes they made if they know that the information they share cannot legally be revealed to anyone. Disclosing mistakes allows environments conducive to errors to be identified, and this facilitates the redesign of systems to create healthcare environments in which it is more difficult to make a mistake.[45]

Nurses and midwives jointly form the largest group of health professionals, so it is hardly surprising that they are also the largest group of reporters of clinical incidents and near misses.[46] Nurses and midwives must become fully conversant with the incident-reporting policy in their workplace. As with all other documentation, the reports submitted are required to be factual and accurate. This can present a challenge at times, as a sentinel or adverse event is most distressing for all concerned, and there can be a tendency for incident reports to be written in emotional language. However, it is most important for the safety and quality process that the reports can be carefully analysed to understand exactly what went wrong so that measures can be put in place to minimise the risk of such an event reoccurring. If nurses or midwives are distressed following an adverse event, it is important that they seek support from their more experienced colleagues. If they do not feel comfortable discussing the matter with their immediate colleagues, all healthcare organisations are required to provide support through some form of employee assistance scheme. Occupational health and safety representatives can provide advice on how to access this support. There is also now a national nurse support system funded through the Nursing and Midwifery Board of Australia.[47]

OPEN DISCLOSURE

A related matter that sits between the recording of adverse events and a patient's right to access their information, if not necessarily their healthcare record, is the movement to inform patients and their families when a person has suffered an adverse event. This process is referred to as 'open disclosure' (OD) and it is published and described by the ACSQHC in *The Australian open disclosure framework*.[48] In the past, often due to legal concerns, health professionals were defensive about admitting that something had gone wrong, even when no fault was necessarily attached to it, usually because of the perceived threat of legal action.

However, it is now considered best practice to explain to people what has happened when things go wrong; this is not necessarily considered to be an admission of liability (see **Chapter 7**). The framework identifies five elements to the process of OD, as follows:

- an apology or expression of regret, which should include the words 'I am sorry' or 'we are sorry';
- a factual explanation of what happened;
- an opportunity for the patient, their family and carers to relate their experience;
- a discussion of the potential consequences of the adverse event;
- an explanation of the steps being taken to manage the adverse event and prevent recurrence.[49]

The framework contains a set of eight principles, many of which are equally relevant to record-keeping:

1 *Open and timely communication. If things go wrong, the patient, their family and carers should be provided with information about what happened in a timely, open and honest manner. The open disclosure process is fluid and will often involve the provision of ongoing information.*

2 *Acknowledgment. All adverse events should be acknowledged to the patient, their family and carers as soon as practicable. Health service organisations should acknowledge when an adverse event has occurred and initiate open disclosure.*

3 *Apology or expression of regret. As early as possible, the patient, their family and carers should receive an apology or expression of regret for any harm that resulted from an adverse event. An apology or expression of regret should include the words 'I am sorry' or 'we are sorry', but must not contain speculative statements, admission of liability or apportioning of blame.*

4 *Supporting, and meeting the needs and expectations of patients, their family and carers. The patient, their family and carers can expect to be:*
   a. *fully informed of the facts surrounding an adverse event and its consequences;*
   b. *treated with empathy, respect and consideration;*
   c. *supported in a manner appropriate to their needs.*

5 ***Supporting, and meeting the needs and expectations of those providing healthcare.*** *Health service organisations should create an environment in which all staff are:*

    a. *encouraged and able to recognise and report adverse events;*

    b. *prepared through training and education to participate in open disclosure;*

    c. *supported through the open disclosure process.*

6 ***Integrated clinical risk management and systems improvement.*** *Thorough clinical review and investigation of adverse events and adverse outcomes should be conducted through processes that focus on the management of clinical risk and quality improvement. Findings of these reviews should focus on improving systems of care and be reviewed for their effectiveness. The information obtained about incidents from the open disclosure process should be incorporated into quality improvement activity.*

7 ***Good governance.*** *Open disclosure requires good governance frameworks, and clinical risk and quality improvement processes. Through these systems, adverse events should be investigated and analysed to prevent them recurring. Good governance involves a system of accountability through a health service organisation's senior management, executive or governing body to ensure that appropriate changes are implemented and their effectiveness is reviewed.*

Good governance should include internal performance monitoring and reporting.

8 ***Confidentiality.*** *Policies and procedures should be developed by health service organisations with full consideration for patient and clinician privacy and confidentiality, in compliance with relevant law (including Commonwealth, state and territory privacy and health records legislation). However, this principle needs to be considered in the context of Principle 1: Open and timely communication.*[50]

Open disclosure is now well established, particularly in the Australian public hospital system, and has the potential to improve relationships between healthcare practitioners and patients.[51] While it does not relate directly to documentation and medical records, it is nevertheless closely related to patients' rights to information, an issue that is also discussed in Chapter 6.

CONCLUSION

It is clear that healthcare records play a most important role in the lives and practice of nurses and midwives. Their good management and meticulous upkeep will protect not only the care and safety of the patient but also the professional standing of the individual nurse or midwife. It is imperative that nurses and midwives keep up to date with the laws and policies relating to documentation and privacy, particularly as the use of electronic records becomes mainstream.

CHAPTER 9 REVIEW QUESTIONS

Following your reading of **Chapter 9**, consider these questions in reaching the objectives of this chapter. Guidance on which part of the chapter will assist you in answering the questions can be found at http://evolve.elsevier.com/AU/Staunton/law/. You may, of course, consider other sources as part of your considerations.

1. For what reasons do we make and retain patient records?

2. What are the safeguards we need to think about in relation to making electronic health records?

3. Why is the requirement for confidentiality so critical in relation to obtaining patient information and making patient records?

4. What rights do patients have to access their own health records?

ENDNOTES

Note: all links were last accessed in March 2023.

1. Inquest into the death of Shona Hookey; NSW Coroner's Court, 22 December 2016 at paras [189]–[190].
2. NSW Health, *Health care records — documentation and management*, policy directive, PD2012_069. December 2012, reviewed June 2019.
3. Inquest into the death of Paul Lau: NSW Coroners Court; 2015/181507, 29 March 2018.
4. *McCabe v Auburn District Hospital* NSWSC, No 11551 of 1982, Grove J 31 May 1980, unreported. See also *Durant v Tamworth Base Hospital* [2003] NSWSC 73, where it was found 'in relation to his relevant complaints of pain [the plaintiff's evidence is] in this regard to be totally outweighed in a probative sense by the notations in the hospital records' (at [31] per Newman AJ).
5. *Spasovic v Sydney Adventist Hospital* [2003] NSWSC 791 (12 September 2003) per James J.
6. Wolf Z R, 'Nurses' stories: discovering essential nursing', (2008) *Medsurgical Nursing*, October, 17(5):324–9.
7. Berry L, 'The research relationship in narrative enquiry', (2016) *Nurse Researcher* 24(1):10–14.
8. Zeitz K and McCutcheon H, 'Observations and vital signs: ritual or vital for the monitoring of postoperative patients?', (2006) *Applied Nursing Research* 19(4):204–11.
9. *Laidlaw v Lion's Gate Hospital* (1969) 70 WWR 727, at 739.
10. Forster S L, Fulde G W O and McCarthy S, 'Emergency department administration, legal matters and quality care', in Fulde G W O and Fulde S (eds) *Emergency medicine: the principles of practice*, Elsevier, Australia, 2009, p 724.
11. *Spasovic v Sydney Adventist Hospital* [2003], op. cit.
12. Ibid, at [388]–[390].
13. Ibid, at [391].
14. Records Principles 2014, made under subsection 96-1(1) of the *Aged Care Act 1997* (Cth).
15. Australian Government, Department of Health, *Aged Care Funding Instrument (ACFI) user guide*, 2017, https://agedcare.health.gov.au/funding/aged-care-subsidies-and-supplements/residential-care-subsidy/basic-subsidy-amount-aged-care-funding-instrument/aged-care-funding-instrument-acfi-user-guide.
16. Australian Government, Department of Health, Aged Care Funding Instrument op. cit., 2017, p 4.
17. Ibid.
18. See for example the websites of the Aged and Community Services Australia, https://acsa.asn.au/ and the Aged Care Industry Association https://acia.asn.au/.
19. Ammenwerth E, Schnell-Inderst P, Machan C and Siebert U, 'The effect of electronic prescribing on medication errors and adverse drug events: a systematic review', (2008) *Journal of the American Medical Informatics Association* 15(5):585–600.
20. Australian Government, Australian Digital Health Agency (ADHA), *Corporate plan 2018–2019 to 2021–2022*, ADHA, Sydney, 2018, p 4, https://www.digitalhealth.gov.au/about-the-agency/corporate-plan/ADHA_Corporate_Plan_2018-2019.pdf.
21. Ibid, p 9.
22. Australian Government, Australian Digital Health Agency (ADHA), My Health Record
23. Australian Government, Australian Digital Health Agency (ADHA), Cancel a My Health Record, nd, https://www.myhealthrecord.gov.au/for-you-your-family/howtos/cancel-my-record.
24. Nursing and Midwifery Board of Australia (NMBA), *Code of conduct for nurses and Code of conduct for midwives*, effective 1 March 2018, https://www.nursingmidwiferyboard.gov.au/Codes-Guidelines-Statements/Professional-standards.aspx.
25. See, for example, the National Health and Medical Research Council's *Principles for accessing and using publicly funded data for health research*, January 2016, https://www.nhmrc.gov.au/about-us/publications/principles-accessing-and-using-publicly-funded-data-health-research.
26. Australian Commission on Safety and Quality in Health Care (ACSQHC), Australian charter of healthcare rights, 2nd ed. 2019
27. Victorian Department of Health, *Confidentiality and privacy in healthcare*, 2018, https://www.betterhealth.vic.gov.au/health/ServicesAndSupport/confidentiality-and-privacy-in-health-care.
28. NSW Health, *Your health care rights and responsibilities*, PD2011_022, reviewed in 2016, https://www.health.nsw.gov.au/patientconcerns/Pages/your-health-rights-responsibilities.aspx.
29. *Privacy Act 1988* (Cth), Schedule 1.
30. Ibid, APP 12.
31. OAIC, 'e-Health records': 2012 and see Australian Privacy Principles quick reference tool: March 2014: issued by the Office of the Australian Information Commissioner.
32. Ibid, APP 12.
33. *Breen v Williams* [1996] HCA 57; (1996) 186 CLR 71.
34. *Breen v Williams* (SC(Eq) (NSW), Bryson J, No. 2363/94, 10 October 1994, unreported).
35. Ibid.
36. *Breen v Williams* (1994) 35 NSWLR 522.
37. *Breen v Williams* [1996], op. cit., Brennan CJ at [7] and [8].
38. Australian Commission on Safety and Quality in Health Care (ACSQHC), *Standards: NSQHS standards*, 2nd ed, 2019, updated May 2021, https://www.safetyandquality.gov.au/standards.
39. Ibid, Action 1.11 *Incident management systems and open disclosure*, https://www.safetyandquality.gov.au/standards/nsqhs-standards/clinical-governance-standard/patient-safety-and-quality-systems/action-111.
40. Victorian Health Incident Management System (VHIMS), *Victorian Health Incident Management System (VHIMS): Minimum Data Set Manual 2021-22*, Issued March 2022.
41. NSW Health, *Incident management policy*, policy directive, PD2020-047, Issued 14 December 2020.
42. Ibid, p 33.

43. *Bray v North Coast Area Health Service* [2009] NSW ADT 93 (4 May 2009).

44. Government of Western Australia, Department of Health, *Qualified privilege: what is qualified privilege?* 2016, https://ww2.health.wa.gov.au/Articles/N_R/Qualified-privilege.

45. Government of Western Australia, Department of Health, *Guidelines for Quality Improvement Committees seeking qualified privilege under the* Health Services (Quality Improvement) Act 1994, pp 2–3.

46. Nuckols T, Bell D and Liu H, 'Rates and types of events reported to established incident reporting systems in two U.S. hospitals', (2007) *Quality and Safety in Health Care* 16:164–8.

47. Nurse and Midwife Support website, https://www.nmsupport.org.au/.

48. Australian Commission on Safety and Quality in Health Care (ACSQHC), *The Australian open disclosure framework*, March 2013, https://www.safetyandquality.gov.au/sites/default/files/migrated/Australian-Open-Disclosure-Framework-Feb-2014.pdf.

49. Ibid, p 11.

50. Ibid, pp 12–13.

51. Iedema R, Jorm C, Wakefield J, Ryan C and Dunn S, 'Practising open disclosure: clinical incident communication and systems improvement', (2009) *Sociology of Health and Illness* 31(2):262–77.

Documentation by Nurses and Midwives

Documentation by nurses and midwives must include the following:

a. Care/treatment plan, including risk assessments with associated interventions.

b. Comprehensive completion of all patient/client care forms.

c. Any significant change in the patient/client's status with the onset of new signs and symptoms recorded.

d. If a change in the patient/client's status has been reported to the responsible medical practitioner, documentation of the name of the medical practitioner and the date and time that the change was reported to him/her.

e. Documentation of medication orders received verbally, by telephone/electronic communication including the prescriber's name, designation and date/time.

Source: NSW Health, *Health care records — documentation and management*, policy directive, PD2012_069, December 2012, reviewed June 2019, https://www1.health.nsw.gov.au/pds/ActivePDSDocuments/PD2012_069.pdf.

SPECIALISED AREAS OF PRACTICE

SECTION OUTLINE

10

MENTAL HEALTH

LEARNING OBJECTIVES

In this chapter, you will:

- gain an understanding of the background to mental health care and legislation in Australia
- become aware of the distinction between civil and forensic patients in the delivery of mental health care and treatment
- examine the common approach taken by the states and territories in the development of mental health legislation that underpins the care and treatment of people with a mental illness
- understand the framework of the mental health legislation in your state or territory, particularly the rights of patients with a mental illness, as well as the admission, care and treatment provisions relating to voluntary or involuntary patients with a mental illness
- be aware of your professional responsibilities in relation to seclusion and restraint if used as part of the inpatient care and treatment of a person with a mental illness.

INTRODUCTION

The approach to the delivery of mental health care and treatment is relatively uniform across the states and territories of Australia. There is, however, differing legislation in each of the states and territories that acts as a starting point when considering the legal requirements inherent in the delivery of mental health care and treatment. Regardless of the differences between the states and territories, there is one important point consistently applied by each of them in the delivery of mental health services. That is, where the person's condition permits, the emphasis is to move from long-term institutional care to community care by providing for a variety of community-oriented care and treatment orders.

The Commonwealth Government has a limited role in the actual delivery of mental health services but does monitor the delivery of such services and, under the auspices of the Australian Institute of Health and Welfare (AIHW), regularly publishes updates on the availability of such services across Australia.

THE ESTABLISHMENT OF PRINCIPLES GOVERNING MENTAL HEALTH CARE AND TREATMENT IN AUSTRALIA

The legislation now in place in each of the states and territories is consistent with the United Nations Principles for the Protection of Persons with Mental Illness and the Improvement of Mental Health Care, the Australian Health Minister's Mental Health Statement of Rights and Responsibilities, and the National Mental Health Plan.

The Principles, adopted by the United Nations General Assembly in 1991, stipulated that all persons requiring mental health care and treatment have the right:

- to the best available mental health care;
- to be treated with humanity and respect for the inherent dignity of the human person;
- to protection from economic, sexual and other forms of exploitation, physical or other abuse, and degrading treatment;

- to be free of discrimination;
- to exercise all civic, political, economic, social and cultural rights.

Where a person, by reason of a mental illness or mental condition, lacks legal capacity, any decision about ongoing care and treatment should be made by an independent and impartial tribunal together with any appointed legal guardian or carer.

Our National Mental Health Statement of Rights and Responsibilities was adopted by all states and territories in 1991 and is consistent with the rights and objectives encompassed within the United Nations Principles. In 1992, to support the Statement the states and territories endorsed the National Mental Health Plan, the aim of that process being:

- to set a clear direction for the future development of mental health services in Australia;
- to promote the mental health of Australians and, where possible, to prevent the development of mental health problems and mental disorders;
- to reduce the impact of mental disorders on individuals, families and the community; and
- to establish a framework to ensure the rights of people with mental illness are protected.

The above process has acted as the impetus for significant changes in mental health legislation in each of the states and territories.

Why There is a Need for Mental Health Legislation

Critical to understanding the rationale behind the mental health legislation of your state or territory is to remember that mental illness, by its very nature, can sometimes interfere with a person's ability to give a valid consent to recommended healthcare and/or treatment. That is because mental illness can sometimes impair a person's ability to understand the nature and effect of their illness and to give informed consent to treatment recommended. When that happens the person is deemed to not have full legal capacity.

At the same time it is important to remember that just because a person has a mental illness does not mean that he/she lacks full legal capacity. It is only when the person's mental illness is compromised, for example, by the presence of acute psychosis with symptoms such as delusions or serious thought disorder, that the issue of the person's legal capacity to give and withhold consent to treatment arises.

As is explored fully in **Chapter 6**, all persons over 18 years of age, barring any symptoms arising from a mental illness or mental condition, are presumed to have full legal capacity. That is, they have the right to give and withhold consent to treatment. In relation to children, that presumption does not apply to a child under 14 years of age where the consent of a parent or guardian is required for treatment proposed for the child. Between the ages of 14 and 18 years the law recognises that young people have full legal capacity to give and withhold consent to treatment on the basis that they understand the nature and effect of the proposed treatment and that it is in their best interests. Generally speaking, however, between the ages of 14 and 16 years, hospitals and health services require the consent of a parent or guardian as well as the child.

Having a mental illness covers a wide spectrum of mental health disorders. For example, an adult person may suffer from severe anxiety or a depressive illness that negatively affects the person's ability to function fully in the community and in their social and family life. In such circumstances, most people will acknowledge that and will voluntarily seek assistance from a health professional, very often a psychologist or a psychiatrist. They may be prescribed a course of psychotherapy or appropriate medication, or a combination of both, which they agree to undertake.

Throughout the above process, the person is no different from a person who seeks treatment for a physical health condition. That is, the person is deemed to have full legal capacity to understand and accept the need for, and consent to, the treatment and/or medication proposed. More often than not the person will undergo treatment while remaining in the community. Hopefully their mental illness will respond to the course of treatment initiated and they will be able to fully resume their life in the community.

Occasionally in the above circumstances, the person may not be able to be treated in the community and may need to be admitted as an inpatient to an appropriate mental health facility. Again, where the person acknowledges and accepts the need for such inpatient treatment and agrees to be admitted and treated, they are deemed to be a **voluntary patient** with full legal capacity, able to give or withhold consent to treatment. Where a child or young person is involved, the consent to treatment is undertaken on their behalf in accordance with the principles outlined above.

It is only when the person's mental illness becomes so severe and deteriorates to an acute psychosis with delusions, hallucinations or serious thought and mood disturbances that the issue of their legal capacity to give and withhold consent to treatment becomes an issue. In those circumstances, the person often has to be detained and treated against their will and, at that point, is deemed to be an **involuntary patient**. When that occurs, it is important to ensure the person is treated and cared for in a safe and proper environment and is not exposed to a risk of harm to himself or herself or others. Such people are, by the very nature of their illness, extremely vulnerable to abuse, neglect and ill treatment.

When such a situation arises, the mental health legislation is designed to provide a framework of protection for mentally ill persons and their families underpinned by an acknowledgment of the civil rights of a person with a mental illness and the importance of including them, as much as possible, in decisions about their care and treatment. In addition, it imposes obligations and responsibilities on mental health professionals when it is considered clinically necessary in the person's best interests and the safety of others to detain, treat and care for a mentally ill person without their consent.

THE LEGISLATIVE FRAMEWORK FOR THE PROVISION AND REGULATION OF MENTAL HEALTH CARE AND TREATMENT IN AUSTRALIA

The framework for the provision and regulation of mental health services in Australia is embodied in the mental health legislation of each of the states and territories. While the overall approach is relatively similar, each state and territory has approached the specific provisions of their respective legislation, often utilising differing terms for the same thing. For example, the term used to permit a person receiving mental health care and treatment to nominate an individual to be consulted in relation to their care is referred to by

diverse titles such as 'designated carer' or 'principal care provider' (NSW); a 'carer' or 'nominated person' (ACT); 'primary carer' (NT); 'nominated support person' (Qld); 'support person' (Tas) and 'nominated person' (Vic and WA). Notwithstanding those and other differences in the terms used, legislation of each of the states and territories follows a similar pattern by making provision, to a greater or lesser degree, under the following relevant subject areas:

■ **objects of the legislation** — that is, what the legislation is designed to achieve. For example, section 4 of the Queensland *Mental Health Act 2000* states, among other objectives, that the purpose of the Act is to make provision for the involuntary assessment, treatment and protection of persons (whether adult or child) who have a mental illness while safeguarding their rights and freedoms and balancing those rights and freedoms with the rights and freedoms of others. Another example along similar lines but expressed a little differently is section 3 of the New South Wales *Mental Health Act 2007*, which states, among other objectives, that the Act is designed to provide for, and facilitate the care and treatment of, persons who are mentally ill or mentally disordered and to protect their civil rights. The mental health legislation of each state and territory details the objects of the Act and are all found within the first few sections of the respective Act;

■ **the principles that should underpin the provision of mental health care and treatment.** In other words, these provisions spell out the principles that health professionals are to apply in the delivery of mental health care and treatment. These provisions are found in each of the respective Acts. For example, section 68(a) of the New South Wales *Mental Health Act* states that people with a mental illness should receive the best possible care and treatment in the least restrictive environment enabling the care and treatment to be effectively given. The *Victorian Mental Health Act* section 11(1) states that the principles that apply require that persons receiving mental health services should have their rights, dignity and autonomy respected and promoted and that

Aboriginal persons receiving mental health services should have their distinct culture and identity recognised and responded to. Again, the respective legislation of each state and territory expresses similar such principles within their legislation and they are applicable to all health professionals who deliver care and treatment under the Act. See s 6 (ACT)); s 68 (NSW); ss 9 and 10 (NT); s 5 (Qld); s 7 (SA); s 15 (Tas) with reference to Mental Health Service Delivery Principles in Schedule 1 of the Act; s 11 (Vic); s 11 (WA) with reference to the Charter of mental health care principles in Schedule 1 of the Act;

■ **the definition of key words and phrases relating to persons who come within the legislation for the purposes of care, treatment and control**. This is very important in understanding the legislation. Each of the states and territories will have a 'definitions' section in their legislation which will either appear at the commencement of the legislation or be listed as a schedule at the end of it. Also, some important definitions will appear as standalone sections within the body of the Act. One such important example is the definition of mental illness **or** mental condition **or** who is a mentally ill person (not all states and territories use the last expression) and they are not defined in identical terms. For example, s 6 of the Western Australia *Mental Health Act* states that a person has a mental illness if the person has a condition that 'is characterised by a disturbance of thought, mood, perception, orientation or memory **and** significantly impairs (temporarily or permanently) the person's judgment or behaviour' whereas s 3 of the South Australian *Mental Health Act* simply states that mental illness is 'any illness or disorder of the mind'. The other states and territories also vary: ss 9 and 10 of the ACT *Mental Health Act* define 'mental disorder' and 'mental illness'; s 4 of the New South Wales *Mental Health Act* defines 'mental illness' and s 14 of the Act defines 'mentally ill'; s 6 of the Northern Territory *Mental Health Act* defines 'mental illness' to be read in conjunction with s 14 of the Act; s 10 of the Queensland *Mental Health Act* defines 'mental illness' as does s 4 of the Tasmania *Mental Health Act*, as well as s 4

of the Victorian *Mental Health Act*. The definitions identified above are set out in detail later in this chapter when the specific legislation of each state and territory is further explained. As is evident by a comparative reading of many relevant definitions as between the states and territories, many are **not** expressed in similar terms and health professionals should be aware of the definition that applies to such phrases in the particular state or territory legislation where they are practising;

■ **the process to be followed to admit, detain and treat a person either as a voluntary patient or as an involuntary patient.** Each state and territory sets out in detail the process that must be observed in order to admit, detain and treat a person either as a voluntary patient able to give a valid consent to treatment **or** as an involuntary patient on the basis they are unable to give a valid consent to treatment because they lack full legal capacity due to their mental illness or condition and require care, treatment and control for their own safety and the safety of others. Again, different expressions are used but essentially the intention is the same. That is, to provide for voluntary patients to give and withhold consent to treatment and inpatient care if required. For involuntary patients, the provisions permit certain persons to take a person to a mental health facility if considered necessary for the person to be 'examined' or 'assessed'. If that is considered necessary, the involuntary patient may be subject to a 'detention' order (or similar such title) for a specified period of hours or days and be subject to further examination, assessment, treatment and detention. Alternatively, if the person's condition permits, they may be subject to a community-based 'treatment order' and be monitored and cared for in the community. Given that the emphasis in the legislation in each of the states and territories is to treat the patient in the least restrictive environment (preferably in the community), those caring for an involuntary patient must view that provision as a paramount objective. At all times the patient's civil rights must be respected and an appropriate person nominated as the patient's 'carer' (howsoever expressed) must be consulted and kept informed of decisions made about the patient's care and treatment;

■ **the types of care and treatment that may be given to a person as a voluntary or involuntary patient.** The legislation permits specific treatment (e.g. ECT) that may be given to a person as a voluntary patient on the basis they have full legal capacity. It also permits specific treatment to be given to an involuntary patient (generally against his or her wishes) on the basis that they lack full legal capacity because of their mental illness or condition. For that to occur, specific steps and safeguards must be observed (e.g. the approval of an independent Tribunal). Some states and territories also specify types of treatment that may **not** be given (e.g. deep sleep and insulin therapy) and also spell out in detail the steps that must be observed by health professionals where seclusion and restraint are implemented as part of inpatient care and treatment;

■ **independent review and appeal mechanisms.** Each state and territory makes provision for independent review and appeal mechanisms to ensure that people with a mental illness or mental condition (or their carers) can challenge treatment or detention decisions made by health professionals on the basis that their civil rights are being impinged. There are also provisions for independent persons (e.g. Official visitors) who are able to visit and inspect mental health facilities to ensure the standard of care and protection required are being maintained.

The Distinction Between Forensic and Civil Patients in the Delivery of Mental Health Care and Treatment

Before considering the mental health care and treatment provisions in more detail, it is important to have a general understanding of the distinction between what are referred to as **forensic** patients and **civil** patients in the care and treatment of persons with a mental illness.

Because of the special nature of forensic patients, some of the states and territories have passed specific legislation to enable the criminal courts to deal with such patients to be considered in conjunction with their mental health legislation[1] whereas the others

incorporate forensic provisions in their mental health legislation.[2]

Forensic Patients

Forensic patients are those people who have committed a criminal act and, having been charged with the criminal offence, are either found by the criminal court to be not guilty on the grounds of mental illness (NGMI) or are found unfit to plead because of an existing mental illness or mental condition. The difference between the two findings is essentially one of timing.

Not Guilty on the Grounds of Mental Illness. To be found NGMI in relation to a criminal offence, the evidence must establish that, *at the time of committing the offence*, the person did not understand the nature and effect of what they were doing and that what they were doing was wrong. For a court to find a person NGMI, it will rely very heavily on the expert evidence of forensic psychiatrists and psychologists together with a comprehensive knowledge of the person's mental health history.

Unfit to Plead. For a person to be found unfit to plead in relation to a criminal offence, the evidence must demonstrate that, *at the time the person comes before the court for trial* and because of a prevailing mental illness or mental condition, the person is unable to understand the offence he or she has been charged with and the role of the judge and jury as part of the court process, and is unable to properly instruct a lawyer to act on his or her behalf.

A good example where a person may be found unfit to plead by a criminal court would be where a person is charged with an offence but, before he or she appears before the court to stand trial, the person sustains severe head injuries in a motor vehicle accident that leaves them significantly intellectually and cognitively impaired. The accident has rendered the person unable to properly enter a plea of guilty or not guilty to the charge, unable to understand and follow the court process and unable to instruct a lawyer to act on their behalf. In such circumstances, the person will generally be found unfit to plead.

In coming to the determination that a person is unfit to plead, a criminal court will rely on the expert evidence of psychiatrists and clinical psychologists as well as the person's relevant medical and mental health history.

Notwithstanding the above distinction, it would be possible for a person to be found NGMI as well as unfit to plead, depending on the expert opinion evidence as to their mental state at the time of committing the offence and when they come before the court for trial.

Forensic Patients Referred to a Mental Health Court or Tribunal. When a person is found NGMI or unfit to plead, they are classified as forensic patients and referred to the nominated mental health court or tribunal of the state or territory to be further dealt with in relation to ongoing care and treatment. It is important to emphasise that, once such a finding is made, the person is a patient and not a convicted inmate.

Not all states and territories use the term 'forensic patient'; for example, Western Australia uses the term 'mentally impaired'.

Forensic patients are reviewed by the mental health court or tribunal of their state or territory, initially every 3 months and then every 6 months.

At those reviews, the tribunal determines ongoing care and placement matters and may, where it is satisfied the person does not represent a risk to his or her own safety or the safety of others, conditionally release the patient on a forensic community treatment order. The tribunal is also empowered to unconditionally release a forensic patient, but will only do so where it is again satisfied the patient does not represent a risk to his or her own safety and the safety of others.

The wider role of mental health tribunals is discussed in more detail later in this chapter.

Civil Patients

Civil patients are those people in the community with a mental illness who may, from time to time, require care, treatment or control for their own protection or for the protection of the community.

Civil patients can be admitted to, treated and detained in a mental health facility without their consent (involuntary patient), or a person with a mental illness may admit himself or herself to a mental health facility for care and treatment (voluntary patient).

With involuntary civil patients, the major emphasis in the mental health legislation is that care and treatment, where appropriate, be given in the 'least restrictive environment'. That is generally achieved by a variety of community-based treatment orders.

The ongoing review and regulation of civil patients, including the approval of community treatment orders, is undertaken by mental health practitioners including psychiatrists together with the mental health court or nominated tribunal of the state or territory.

The Role and Function of Mental Health Courts or Nominated Tribunals in the Review and Regulation of Persons with a Mental Illness or Mental Condition

Each state and territory has a relevant mental health court or nominated tribunal to deal with the review and regulation of those patients (forensic and civil) receiving mental health care and treatment under the legislation.

In **New South Wales** and the **Northern Territory** the relevant tribunal is titled the Mental Health Review Tribunal. In **Tasmania**, **Victoria** and **Western Australia**, it is titled the Mental Health Tribunal. In **South Australia** the role is undertaken by a division of the Civil and Administrative Tribunal of South Australia, and in the **Australian Capital Territory** it is undertaken by the ACT Civil and Administrative Tribunal (referred to as ACAT). **Queensland** has both a Mental Health Review Tribunal and a Mental Health Court.

The role and function of these bodies are set out in the mental health legislation of the states and territories and can vary somewhat, but overall their role is the same. In **New South Wales**, for example, the role of the tribunal in dealing with **civil patients** encompasses:

- conducting mental health inquiries and making involuntary patient orders authorising the continued involuntary detention of a person in a mental health facility;
- reviewing involuntary patients in mental health facilities, usually every 3 or 6 months, and in appropriate cases every 12 months;
- reviewing voluntary patients in mental health facilities, usually every 12 months;
- hearing appeals against an authorised medical officer's refusal to discharge an involuntary patient;
- making, varying or revoking community treatment orders;

- approving the use of electroconvulsive therapy (ECT) for involuntary patients;
- determining whether voluntary patients have consented to ECT;
- approving surgery for an involuntary patient detained in a mental health facility;
- approving special medical treatment (sterilisation) for involuntary patients; and
- making and revoking orders under the *Trustee and Guardian Act 2009* (NSW) for a person's financial affairs to be managed by the New South Wales Trustee.

In addition, the tribunal regularly reviews and determines care and placement provisions, including, where appropriate, approving community treatment orders for all **forensic patients** who:

- have been found not guilty by a court by reason of mental illness;
- have been found unfit to be tried by reason of mental illness; or
- have been transferred from prison to hospital because of mental illness.

Understanding the Legal and Professional Obligations that Arise for Nurses Caring for Patients Under the Mental Health Legislation of the State or Territory

As in any area of healthcare, the law imposes a duty and standard of care expected of nurses and other health professionals working in the field of mental health. That issue is explored fully in **Chapter 7** but it is important to emphasise when considering the delivery of mental health care, be it in a mental health facility or in the community.

Ultimately, the adequacy or otherwise of professional nursing care in mental health will be assessed against the legal test applying to all fields of professional endeavour. That is, in considering any situation, the test to be applied is to ask whether the manner in which the particular care was delivered would be 'widely accepted in Australia by peer professional opinion as competent professional practice'.

The practical application of that test means that every aspect of nursing care in mental health is subject to objective professional standards complemented by clinical protocols and policies. Some of those professional standards are also embodied in legislation. The most obvious examples of this are in the specific domain of seclusion and restraint, which are acknowledged as acceptable forms of intervention treatment in certain circumstances in relation to the care of a person with a mental illness.

The use of such procedures is very strictly controlled, either by legislative provision or by detailed policy and clinical protocols issued by the employer. For example, the Northern Territory, Queensland, Tasmania, Victoria and Western Australia all make provision in their respective mental health legislation detailing provisions that must apply when seclusion and restraint are implemented. The Australian Capital Territory makes limited provision in relation to 'minimum confinement and restraint', whereas New South Wales and South Australia have no specific legislative provision but do have detailed mandatory policies.

The upshot of the above provisions is that when a person is held in seclusion or is restrained contrary to the legislative provisions of the state or territory, or in contravention of mandated policy, it would almost certainly result in a finding that the care of the patient was not in accordance with care that 'would be widely accepted in Australia by peer professional opinion as competent professional practice'.

A recent example of the above is to be found in **Case example 10.1**.

CASE EXAMPLE 10.1

Inquest into the death of Miriam Merten[3]

Mrs Merten was being cared for in the mental health unit of the Lismore Base Hospital. She had had numerous admissions to the unit over many years and could be difficult to manage. On 26 May 2014, she again presented to the hospital and, due to management issues, was placed in seclusion in the mental health unit. That seclusion commenced at 11.50 pm on 1 June 2014 and ended at approximately 6 am on 2 June 2014, when she was released to go to the toilet. Between the hours of 11.50 pm on 1 June and 6.49 am on 2 June, the CCTV footage disclosed that the patient had at least 24 falls. She also had sustained 'self-beatings of her head'. None of those incidents were detailed in her observation charts or clinical records.

Inquest into the death of Miriam Merten (Continued)

Mrs Merten was admitted to the intensive care unit of the hospital on 2 June 2014 at approximately 8 am. She died the following day as a result of traumatic and hypoxic brain injury that the court found was 'caused by numerous falls and the self-beating of her head on various surfaces the latter not done with the intention of taking her own life'.

Comments and Relevant Considerations Relating to the Coroner's Inquest and the Professional Standards Inquiry that Followed

At the inquest to determine the manner and cause of Mrs Merten's death, the coroner stated that the treatment afforded her by the nursing staff 'falls significantly below the standard expected'. He particularly highlighted the policies and protocols that were in place that clearly stated how Mrs Merten should have been managed. For example, the NSW Health policy in relation to seclusion provided for actual observations on a regular basis to be taken and recorded as well as communication with the patient 'to ensure the patient's physical safety and continually assess behaviour with the view to ceasing the intervention as soon as possible'. The coroner stated: 'The senior nurse deliberately made a decision not to comply with this protocol leading, together with other conduct, to conclude that there was no intention to cease seclusion during her shift'.

In separate legal proceedings,[4] the registered nurse in charge of the night shift was charged with unsatisfactory conduct as well as professional misconduct in relation to her conduct on the night in question. In their findings upholding those charges, the Tribunal said, *inter alia*, as follows:

> *Ms Borthistle's conduct in not undertaking adequate observations (of the patient) throughout the first hour of seclusion demonstrated poor judgment. It demonstrated judgment possessed and care exercised that, in our view, fell grossly below the relevant standard because Mrs Borthistle's primary responsibility once (the patient) was in seclusion was to ensure her safety. The relevant policy sets out the means by which the responsibility is to be met:*
>
> *maintenance of 1:1 observations for the first hour and thereafter at set intervals. By refusing to comply with that policy, she placed the patient at predictable risk of harm, which, because she ignored it, came to pass.*

While the above example may appear extreme when one has regard to its facts and circumstances, it highlights to nursing staff that, when caring for people in the mental health system, they must do so in accordance with the legal and professional standards expected of them.

Nurses working in the area of mental health care and treatment should take the time to become familiar with the mental health legislation relevant to their state or territory as well as all relevant policies and protocols relating to the delivery of care. Also, employers have an obligation to ensure nursing staff members are provided with appropriate in-service education to familiarise them with all relevant legislative provisions, policies and protocols.

OVERVIEW OF THE MENTAL HEALTH LEGISLATION OF EACH STATE AND TERRITORY

The intention in this chapter is to provide nurses with an overview of the relevant mental health legislation in each state and territory. Such legislation is available online and, at first glance, may appear daunting to follow. Accordingly, the following overview of the legislation is intended to provide nurses working in the area with relevant information about the mental health legislative provisions that apply in each state and territory. The overview is not intended to be an exhaustive consideration of every provision of the mental health legislation of each state or territory but rather to highlight those sections of the legislation that would generally arise for consideration by nursing staff on a day-to-day basis in the course of their work.

The overview is addressed in the following four discrete sections:

1. **The objectives, principles and rights under the Act.** For example, these sections ensure that the mental health legislation provides suitable protection for persons who are treated within its provisions by emphasising the person's civil and human rights, the right to be provided with the

best possible mental health care and the right to be included in decisions about their care wherever possible.

2. **Relevant definitions under the Act.** For example, these sections define specific words or phrases used in the legislation: how is mental illness defined, who is a carer under the legislation, who is an involuntary patient, what is meant by reference to a mental health facility as well as many others. Generally speaking, such definitions as well as many others may be found at the beginning of the legislation or in a schedule or dictionary at the end of the legislation. Before considering the legislation in detail, it is always helpful to scrutinise the definitions applied to words or phrases that appear in the legislation.

3. **Admission, detention, care and treatment of persons under the Act.** For example, these sections detail who may admit a person to a mental health facility as an involuntary patient, what processes must be followed when a person is admitted and detained as an involuntary patient and who must be notified. Provision is also made in the legislation as to what treatments are specifically approved — for example, electroconvulsive therapy — and which treatments are prohibited — for example, deep sleep or insulin coma therapy. Also, most of the states and territories make specific provision as to the definition of, and procedure to be observed when, restraint and seclusion are to be implemented as part of a person's treatment and care.

4. **Review of care and appeal provisions under the Act.** For example, when a tribunal is required to review a person detained under the legislation and what appeal rights a patient has if they are unhappy with the decision of a tribunal or court in relation to their care and detention, particularly as an involuntary patient.

AUSTRALIAN CAPITAL TERRITORY: *MENTAL HEALTH ACT 2015*

1. Objectives, Principles and Rights Under the Act

The objects of the Act are set out in **section 5**. For example, one of the objects is to promote the recovery of people with a mental disorder or mental illness (s 5(a)).

Section 6 sets out the principles that must apply when exercising any functions under the Act in relation to a person with a mental disorder or mental illness. For example, section 6(a) states that a person with a mental disorder or mental illness has the same rights and responsibilities as other members of the community and is to be supported to exercise those rights and responsibilities without discrimination.

Section 15 requires that a person who is to receive treatment, care or support in a mental health or community care facility is to be orally advised of their rights under the Act and given a written statement of those rights that must include those matters detailed in the section including, for example, the right to obtain legal advice and seek a second opinion from an appropriate mental health professional. Section 15 also requires that such information be provided in a way that the person is most likely to understand. A copy of the written information must be given to the person's legal representative and nominated person, among others.

Section 16 requires the person responsible for a mental health or community care facility to ensure that relevant information is available and readily accessible to people who are admitted for care and treatment. Relevant information includes copies of the *Mental Health Act* and any explanatory information about the Act printed in different languages, as well as the names, addresses and telephone numbers of relevant mental health entities that the person may wish to contact for advice and assistance.

Section 17 requires the person responsible for a mental health or community care facility to ensure that a person admitted to that facility is given the opportunity and facilities to communicate with people of the person's choice (unless otherwise prohibited under the Act).

2. Relevant Definitions Under the Act

The **Dictionary** at the end of the Act contains relevant definitions, but the definitions of mental disorder and mental illness are found in the Act itself.

Section 9 states that **mental disorder** means 'a disturbance or defect, to a substantially disabling degree, of perceptual interpretation, comprehension, reasoning, learning, judgment, memory, motivation or emotion' but does not include a condition that is a mental illness.

Section 10 states that **mental illness** means a condition that seriously impairs (either temporarily or permanently) the mental functioning of a person in one or more areas of thought, mood, volition, perception, orientation or memory, and is characterised by:

a. *the presence of at least 1 of the following symptoms:*
   i. *delusions;*
   ii. *hallucinations;*
   iii. *serious disorders of streams of thought;*
   iv. *serious disorders of thought form;*
   v. *serious disturbance of mood; or*
b. *sustained or repeated irrational behaviour that may be taken to indicate the presence of at least 1 of the symptoms referred to in paragraph (a).*

Note: given the definition of mental disorder, the Act would deal with persons with an intellectual disability as well as a mental illness.

Section 11 provides that a person is **not** to be regarded as having a mental disorder or mental illness only if the person expresses, or refuses or fails to express, an opinion in relation to politics, religion, law or morals, or engages, or refuses or fails to engage, in a particular political, religious, illegal or immoral conduct or anti-social behaviour or takes alcohol or any other drug.

The Act gives particular primacy to a person's **decision-making capacity** when decisions are made about the provision of treatment, care or support to a person with a mental disorder or mental illness. **Section 7** provides that a person has decision-making capacity if the person, with assistance if needed:

■ understands when a decision about treatment, care or support needs to be made; and
■ understands the facts that relate to that decision; and
■ understands the main choices available to them in relation to the decision; and
■ can weigh up the consequences of the main choices; and
■ understands how the consequences affect them; and, on the basis of the above factors, can make the decision; and

■ communicates the decision in whatever way they can.

Section 12(1) provides that a person is a **carer** under the Act 'if the person provides personal care, support or assistance to a person who has a mental disorder or mental illness'. However, section 12(2) provides that a person is not a carer who provides care or assistance subject to a commercial arrangement, as a volunteer, as part of a course of training or education, is a domestic partner, parent, guardian, relative or lives with the person.

Section 19 permits a person with a mental disorder or mental illness who has decision-making capacity to nominate someone to be their **nominated person**. The main function of such a person is to help the person with a mental disorder or mental illness by ensuring that their interests are respected if the person requires treatment, care or support. The nominated person is able to receive information and be consulted about decisions in relation to treatment, care or support for the person with a mental disorder or mental illness (**s 20**).

The **Dictionary** defines a **mental health facility** as 'a facility for the treatment, care or support, rehabilitation or accommodation of people with a mental illness', including 'a psychiatric facility'. The **Dictionary** defines a **mental health order** as 'a psychiatric treatment order, a community care order or a restriction order'.

References to **ACAT** throughout the Act are references to the ACT Civil and Administrative Tribunal. ACAT is the tribunal that hears and determines applications and reviews in relation to both mentally disordered and mentally ill persons.

3. Admission, Detention, Care and Treatment of Persons Under the Act

Voluntary Assessment Order

Section 33 allows a person who believes themselves to be, because of mental illness or mental disorder, unable to make reasonable judgments about their own health and safety and likely to do serious harm to others, to apply to ACAT for an assessment order on their own behalf. In voluntarily making such an application, the person is submitting themselves to the powers of ACAT to make such an order.

Involuntary Assessment Order (other than Emergency Admission and Detention)

Sections 34 and **35** permit a person, the person referred to as the **applicant** (s 34) or the **referring officer** (s 35), to apply to the tribunal for an assessment order to be made in respect of another person if the applicant or referring officer believes on reasonable grounds that the health and safety of the person is at risk because the person, due to mental disorder or mental illness:

- is unable to make reasonable judgments about matters relating to his or her own health or safety; or
- is unable to do anything necessary for his or her health or safety; or
- is likely to do serious harm to others.

Note: the definition of 'referring officer' is in the Dictionary of the Act and includes a police officer or a member of staff of the Director of Public Prosecutions.

Assessment Orders

Once the tribunal makes an assessment order, the person must be assessed and the tribunal is required to consider that assessment (**s 37**).

An **assessment order** may be made by the tribunal if it is satisfied that the person appears to have a mental disorder or mental illness and the person's health or safety is likely to be at risk and the person is likely to do serious harm to others (**s 37(a)**).

Section 38 requires that ACAT must, if considering ordering an assessment order, tell the person in writing of its intention, find out the person's opinion in relation to such an assessment and obtain the person's consent to the assessment.

Section 39 permits ACAT to make an emergency assessment order if it has a serious concern about the immediate safety of the applicant for the order or other persons. In such circumstances, ACAT must give the Chief Psychiatrist written notice of those concerns and may, if it is necessary and reasonable, make an assessment order without requiring the person's consent, as required in section 38.

Section 40 requires that an assessment order must contain details of where and, if appropriate, by whom the assessment is to be conducted. A person may be admitted to a mental health facility for an assessment to be undertaken. If required, ACAT may make a removal order to have a person taken to a mental health facility to conduct an assessment (**s 43**).

Section 41 provides that ACAT must tell the Public Advocate in writing about making an assessment order immediately after it is made. Also, if a person is admitted to a mental health facility for an assessment to be made, the Public Advocate and the person's lawyer may have access to the person at any time (**s 46**).

Mental Health Orders

Before making a mental health order, ACAT must consider the outcome of an assessment conducted under an assessment order (**s 53**).

Section 55 requires that before making a mental health order, the tribunal is required to hold an inquiry.

Section 56 provides a comprehensive list of matters the tribunal must take into account in making a mental health order. For example, section 56(1)(b) provides that the tribunal must consider 'whether the person consents, refuses to consent or has the decision-making capacity to consent, to a proposed course of treatment, care or support'. Once it has considered all the matters identified in section 56, the tribunal, as it considers appropriate, may make one of three types of mental health order:

1. psychiatric treatment order;
2. restriction order;
3. community care order.

Under **section 58** a **psychiatric treatment order** permits the tribunal to order the involuntary psychiatric treatment of a person if it considers:

- the person has a mental illness; and
- the person does not have decision-making capacity to consent to care, treatment or support and refuses to receive the treatment, or the person has decision-making capacity but refuses to consent to care, treatment or support; and
- the person is likely to harm himself or herself or others; and
- the tribunal is satisfied the treatment will help reduce the risk of further deterioration in the person's condition; and
- the treatment cannot be provided in a less restrictive environment.

The psychiatric treatment order:

- may stipulate the mental health facility the person is to be taken to; and
- state the treatment (other than ECT and psychiatric surgery), counselling, training, therapeutic or rehabilitation programs the person should receive;
- place limits on who the person may communicate with; and
- must include a statement indicating that the person who is the subject of the order has the capacity to consent to the making of the order and does so, or has the capacity to consent but refuses to do so, or does not have the capacity to consent.

Before any treatment, care or support is given to a person under the psychiatric treatment order, the Chief Psychiatrist must explain to the person the nature and effect of the proposed care and treatment in a way the person is most likely to understand (**s 63**).

A **restriction order** may be made concurrent with a psychiatric treatment order and permits the tribunal to order where the person is to live or a place where he or she is to be detained (**s 61**). A restriction order may be made in conjunction with a community care order, requiring the person to live in a community care facility or another place (**ss 68** and **69**).

Section 67 specifies what information a **community care order** may contain, for example, that the person is to undertake a counselling, training, therapeutic or rehabilitation program (s 67(1)(c)).

Section 76 provides that a psychiatric treatment order or a community care order has effect for 6 months or a shorter period, if so specified. A restriction order has effect for 3 months or a shorter period, if so specified.

Section 79 provides that the tribunal has the power, on application or on its own initiative, to review a mental health order. In doing so, the tribunal may vary or revoke an order, make an additional mental health order, or order a further assessment of the person.

Emergency Admission and Detention

Section 80 provides that a police officer or authorised ambulance paramedic, or a doctor or mental health officer may take a person to an approved health facility for admission if they have reasonable grounds for believing the person has a mental disorder or mental illness and requires immediate care, treatment or support, or if they believe the person's condition will deteriorate within 3 days if immediate treatment and care is not given, or if the person has refused treatment and care which is necessary to protect the person's own safety or that of the public.

A **mental health officer** for the purposes of the Act is a person appointed as such by the Minister and is a nurse, an authorised nurse practitioner, a psychologist, an occupational therapist or a social worker (s 201 of the Act).

Where a person is taken to an approved mental health facility, they may be detained by the person in charge of the facility. **Section 81** states that the person in charge:

a. *may keep the person in such custody as the person in charge thinks appropriate; and*
b. *may subject the person to such confinement as is necessary and reasonable —*
   i. *to prevent the person from causing harm to himself or herself or to another person; or*
   ii. *to ensure that the person remains in custody; and*
c. *may subject the person to minimum confinement or restraint as is necessary and reasonable —*
   i. *to prevent the person from causing harm to himself or herself or to another person; or*
   ii. *to ensure that the person remains in custody. [emphasis added]*

Unlike the legislation in some of the other states and territories, the *Australian Capital Territory Act* does not set out detailed provisions that must be adhered to by nursing staff when implementing **minimum confinement and restraint**. There are a number of circumstances in the Act that permit minimum confinement and restraint to be implemented — for example, **section 65(2)** in relation to the making of a psychiatric treatment order, **section 73(2)** in relation to community care orders and **section 88** in relation to treatment during detention. Specifically, section 88(5) provides that, if a detained person is subjected to confinement, restraint, involuntary seclusion or forcible giving of medication, the person in charge of the facility must:

a. *enter in the detained person's record the fact of and the reasons for the confinement, restraint, involuntary seclusion or forcible giving of medication; and*
b. *tell the public advocate in writing of the restraint, involuntary seclusion or forcible giving of medication; and*
c. *keep a register of the restraint, involuntary seclusion or forcible giving of medication.*

It would be expected that there would be clear written policies in place to ensure the use of confinement and restraint are safely implemented, regularly monitored and relevant observations recorded.

Section 83 requires any police officer, authorised ambulance paramedic, doctor or mental health officer who takes a person to an approved mental health facility to provide a written statement containing a description of actions taken, including the application of any restraint and seclusion, in bringing the person to the facility and the reasons for taking the actions. The person in charge of the facility is responsible for filing the statement with the person's clinical records.

Continued Detention Following Emergency Admission

Following an emergency admission to an approved mental health facility, the person admitted must be examined by a doctor within 4 hours (**s 84**). Where the doctor believes that further detention is necessary, he or she may authorise involuntary detention and care for a period not exceeding 3 days (**s 85**).

Section 89 requires that within 12 hours of admission the Public Advocate and the tribunal are to be notified. If a further period of involuntary detention is required beyond the initial 3 days, the tribunal must extend that period of detention and can only do so in the first instance for a further 11 days (**s 85(3)**).

Following the initial period of involuntary detention after an emergency admission, the tribunal is required to have the person assessed before holding an inquiry and making any mental health order.

The Obligation of the Tribunal When Making Orders Under the Act

In making orders under the Act, the tribunal must, in the first instance, particularly consider the overriding objectives and principles of the Act as set out in **sections 5** and **6** respectively. For example, **section 5** states that one of the objectives is to 'ensure that people with a mental disorder or mental illness receive assessment and treatment, care or support in a way that is least restrictive or intrusive to them' (s 5(c)).

Section 56 sets out those matters the tribunal must take into account in making a mental health order. For example, section 56(1)(g) states that 'any restrictions placed on the person should be the minimum necessary for the safe and effective care of the person'. The power of the tribunal to make a community care order facilitates such an objective.

Electroconvulsive Therapy and Psychiatric Surgery

Part 9 of the Act deals with what is referred to as ECT and psychiatric surgery. Those terms are defined as follows:

■ *electroconvulsive therapy means a procedure for the induction of an epileptiform convulsion in a person (**s 145(1)**);*
■ *psychiatric surgery means specialised neurosurgery for psychiatric conditions (**s 145(1)**);*
■ *neurosurgery means surgery on the brain of a person for the purpose of treating a pathological condition of the physical structure of the brain (**s 145(2)**).*

Section 148 provides that consent to one of the above procedures must be given in writing and signed by the person giving the consent and appropriately witnessed.

For the purposes of giving consent to a procedure, the Act distinguishes between an adult with decision-making capacity and one who does not have decision-making capacity, and likewise for a young person (a person older than 12 years but under 18 years of age).

The Administration of ECT to an Adult with Decision-Making Capacity. Under section 148:

■ ECT may be administered where the person is an adult; and

- has decision-making capacity to give consent, has given that consent and the consent has not been withdrawn either orally or in writing; and
- ECT has not been administered on nine or more occasions since the consent was given.

The Administration of ECT to an Adult Without Decision-Making Capacity. Under **section 149**:

- ECT may be administered where the person is an adult; and
- where the person does not have decision-making capacity, but has given an advance consent direction, and the ECT is administered in accordance with the direction and the person does not refuse or resist; and
- ECT may also be administered if an emergency ECT order is in force in relation to the person, and either the person does not resist or refuse, or a psychiatric treatment order or a forensic treatment order is in place in relation to the person.

Similar provisions are in place in relation to a young person with or without decision-making capacity (**ss 150** and **151**).

The Chief Psychiatrist or a doctor may apply to ACAT if they believe 'on reasonable grounds' that such an order should be made in relation to a person (**s 153**).

Sections 156 and **157** of the Act set out those matters ACAT must take into account in making an ECT order, such as:

- the administration of the therapy is likely to substantially benefit the person; and
- it is the most appropriate form of treatment reasonably available; and
- all other forms of treatment have been tried and have not been successful.

Psychiatric Surgery. **Section 169** requires a doctor to seek approval by the Chief Psychiatrist in writing to undertake psychiatric surgery. The doctor must be a psychiatrist and the application must be accompanied by evidence of the consent of the person or an advance consent direction or a copy of an order from the Supreme Court pursuant to the provisions of **section 173** authorising the proposed psychosurgery. An application

to the Supreme Court is required if the person who is to have the proposed surgery does not have decision-making capacity or an advance consent direction has not been given.

On receipt of that application, the Chief Psychiatrist is required to submit it to a committee, appointed by the Minister of Health, for consideration (**s 170**). The committee is appointed by the Minister and consists of a psychiatrist, a neurosurgeon, a lawyer, a clinical psychologist and a social worker (**s 175**).

A person who has given consent to the performance of psychiatric surgery or who is the subject of a Supreme Court order in respect of such a procedure may withdraw that consent at any time orally or in writing (**s 174**).

4. Review of Care and Appeal Provisions Under the Act

The role of ACAT is to hear and determine applications for mental health orders under the Act — that is, a psychiatric treatment order, a restriction order or a community care order.

Appeal Rights

Section 267 provides for a right of appeal from an order made by ACAT to the Supreme Court of the Australian Capital Territory. Appeals may be brought by:

- someone in relation to whom the decision was made;
- a person who appeared or who was entitled to appear before ACAT in the proceedings under appeal;
- the discrimination commissioner;
- anyone else with leave of the Supreme Court.

Official Visitors

Sections 208 and **209** provide for the appointment of Official visitors. The ACT *Official Visitors Act 2012* creates the generic position of Official visitor. However, for the purposes of the *Mental Health Act*, the specific suitability requirements for the appointment of Official visitors in relation to mental health services and facilities (referred to as 'visitable' places) are to be found in sections 208 and 209 of the *Mental Health Act*. Likewise, the functions of Official visitors are set out in **sections 211** and **214**, and require Official visitors to visit and inspect mental health facilities (a visitable place) and inquire into:

- *the adequacy of services provided at the visitable place for the assessment and treatment of persons with a mental disorder or mental illness; and*
- *the appropriateness and standard of facilities at the visitable place for the recreation, occupation, education, training and rehabilitation of persons receiving treatment or care for a mental disorder or mental illness; and*
- *the extent to which people receiving treatment, care or support for mental disorder or a mental illness are being provided the best possible treatment, care or support appropriate to their needs in the least possible restrictive environment and least possible intrusive manner consistent with the effective giving of that treatment or care; and*
- *any other matter that an Official visitor considers appropriate [in light of the principles in section 6 of the Act] (s211); also*
- *any complaint made to an Official visitor by a person receiving treatment, care or support for a mental disorder or mental illness (s 214).*

In addition to the specific functions set out in section 211 of the *Mental Health Act*, an Official visitor also has the generic powers granted under **section 14** of the *Official Visitors Act 2012*. Under **section 15** of that Act, in exercising their powers and functions, Official visitors may enter any 'visitable place' at any reasonable time after receiving a complaint and on their own initiative. When at a visitable place, an Official visitor may inspect any part, see any person receiving care, make any inquiries about people in care and inspect a person's health record if consent has been given either orally or in writing.

It is an offence, without reasonable excuse, to refuse to assist or to obstruct an Official visitor exercising his or her powers under **section 19** of the *Official Visitors Act*. An Official visitor is required to provide a report to the Minister and may provide a copy of the report to the Public Advocate in relation to complaints investigated.

Chief Psychiatrist and Care Coordinator

Section 196 provides for the appointment of a public servant as Chief Psychiatrist. The primary function of the Chief Psychiatrist is to provide treatment, care, rehabilitation and protection for persons who have a mental illness and to make reports and recommendations to the Minister in relation to matters affecting the provision of treatment, care and support for those people (**s 197**).

The Chief Psychiatrist is able to delegate his or her functions under the Act to 'a psychiatrist who is a public employee or is engaged by the Territory' (**s 200**).

Section 204 provides for the appointment of a public servant as Care Coordinator. The primary function of the Care Coordinator is to coordinate the treatment, care or support, together with the necessary associated staff and facilities, for people with a mental disorder in accordance with a community care order, with or without a restriction order or a forensic community care order made by ACAT (**s 205**).

Inspectors Appointed in Relation to Private Mental Health Facilities

The Act allows for the appointment of people known as **inspectors** in relation to the control and licensing of private mental health facilities.

Section 234 provides that the Director-General may appoint such inspectors as are considered necessary. **Section 236(1)** provides that an inspector may, at any reasonable time, enter any licensed premises and do one or more of the following:

a. *inspect the premises and equipment used at the premises in connection with the treatment, care or support of a person;*
b. *inspect any book, document or other record that is in the possession of the occupier of the premises, or to which the occupier has access, relating to the conduct of the private psychiatric facility at the premises;*
c. *require the occupier of the premises to give the inspector, within a reasonable time, a copy of any information, book, document or other record that is in the possession of the occupier, or to which the occupier has access, relating to the conduct of the private psychiatric facility at the premises.*

Any person who, within a specified time, fails to comply with a request from an inspector to provide a copy of a document, book, information or other record is liable to a penalty under the Act (**s 237**).

Mental Health Advisory Council

A Mental Health Advisory Council was established under the Act (**s 238**). The functions of the council are to advise the Minister generally about emerging mental health issues, mental health service reforms and mental health policy requiring legislative change (**s 239**).

The composition of the council is to include people who have or have had a mental illness or mental disorder as well as professionals with current knowledge of mental health treatment, care or support (**s 240**).

NEW SOUTH WALES: *MENTAL HEALTH ACT 2007*

1. Objectives, Principles and Rights Under the Act

Section 3 sets out the objectives of the Act which, among others, are to facilitate the care and treatment of persons who are mentally ill or mentally disordered and to protect their civil rights and to facilitate that care and treatment through community care facilities.

Section 68 details the principles of care and treatment that are to be given effect with respect to caring for and treating people with a mental illness or mental disorder including, for example, that the provision of care and treatment under the Act 'should be designed to assist people with a mental illness or mental disorder, wherever possible, to live, work and participate in the community' (s 68(c)).

Section 105 sets out the objectives of the New South Wales public health system in relation to the provision of mental health services in the state. For example, section 105(b) provides that the role of the New South Wales public health system in relation to mental health services is to 'promote the establishment of community mental health services for the purpose of enabling the treatment in the community wherever possible of persons who are mentally ill or suffering from the effects of mental illness or who are mentally disordered'.

Section 74 requires a person admitted to or detained in a mental health facility to be given both an oral explanation and a written statement of their legal rights and entitlements. The section also requires the information to be in a language the person understands. **Section 74(a)** requires a similar such statement to be given to a voluntary patient.

Schedule 3 at the end of the Act sets out the Statement of Rights that must be given to a person admitted to or detained in a mental health facility. **Schedule 3A** sets out the statement to be given to voluntary patients.

Section 71 provides for the nomination by a mentally ill or mentally disordered person (who becomes a patient) of a **designated carer**. The person nominated is required to be consulted and notified in relation to the mentally ill or mentally disordered person's care and treatment and also has appeal rights on behalf of the person. **Section 72** allows the person to nominate up to two people to be his or her designated carer.

Section 72A provides for a person to be designated as **principal care provider** of a mentally ill or mentally disordered person. A principal care provider is stated to be 'the individual who is primarily responsible for providing support or care to the person'. A person may be both a 'designated carer' and a 'principal care provider'.

2. Relevant Definitions Under the Act

The majority of definitions are set out in **section 4** of the Act, where **mental illness** is defined in the following terms:

> **mental illness** *means a condition that seriously impairs, either temporarily or permanently, the mental functioning of a person and is characterised by the presence in the person of any one or more of the following symptoms:*
> a. *delusions,*
> b. *hallucinations,*
> c. *serious disorder of thought form,*
> d. *a severe disturbance of mood,·*
> e. *sustained or repeated irrational behaviour indicating the presence of any one or more of the symptoms referred to in paragraphs (a)–(d).*

Section 14, however, defines a **mentally ill** person as follows:

> 1. *A person is a mentally ill person if the person is suffering from mental illness and, owing to that illness, there are reasonable grounds for believing*

that care, treatment or control of the person is necessary:

    a. for the person's own protection from serious harm, or

    b. for the protection of others from serious harm.

2. *In considering whether a person is a mentally ill person, the continuing condition of the person, including any likely deterioration in the person's condition and the likely effects of any such deterioration, are to be taken into account.*

Given the two definitions above, the Act distinguishes between a person who has a 'mental illness' and a person who is 'mentally ill'. What this means is that a person who has a mental illness cannot be automatically classified as being mentally ill because the definition of mental illness has to be read in conjunction with the definition of a mentally ill person.

For a person to be deemed mentally ill in New South Wales the following criteria have to be addressed:

    a. *the person must be suffering from a mental illness as per the definition in section 4 of the Act; and*

    b. *there are reasonable grounds for believing that care, treatment and control of the person is necessary for the protection of the person or others from serious harm; and*

    c. *the continuing condition of the person including any likely deterioration and the likely effects of such deterioration is to be taken into account as provided in section 14 of the definition of 'mentally ill person'; and*

    d. *there is no less restrictive environment in which appropriate care, treatment and control can be safely and effectively provided.[5] [emphasis added]*

It is also relevant to note that the definition of **mental illness** does not include any reference to dementia or developmental disability. The intention is that such conditions are not recognised as a mental illness for the purposes of the New South Wales Act, unless they are accompanied by any of the symptoms identified in the definition of mental illness in section 4.

If there is no evidence of mental illness, such people are provided for under the *Guardianship Act 1987* (NSW). That Act and the *Mental Health Act* are intended to be complementary, and a guardianship order can coexist with an order under the *Mental Health Act*. However, the *Mental Health Act* takes precedence where there is an inconsistency.[6]

Section 15 defines a mentally disordered person as follows:

> *A person (whether or not the person is suffering from mental illness) is a mentally disordered person if the person's behaviour for the time being is so irrational as to justify a conclusion on reasonable grounds that temporary care, treatment or control of the person is necessary:*
>
>   *a. for the person's own protection from serious physical harm, or*
>
>   *b. for the protection of others from serious physical harm.*

Emphasis is given in this definition to irrational behaviour 'for the time being' such that 'temporary' care, treatment or control is necessary.

This definition is intended to deal with those people who are not mentally ill as defined in the Act (though they may have a mental illness), but whose behaviour is temporarily irrational and presents a danger to themselves or others.

The best example of a mentally disordered person would be a person suffering a severe personal traumatic crisis in a social or domestic situation where they are unable to control their emotions and may become suicidal.

Section 16 identifies certain words or conduct that in themselves may not indicate mental illness or disorder — for example, holding or expressing particular political, religious or philosophical beliefs. The intention of section 16 is to ensure that a person whose beliefs or behaviour might be considered socially unacceptable or generally not tolerated is not a mentally ill person and therefore cannot be involuntarily detained in a hospital. It should be noted, however, that section 16(2) does provide that a person who suffers 'serious or permanent physiological, biochemical or psychological effects' as a result of long-term drug or alcohol intake can be deemed to have a mental illness within the meaning of the Act.

Section 4 states that a **declared mental health facility** is any premises declared to be so by the

'Secretary' of NSW Health in accordance with the procedure under section 109 of the Act and would include any private mental health facility so declared.

Section 17 defines **assessable person** as 'a person detained in a declared mental health facility for whom a mental health inquiry is required to be held'. This situation normally arises when a person is admitted as an involuntary patient on the basis that he or she is believed to be a mentally ill or mentally disordered person.

3. Admission, Detention, Care and Treatment of Persons Under the Act

Admission as a Voluntary Patient

Section 5 of the Act permits a person to be admitted to a mental health facility at his or her own request subject to the provision that an authorised medical officer agrees that the person is likely to benefit from care and treatment in that facility.

Section 8 provides that the person may leave when they want to or when they are well enough to be discharged.

Care has to be taken in dealing with the voluntary admission of persons under 16 years of age and those people who are under guardianship within the *Guardianship Act 1987*. **Sections 6–8** provide for such an occurrence.

Section 11 provides that a person who requests and is refused admission as a voluntary patient or who believes they have been inappropriately discharged may seek a review of that decision. This is not a formal appeal mechanism but simply a provision requiring the medical superintendent to review the decision of another medical officer.

Section 9 provides that should a voluntary patient remain in a mental health facility for a continuous period in excess of 12 months their case must be reviewed by the Mental Health Review Tribunal. In undertaking that review, the tribunal may order the discharge of the patient but may defer the discharge for a period not exceeding 14 days, or make no order at all, thereby continuing the patient's care and treatment as a voluntary patient.

Admission as an Involuntary Patient

An involuntary patient is a person who is admitted and detained in a mental health facility for the purposes of receiving care, treatment and control either against the person's wishes or on the request of a specified other person or a court order. A person may be admitted and detained as an involuntary patient on the grounds that the person is either a mentally ill person or a mentally disordered person as defined in the Act.

Regardless of whether the person is mentally ill or mentally disordered, admission of an involuntary patient to a hospital for care and treatment can be done in one of these ways:

- on the certificate of a medical practitioner or accredited person (s 19);
- on the information of an ambulance officer (s 20);
- after apprehension by police (s 22);
- following an order for medical examination (s 23);
- on order of the court (s 24);
- on transfer from another health facility (s 25);
- on request of the person's designated carer, principal care provider, relative or friend (s 26).

Examination Requirements Following Admission as an Involuntary Patient

Once a person has been brought to the declared mental health facility for admission as an involuntary patient, a number of medical examinations must be undertaken under the Act to permit the person's ongoing detention in that facility. **Section 27** sets out the requirements for these examinations. If, following the requisite examinations, the person is found not to be mentally ill or mentally disordered, the person must not be detained.

Tribunal Inquiry for a Mentally Ill Person Under the Act

If a person is found to be mentally ill following admission and examination, he or she is then known as an **assessable person** and is subject to an inquiry by the tribunal. **Section 27(d)** requires that steps be taken to bring the person before the tribunal 'as soon as practicable'.

Specific provisions in the Act must be followed preparatory to bringing a person before a tribunal inquiry. They may be summarised as follows:[7]

- the mental health facility must notify the person's designated carer of the tribunal inquiry (s 76);
- the person must be given an explanation about the proposed inquiry in a language he or she can understand;

- the person must be given a clear explanation of their rights as well as an explanation of the order the mental health facility will be seeking from the tribunal inquiry;
- the person is entitled to have the opportunity to ask questions about the inquiry process and, if need be, a competent interpreter should be arranged and be present to assist as required;
- the person is entitled to independent legal representation at the inquiry and, where appropriate, that should also be organised. Steps should be taken to ensure the person has the opportunity to talk with their legal representative in private and with confidentiality;
- where reasonably practicable, the person should appear in street clothes for the inquiry hearing (s 34); and
- steps should be taken to ensure the minimum of medication, consistent with proper care, is prescribed, to ensure the person is able to communicate adequately with their legal representative before the inquiry hearing (s 29).

At the inquiry, the tribunal is required to determine, on the balance of probabilities, whether the person is mentally ill; that is, whether it is more likely than not that the person is mentally ill.[8]

Section 35 provides that if the tribunal comes to the decision that the person is a mentally ill person, the following care provisions are available for the tribunal to consider:

- discharge the person into the care of their designated carer; or
- discharge the patient on a community treatment order (CTO); or
- make an involuntary patient order (IPO) directing that the person be detained for a period not exceeding 3 months.

Conversely, if the tribunal is not satisfied that the person is mentally ill, **section 35** allows the tribunal to consider:

- discharging the person; or
- discharging the patient but deferring the discharge for a period not exceeding 14 days if it is considered to be in the person's best interests.

It is worth noting that once the tribunal has made an IPO to detain the person, it must consider the person's capacity to manage their financial affairs. If the tribunal considers the person is not capable of managing his or her financial affairs, it must make an order for financial management under section 44 of the *Trustee and Guardian Act 2009* (NSW). Such an order can be revoked by the tribunal at a later time if the person is discharged and the tribunal is satisfied the person can manage their own financial affairs (*Trustee and Guardian Act 2009* s 88).[9]

Limited Detention of a Mentally Disordered Person as an Involuntary Patient

Section 31 outlines the relevant detention provisions applying to a person found to be mentally disordered. They are summarised as follows:

- a mentally disordered person must not be detained for a continuous period of more than 3 days (not including weekends and public holidays);
- the person must be examined at least once every 24 hours by an authorised medical officer;
- the person must not be detained if, following such examination, the authorised medical officer believes the person is not mentally disordered or mentally ill or that care of a less restrictive kind is appropriate and available;
- a person must not be admitted or detained as a mentally disordered person on more than three occasions in any one month.

Forms and Types of Treatment Under the Act

Community Treatment Orders. A Community Treatment Order (CTO) is an order made by the Mental Health Review Tribunal that requires a person to live at a designated address and visit a community mental health facility or be at a specified place at certain times to receive treatment as contained in the treatment plan that is an integral part of a CTO.

Section 53 provides that, in deciding to approve a CTO, the tribunal is required to consider these provisions:

- Has an appropriate treatment plan been drawn up by the community mental health facility?

- Will the person benefit from a CTO as the least restrictive alternative consistent with safe and effective care?
- Is the community mental health facility capable of implementing the plan?
- Does the person have a prior diagnosis of a mental illness and, if so, is there a history of refusing to accept appropriate treatment?

It is worth noting that in making an application for a CTO, a treatment plan must accompany it. **Section 65** allows the tribunal to vary or revoke a CTO as part of its regular review process.

Electroconvulsive Therapy (ECT). The Act makes provision for ECT and the conditions required to apply when ECT is proposed.

WHO CAN ADMINISTER ECT? Two medical practitioners must be present — one experienced in administering ECT, the other experienced in administering anaesthesia (**s 88**).

ADMINISTERING ECT TO A VOLUNTARY PATIENT. ECT may be given to a voluntary patient once their informed and freely given consent has been obtained and the patient has been given the information as set out in **section 91**.

It is important to know that voluntary patients cannot be given ECT without their written informed consent. If the voluntary patient lacks the capacity to consent, no other person may consent on their behalf. Where an authorised medical officer is unsure whether a voluntary patient is capable of giving informed consent, an application must be made to the tribunal for determination.

ADMINISTERING ECT TO AN INVOLUNTARY PATIENT. Section 94 requires that an authorised medical officer must apply to the tribunal for permission to administer ECT to an involuntary patient or any other person detained in a mental health facility. The application must be accompanied by a certificate from two medical practitioners (one of whom is a psychiatrist) stating that ECT is a reasonable and proper treatment in all the circumstances and is necessary or desirable for the safety or welfare of the patient.

MAXIMUM NUMBER OF TREATMENTS AND DURATION OF AN ECT ORDER. Section 96 provides that the maximum number of ECT treatments the tribunal may order must not exceed 12 except in special circumstances. When an order for ECT is made, it is valid for 6 months unless a shorter period is specified *or* until the patient is no longer an involuntary or detained patient.

Surgery or Special Medical Treatment. **Section 98** of the Act defines a **surgical operation** as any 'surgical procedure, a series of related surgical operations or surgical procedures, and the administration of an anaesthetic for the purpose of medical investigation'.

SURGICAL OPERATIONS FOR A VOLUNTARY PATIENT. Where a condition arises requiring surgical intervention, a voluntary patient is generally capable of consenting to whatever procedure is necessary — for example, an appendicectomy or repair of an inguinal hernia. However, if it is an emergency and, for whatever reason, a voluntary patient is not able to give informed consent, the Director-General of Health or the tribunal may give consent on their behalf if it is considered necessary, as a matter of urgency, to save life or prevent serious harm to the patient.

SURGICAL OPERATIONS FOR AN INVOLUNTARY PATIENT. In relation to an involuntary patient, surgery can be undertaken if the patient is able to give informed consent. Where that is not possible, the patient's designated carer is to be advised in writing and permission requested.

Section 99 details the steps that must be taken to secure consent for emergency surgery for an involuntary patient if the patient is incapable of giving consent. Again the designated carer must be notified.

Section 101 permits an authorised medical officer to apply to the tribunal for consent to surgery for an involuntary patient if the designated carer does not agree to the proposed surgery or cannot be located.

SPECIAL MEDICAL TREATMENT. Section 98 defines **special medical treatment** as any treatment, procedure, operation or examination that is carried out on a person that is intended, or is reasonably likely, to have the effect of rendering the person infertile.

Section 102 prohibits special medical treatment for a patient unless it is necessary, as a matter of urgency, to save the patient's life or prevent serious damage to the patient's health or if consent has been given by the tribunal.

Section 103 permits the tribunal to give consent to the procedure if satisfied it is necessary to prevent serious damage to the patient's health and the patient is over 16 years of age.

Seclusion and Restraint

The New South Wales Act does not include specific provisions in relation to the use of **seclusion** and **restraint** as treatment options to manage aggressive behaviour in its mental health facilities. However, NSW Health does have a detailed policy directive (PD2020_004) titled *Seclusion and restraint in NSW Health settings*. That document, issued in March 2020, outlines the 'principles, values and procedures that underpin efforts to prevent, reduce and, where safe and possible, eliminate the use of seclusion and restraint in NSW Health settings. It promotes a human rights approach and the use of least restrictive practices'. The policy defines a number of terms including 'restraint' (the restriction of an individual's freedom of movement') encompassing 'chemical restraint' (the use of a medication or chemical substance in order to restrict a person's movement), 'mechanical restraint' (the application of devices to a person's body to restrict movement) and physical restraint ('hands-on' immobilisation), as well as 'seclusion' (the confinement of a person alone in a room or area from which free exit is prevented). Specifically in relation to mental health units it requires (at p 17) 'each seclusion and restraint (currently physical and mechanical) episode must also be recorded in a dedicated Register to allow for reporting' as well as specifying the details the Register must include, for example, the date and type of seclusion or restraint as well as time started and time ended. A similar Register must also be kept in relation to the 'seclusion and restraint of mental health consumers in declared emergency departments'.

It would be expected that the detailed policy including the dedicated Register would be published and enforced in all mental health units and emergency departments.

Specific Treatments Prohibited Under the Act

Section 83 specifically prohibits the administration or performance on another person of psychosurgery, deep sleep therapy or insulin coma therapy.

4. Review of Care, Treatment and Appeal Provisions Under the Act

The Act provides ongoing mechanisms for the review of treatment orders as well as standards of care provided in both mental health facilities and associated centres overseeing community care, treatment and orders under the Act.

Mental Health Review Tribunal

Section 140 of the Act establishes the tribunal in New South Wales. The functions of the tribunal in relation to civil and forensic patients are detailed earlier in this chapter; essentially, the tribunal reviews and determines relevant treatment orders and may revoke such orders as necessary. It also determines applications for ECT and other treatment as required under the Act and determines appeals by a person against the refusal of a medical superintendent to discharge the person from a mental health facility.

Authorised Officers

Section 137 provides for the appointment of authorised officers by the Secretary of NSW Health. Their role is to visit and inspect mental health facilities and conduct investigations about care, treatment or control of persons in mental health facilities. **Section 138** provides such persons with wide-ranging powers of inquiry who may request the production of books, documents and records and cross-examine employees under oath.

Official Visitors

Section 129 provides for the appointment of Official visitors by the Minister for Health and **sections 131–134A** detail their powers and obligations. Essentially, they are required to visit mental health facilities at least once every month. They may or may not give notice of their intention to do so.

Official visitors are able to inspect premises and examine patient records. They are also to make themselves available to speak with patients or designated carers who have the right to bring to the attention of the Official visitor any matter they are unhappy about in relation to care and treatment. Official visitors report to a person appointed as the Principal Official Visitor who in turn reports to the Minister for Health on a regular basis.

Appeal Provisions

Section 163 allows 'a person' to appeal to the Supreme Court of New South Wales against a determination made by the tribunal with respect to a person or the failure or refusal of the tribunal to make an order with respect to the person.

Specific Standards Relating to the Administration of Medication

Section 85 provides that a medical practitioner must not administer or cause to be administered to a person a dosage of drugs for any mental illness or condition from which the person is or is suspected to be suffering that, in light of proper professional standards, would be considered excessive or inappropriate.

***Usage of Medication to be Reviewed.* Section 86** provides that the medical superintendent or the director of community treatment at a mental health facility is to establish and maintain an internal review system to monitor and review the prescription and use of drugs within the mental health facility in terms of frequency of administration, dosage, intended and unintended effects, and appropriateness of use.

NORTHERN TERRITORY: *MENTAL HEALTH AND RELATED SERVICES ACT 1998* (INCORPORATING AMENDMENTS ARISING FROM NORTHERN TERRITORY *MENTAL HEALTH AND RELATED SERVICES AMENDMENT ACT 2007*)

1. Objectives, Principles and Rights Under the Act

Section 3 sets out the objects of the Act. For example, section 3(a) provides for a commitment to the proper care, treatment and protection of people with mental illness while protecting their civil rights.

Section 7A provides for the nomination of a person to be a primary carer to provide care and support to the mentally ill person. That person may be a relative or someone closely involved in the care of, or support to, the person. A relative may be a person where the relationship arises through common ancestry, adoption or de facto relationship or any customary law or tradition (including Aboriginal customary law or tradition).

Section 8 requires that the Act be interpreted in a way that best protects the person with a mental illness — for example, that they should receive 'the best possible care and treatment in the least restrictive and least intrusive environment' (s 8(a)). Section 8AA provides that a treatment order may be made for a person with a complex cognitive impairment under the *Disability Services Act 1993*.

Section 9 contains the principles that must apply in the provision of care and treatment to a person with a mental illness, mental disturbance or complex cognitive impairment — for example, where possible, the person is to be treated in the community (s 9b)).

Section 10 contains the principles that must apply when admitting and treating a person as an involuntary patient — for example, the person should be admitted only after every effort to avoid the person being admitted as an involuntary patient has been taken (s 10(a)).

Section 11 contains the principles that must apply relating to the admission, care and treatment of Aboriginal and Torres Strait Islander persons — for example, that, as far as possible, treatment and care to a person of such a background should be 'consistent with the person's cultural beliefs, practices and mores, taking into account the views of the person's family and community' (s 11(a)).

Section 12 sets out the principles relating to the rights of carers and families — for example, as far as practicable and appropriate, family members should be consulted and involved in the person's treatment and care (s 12(c)).

Section 13 sets out the principles relating to the rights and conditions of a person with a mental illness, mental disturbance or complex cognitive impairment who is being treated in an approved treatment facility — for example, that the person's legal rights and his or her right to privacy and to religious freedom are to be respected (s 13(a)).

Sections 87–99 set out the rights of patients and carers, where a person is admitted to an approved treatment facility or is subject to a community management order, to be given certain information including information concerning the person's treatment and medication as well as specifying a person's rights and entitlements under the Act. Such information is to be given in a language the person understands.

2. Relevant Definitions Under the Act

Section 4 contains most of the relevant definitions of words or phrases used in the Act but some are defined in a specific section.

Section 6 of the Act defines mental illness as follows:

1. *A **mental illness** is a condition that seriously impairs, either temporarily or permanently, the mental functioning of a person in one or more of the areas of thought, mood, volition, perception, orientation or memory and is characterised:*
   a. *by the presence of at least one of the following symptoms:*
      i. *delusions;*
      ii. *hallucinations;*
      iii. *serious disorders of the stream of thought;*
      iv. *serious disorders of thought form;*
      v. *serious disturbances of mood; or*
   b. *by sustained or repeated irrational behaviour that may be taken to indicate the presence of at least one of the symptoms referred to in paragraph (a). [emphasis added]*

It is important to know that having a 'mental illness' by itself is not sufficient to justify a person's admission to a treatment facility as an involuntary patient under the Act. For that to occur, **section 14** requires the presence of a mental illness as defined and that, as a result, the person requires care, treatment and control for their safety and the safety of others. That issue will be discussed further in this chapter.

Section 6(3) provides that a person is not considered to have a mental illness merely because he or she expresses particular political or religious beliefs or has engaged in illegal conduct or anti-social behaviour as well as other denoted conduct. In addition, section 6(3) also provides that a person is not considered to have a mental illness merely because the person has an intellectual disability, a personality disorder, a habit or an impulse disorder, has been admitted on the grounds of mental disturbance or complex cognitive impairment or has acquired brain injury.

Section 6A(1) states that a person has a **complex cognitive impairment** if the person has a 'cognitive impairment with a behavioural disturbance' whereas **Section 6A(2)** states that a person has a **cognitive impairment** if the person has an intellectual impairment, neurological impairment or acquired brain injury (or any combination of these) that:

a. *is, or is likely to be, permanent; and*
b. *results in substantially reduced capacity in at least one of the following:*
   i. *self-care or management;*
   ii. *decision making or problem solving;*
   iii. *communication or social functioning.*

Section 6A(3) states that a person has a **behavioural disturbance** if the person's mental condition has deteriorated to the extent that the person is behaving in an aggressive manner or engaging in seriously irresponsible behaviour.

Section 4 includes a definition of **mentally disturbed** as being the behaviour of a person 'that is so irrational as to justify the person being temporarily detained' under the Act. The emphasis in the definition is clearly on the need for 'temporary' detention based on the person's 'irrational' behaviour. Such circumstances may arise in severe personal traumatic crisis in a social or domestic situation where the person may be unable to control his or her emotions and may become suicidal. The circumstances in which a person may be admitted as an involuntary patient on the grounds of mental disturbance or complex cognitive impairment are further detailed in **sections 15** and **15A** of the Act respectively.

Section 4 defines **approved treatment facility** as a place or premises declared as such in accordance with the provisions of **section 20** of the Act. Section 20 requires the Minister to declare named places or premises as an 'approved treatment facility'.

Section 7(2) defines **informed consent** as consent freely and voluntarily given by a person capable of understanding the effect of giving consent and that the person communicates his or her consent on the approved form. Section 7(3) lists the information that must be provided to a person to enable informed consent to be given and using a 'competent interpreter' if required.

Section 7A defines **primary carer** as someone providing care and support as a relative or someone close to the person, or someone closely involved in the treatment or care of, or support to, the person. A relative of the person includes anyone related to the person through common ancestry, adoption, marriage, de facto relationship or any customary law or tradition (including Aboriginal law or tradition).

Section 23 provides that a **designated mental health practitioner** is appointed and must be a psychologist, registered nurse, occupational therapist, Aboriginal and Torres Strait Islander health practitioner, social worker or paramedic, all of whom must have two years' experience and have undergone approved training.

3. Admission, Detention, Care and Treatment of Persons Under the Act

Admission as a Voluntary Patient

Section 25 permits a person who is aged 14 or over to apply to be admitted to an approved treatment facility as a voluntary patient. There are also specific provisions in **sections 26** and **27** to permit the admission of persons under 18 years as a voluntary patient as well as persons under guardianship.

Section 29 permits a voluntary patient to leave an approved treatment facility at any time, who must be advised of that right when admitted as a voluntary patient.

Admission as an Involuntary Patient

A person may be admitted as an involuntary patient on the grounds of mental illness, mental disturbance or complex cognitive impairment

Admission as an Involuntary Patient on the Grounds of Mental Illness. **Section 14** sets out the criteria for the involuntary admission of a person on the grounds of mental illness as follows:

a. *the person has a mental illness;* and
b. *as a result of the mental illness:*
 i. *the person requires treatment that is available at an approved treatment facility;* and
 ii. *without the treatment the person is likely to:*
   A. *cause serious harm to himself or herself or to someone else;* or
   B. *suffer serious mental or physical deterioration;* and

iii. *the person is not capable of giving informed consent to the treatment or has unreasonably refused to consent to the treatment;* and
c. *there is no less restrictive means of ensuring that the person receives the treatment. [emphasis added]*

What is important to remember is that, for a person to be admitted as an involuntary patient, the person must have a mental illness as defined in section 6 of the Act and satisfy the need for detention, care and treatment for their own safety and the safety of others as required in section 14 of the Act.

ASSESSMENT TO BE UNDERTAKEN. In the first instance, **section 32** requires an **assessment** to be undertaken. A person may request that he or she be assessed to determine whether they need treatment under the Act (s 32(1)), or another person with a genuine interest or concern about the person may request such an assessment (s 32(2)). A request for assessment may be made to a medical practitioner, an authorised psychiatric practitioner or a designated mental health practitioner (s 32(3)), who must assess the person (s 32(4)) unless they decline the request because they believe the person does not need treatment (s 32(5)).

Section 32A also permits a police officer to apprehend and bring a person to an authorised psychiatric practitioner, medical practitioner or designated mental health practitioner for assessment if the police officer believes the person may require treatment under the Act and is likely to cause harm to himself, herself or others. If necessary, the police officer may enter premises without a warrant to apprehend the person and use any reasonable force and assistance required.

PSYCHIATRIC EXAMINATION RECOMMENDED FOLLOWING ASSESSMENT. **Section 34** provides that, following assessment, a recommendation may be made by the assessing practitioner for a psychiatric examination to be undertaken if they are satisfied that the person meets the criteria for involuntary admission on the grounds of mental illness or mental disturbance. When that occurs, the person is taken to an approved treatment facility or hospital.

A recommendation for a psychiatric examination remains in force for 14 days (**s 34(7)**).

EXAMINATION AT AN APPROVED TREATMENT FACILITY. Section 38 provides the alternatives available to an authorised psychiatric practitioner following examination and assessment, which are:

- admit the person as an involuntary patient on the grounds of mental illness;
- admit the person as an involuntary patient on the grounds of mental disturbance;
- place the person under an involuntary community management order;
- if the person does not fit any of the above criteria, the person must be released.

ADMISSION AND DETENTION FOR PSYCHIATRIC ASSESSMENT. Section 39 allows a person, on the grounds of mental illness, to be detained for 24 hours as an involuntary patient following a recommendation for psychiatric examination. If, following the examination, an authorised psychiatric practitioner is satisfied that the person fulfils the criteria for involuntary admission, the person may be detained initially for 14 days. The person cannot be detained beyond that time unless an authorised psychiatric practitioner is satisfied that the person fulfils the criteria for involuntary admission on the grounds of mental illness.

Section 40 requires that once a person is admitted as an involuntary patient he or she must be examined by an authorised psychiatric practitioner not less than once every 72 hours and a record of each examination is to be made in the person's case notes.

Section 41 contains requirements to notify the person, their decision-maker, primary carer or guardian as well as the Mental Health Review Tribunal of the person's admission on the grounds of mental illness.

Admission as an Involuntary Patient on the Grounds of Mental Disturbance. As set out above, **section 4** defines what is meant by a **mentally disturbed** person. **Section 15** provides a more detailed description of what is meant by mental disturbance and sets out the criteria for a person's involuntary admission on the grounds of mental disturbance, predominantly that:

- the person does not fulfil the criteria for involuntary admission on the grounds of mental illness; *and*

- the person's behaviour is, or within the immediately preceding 48 hours has been, so irrational as to lead to the conclusion that the person is not able to function in a socially acceptable and culturally appropriate manner; *and*
- the person is behaving in an abnormally aggressive or irresponsible manner or is engaging in seriously irresponsible conduct that justifies psychiatric assessment, treatment and care; *and*
- unless the person receives treatment and care at an approved treatment facility, he or she is likely to cause harm to himself or herself or others; *and*
- there is no less restrictive means of ensuring that the person receives the treatment and care required.

Section 42 provides that, where a person is detained as an involuntary patient on the grounds of mental disturbance, he or she may be initially detained for 72 hours. The person may be detained for a further 7 days if, after examining the person, two authorised psychiatric practitioners believe the person needs care and treatment and that the person is not capable of consenting or unreasonably refuses to give such consent and there is no less restrictive way to provide the necessary care and treatment.

Section 43 requires notification to be given to the person, their decision-maker, guardian or primary carer as well as the Mental Health Review Tribunal of the person's admission as an involuntary patient on the grounds of mental disturbance.

Section 44 requires that, during the period of detention, the person must be examined by an authorised psychiatric practitioner every 24 or 72 hours depending on the basis for detention. Before the 7-day period expires, the person may be admitted as a voluntary patient, admitted as an involuntary patient on the grounds of mental illness, placed on an interim community management order, or released.

Admission as an Involuntary Patient on the Grounds of Complex Cognitive Impairment. **Section 44C** provides that, where an authorised psychiatric practitioner and authorised officer are of the opinion a person has a complex cognitive impairment, they must apply to the tribunal for the person's involuntary admission and detention. If the person is already an involuntary patient admitted on the grounds of mental disturbance, an application must be made to the Mental Health Review Tribunal within the specified time.

Section 44E provides that if, after reviewing the application, the tribunal is satisfied that the person has a complex cognitive impairment, the tribunal must order the person to be admitted and detained as an involuntary patient subject to a prepared treatment management plan drawn up in accordance with s 44A of the Act. If the tribunal is not satisfied the person has a complex cognitive impairment, the person must be discharged from detention.

Review by the Tribunal After Involuntary Admission

Section 123 requires the Mental Health Review Tribunal to review within 14 days a decision of an authorised psychiatric practitioner to involuntarily detain a person on the grounds of mental illness, mental disturbance or complex cognitive impairment or make the person subject to an involuntary interim community management order.

In undertaking its review, the tribunal may uphold the decision of the practitioner or substitute its own decision including revoking the admission of the person as an involuntary patient or as subject to an involuntary interim community management order (s 123(5) and (7)).

Community Management Orders (CMOs)

The Act makes provision for persons to be treated in the community rather than having to be admitted to an approved treatment facility. In the first instance, this is by way of an interim community management order that, if confirmed by the tribunal, is renewed as a community management order.

Section 45 permits an authorised psychiatric practitioner to make an **interim community management order** in the first instance where the practitioner is satisfied that the person fulfils the criteria for involuntary treatment in the community.

An interim community management order remains in force for 14 days, and the following treatment may be administered under such an order (s 45(4)):

- treatment that will prevent the person causing serious harm to himself or herself or someone else;

- treatment that will prevent behaviour of the person that is likely to cause serious harm to himself or herself or someone else;
- treatment that will prevent any further physical or mental deterioration of the person;
- treatment that will relieve acute symptomatology.

Section 46 states that an interim community management order must contain specific provisions including the approved treatment agency that is to supervise it, where the treatment is to occur and details of the treatment to be given.

Section 123 provides that, once the Mental Health Review Tribunal has been notified that an interim community management order has been made, it must review that order as soon as practicable within 14 days. Having done that, the tribunal may confirm a **community management order** in relation to the person for no longer than 6 months and, where it does so, must fix a date for the order to be reviewed again.

Section 49 requires a community management order to be in writing and contain specific provisions as detailed in the section.

The Prohibition of Certain Forms of Treatment Under the Act

Psychosurgery, Deep Sleep Therapy, Insulin Therapy and Sterilisation. Psychosurgery as defined in **section 58**, deep sleep therapy, insulin coma or sub-coma therapy (**s 59**) and sterilisation as a treatment for mental illness, mental disturbance or complex cognitive impairment (**s 60**) are all prohibited under the Act. Any person who performs any of those treatments on a person is liable to a monetary penalty.

The Regulation of Certain Forms of Treatment under the Act

Mechanical Restraint. Section 61 defines **mechanical restraint** and the specific conditions that must apply before it may be used. This is an important issue for nurses working in mental health units where dealing with aggressive patients is often a real problem. Mechanical restraint is defined as the application of a device (including a belt, harness, manacle, sheet and strap) on a person's body to restrict the person's movement, but does not include the use of furniture (including a bed with sides and a chair with a table fitted on its arms) that restricts the person's capacity to get off the furniture (s 61(1)).

Mechanical restraint of a person in an approved treatment facility may be applied only where:

- no other less restrictive method of control is applicable; and
- it is necessary for the purposes of medical treatment to prevent the person from causing injury to himself or herself or others; and
- to prevent the person from persistently destroying property or absconding from the facility.

Mechanical restraint cannot be applied unless it is approved by an authorised psychiatric practitioner or, in the case of an emergency, the senior registered nurse on duty (s 61(4)). The form of the mechanical restraint to be used and the duration of its application must be determined by the authorised psychiatric practitioner or senior registered nurse who approves it and such restraint may be applied without the person's consent (s 61(6) and (7)).

Section 61(8)–(13) sets out the detailed provisions that must be observed when mechanical restraint is applied and includes provisions that require continuous observation by a registered nurse or medical practitioner and the patient must be reviewed at intervals not longer than 15 minutes as well as being provided with adequate food and drink and access to toilet facilities.

Seclusion. Section 62 details the provisions that must be observed when a person has been placed in seclusion, including the circumstances in which it may be used, who has the authority to order it and the records that must be kept of that process. They are in relatively similar terms to those applying to the use of mechanical restraint.

Electroconvulsive Therapy

ECT AS A VOLUNTARY PATIENT. Section 66 of the Act permits ECT to a voluntary patient where the person's informed consent is obtained or the person's adult guardian consents.

ECT AS AN INVOLUNTARY PATIENT. Where a person is unable to give informed consent, **section 66(2)** allows the tribunal to authorise ECT where

two psychiatric practitioners report that the person's condition is such that ECT is reasonable and proper treatment and the person's primary carer cannot be located.

Section 66(3) permits ECT to be performed on an involuntary patient without the tribunal's consent where two authorised psychiatric practitioners are satisfied that it is immediately necessary to save the person's life, to prevent the person suffering serious mental or physical deterioration or to relieve severe distress. Where ECT is performed without the authority of the Mental Health Review Tribunal, the tribunal is required to be advised as soon as practicable after it is performed.

Section 66(6) requires that at least two medical practitioners be present when ECT is performed.

Non-Psychiatric Treatment

Section 63(1) defines what is meant by **non-psychiatric treatment**. Where necessary, medical or surgical treatment that is unrelated to a mental illness, mental disturbance or complex cognitive impairment may be administered to a person where the consent of the person or the person's guardian is obtained or it is approved by the tribunal. For example, a person may require surgery to repair a hernia or medication for hypertension. Such treatment would be considered 'non-psychiatric'.

4. Review of Care and Appeal Provisions Under the Act

Community Visitors

Section 103 of the Act provides for the appointment of persons known as Community visitors. **Section 104** provides that their role is to inquire into and make recommendations relating to:

- the adequacy of services for accessing and treating persons in approved treatment facilities or by approved treatment agencies;
- the standard and appropriateness of facilities for the accommodation, physical wellbeing and welfare of persons receiving treatment or care at approved treatment facilities or by approved treatment agencies;
- the adequacy of information relating to the rights of persons receiving treatment at approved

treatment facilities or by approved treatment agencies and the complaint procedures under the Act;

- the accessibility and effectiveness of complaint procedures under the Act;
- the failure of persons employed in approved treatment facilities or by approved treatment agencies to comply with the provisions of the Act;
- any other matter that a Community visitor considers appropriate having regard to the principles and objectives of the Act; and
- any other matter as directed to the Principal community visitor by the Minister for Health.

Section 108 empowers Community visitors to visit approved treatment facilities or approved treatment agencies and provide reports arising from their visits, including any findings or recommendations, to the Principal community visitor.

Any person who is receiving treatment or care at an approved treatment facility or by an approved treatment agency must be able to access the Community visitors when they visit that facility on a regular basis.

Mental Health Review Tribunal

Section 118 establishes the tribunal, and its major functions are to:

- review long-term voluntary admissions (**s 122**);
- review involuntary admissions and community management orders (**s 123**);
- review reports as provided to it (**s 125**);
- hear appeals against decisions of a medical practitioner or an authorised psychiatric practitioner under certain sections of the Act (**s 127**).

An application may be made to the tribunal by the person who is the subject of the tribunal's decision. In addition, an application may be made on the person's behalf by the person's adult guardian, representative, legal practitioner, or a person with a genuine interest in and concern for the person (s 127(3)).

The tribunal has the power to make orders and to vary, affirm or set aside orders already made.

Appeals to the Supreme Court of the Northern Territory

Section 142 provides that a person aggrieved by a decision or refusal of the tribunal to make a decision within a reasonable time may appeal to the Supreme Court against that decision or refusal. Also, a person who has a sufficient interest in the matter which is the subject of a decision or refusal of the tribunal may, with the leave of the Supreme Court, appeal to the court against that decision or refusal. Any such appeal is by way of a rehearing and, in determining the appeal, the Supreme Court may (**s 143**):

- affirm, vary or set aside the decision or order of the tribunal;
- make any decision or order that the tribunal may have made;
- remit the matter to the tribunal for further consideration;
- make any other order that it thinks fit.

QUEENSLAND: *MENTAL HEALTH ACT 2016*

1. Objectives, Principles and Rights Under the Act

Section 3(1) states that the objects of the Act are to maintain the health and wellbeing of persons who have a mental illness and who do not have the capacity to consent to be treated. Also the Act is intended to make provision for a person to be treated as a forensic patient by diverting the person from the criminal justice system if he or she is found to have been of unsound mind at the time of committing an unlawful act or is unfit to be tried, and to protect the community from such persons who may be at risk of harming others.

Section 3(2) states that the main objects of the Act are to be achieved in a way that safeguards the rights of persons, is the least restrictive of the person's rights and liberties and promotes the person's recovery and ability to live in the community without the need for involuntary treatment.

Section 5 sets out the general principles that must apply to the way in which the Act is administered; for example, a person with a mental illness must be recognised as having the same basic human rights as exist for all persons; furthermore, his or her human worth and dignity as an individual is to be recognised and taken into account (s 5(a)). Further **Section 7** requires that any person performing or exercising a power under the Act must have regard to the principles mentioned in s 5.

To the extent that the Act applies to a person who has an intellectual disability, **section 8** extends the provisions of the Objects of the Act (s 3) and the Principles of the Act (s 5) to that person.

Section 25 provides for a statement of rights to be given to involuntary patients and others, and that a person who becomes an involuntary patient may appoint one or two nominated support persons to support him or her while receiving care and treatment under the Act.

Sections 223–224 permit an involuntary patient to appoint no more than two nominated support persons. The role of such a person is to support the person and represent the patient's views, wishes and interests in relation to the patient's care and treatment.

Section 291 provides that a patient's nominated support person, family, carers and other support persons may contact the patient while he or she is receiving care and treatment, participate in decisions about the patient's care and treatment and receive appropriate information about the patient's care and treatment.

Sections 277–279 provide for a statement of rights to be prepared by the Chief Psychiatrist (s 277) and given to all patients and to the patient's nominated support person, family and carers (s 278). Also, signs must be displayed in all authorised mental health services advising that a copy of a statement of rights is available on request (s 279).

Sections 281–290 confirm a number of rights of patients under the Act including the right of a patient to be visited by his or her nominated support person, family and carers; the right to have access to legal representatives; and the right to have information about care and treatment given in a way and in a language the patient best understands.

Sections 293–295 provide for the appointment by an authorised mental health service of an independent patient rights adviser to ensure that a patient and the patient's support persons are advised of their rights and responsibilities; to help the patient and the patient's support persons to communicate their views about the patient's treatment and care; to consult with relevant mental health professionals about the rights of patients under the Act; to advise the patient of their rights in relation to tribunal hearings and, if requested, help the patient

engage representation for the hearings; to identify the need for the appointment of a personal guardian or attorney for the patient and to assist where appropriate.

2. Relevant Definitions under the Act

Section 9 refers to the **Dictionary** in Schedule 3 at the end of the Act that details the meaning of key words used in the Act. While reference should be made to it prior to any detailed consideration of the Act, a number of relevant definitions are found within the Act itself and will be referred to where appropriate in the text.

Section 10 defines **mental illness** as being 'a condition characterised by a clinically significant disturbance of thought, mood, perception or memory'. **Section 10(2)** provides that a person is not to be considered to have a mental illness merely because of one or more of the following:

a. *the person holds or refuses to hold a particular religious, cultural, philosophical or political belief or opinion; or*
b. *the person is a member of a particular racial group; or*
c. *the person has a particular economic or social status; or*
d. *the person has a particular sexual preference or sexual orientation; or*
e. *the person engages in sexual promiscuity; or*
f. *the person engages in immoral or indecent conduct; or*
g. *the person takes drugs or alcohol; or*
h. *the person has an intellectual disability; or*
i. *the person engages in anti-social or illegal behaviour; or*
j. *the person is or has been involved in family conflict; or*
k. *the person has previously been treated for mental illness or been subject to involuntary assessment or treatment.*

Section 10(3) provides that a person with the characteristics listed in section 10(2) can still have a mental illness. Examples of where subsection (3) would be relevant include where:

■ a person may have a mental illness caused by taking drugs or alcohol

- a person may have a mental illness as well as an intellectual disability.

Section 10(4) provides that, on an assessment, a decision that a person has a mental illness must have been made in accordance with internationally accepted medical standards.

An **authorised mental health service** has a diverse definition. The **Dictionary** states that it is (a) a service declared as such under section 329 of the Act, (b) an authorised mental health service (rural or remote) declared as such under section 331 of the Act or (c) a high-security unit.

Section 11 provides that an involuntary patient is any person subject to an examination authority, a recommendation for assessment, a treatment authority, a forensic order, a treatment support order or a judicial order.

3. Admission, Detention, Care and Treatment of Persons Under the Act

The Act provides for the voluntary and involuntary admission of people to an authorised mental health service as follows.

The first step is for an examination to be carried out to determine whether to make a recommendation for assessment. **Section 31** permits an examination to be undertaken by a doctor or an authorised mental health practitioner where the person asks for such an examination (voluntarily) **or** is subject to an examination authority **or** an emergency examination authority.

An **examination authority** is issued by the tribunal pursuant to **sections 502–504** of the Act. Generally speaking, the tribunal will issue an examination authority if it considers the person may have a mental illness.

In order to undertake an examination a doctor or authorised mental health practitioner may enter a person's place without the person's consent (s **32**) and, if need be, may use reasonable force to do so (s **33**) and may request the assistance of police (s **34**).

An **emergency examination authority** is issued pursuant to the provisions of section 157D of the Queensland *Public Health Act 2005* by a police officer or ambulance officer who takes a person to a public sector health service facility for treatment and care and issues an emergency examination authority. When that

occurs, the person may be detained for up to 6 hours (s 157E of the *Public Health Act*) and the person is to be examined by a doctor or an authorised mental health practitioner to determine whether to make a recommendation for assessment pursuant to the *Mental Health Act* (section 157F of the *Public Health Act*).

In conducting an examination, **section 39** provides that a doctor or authorised mental health practitioner may make a recommendation for assessment if they are satisfied that:

- the treatment criteria apply to the person; and
- there is no less restrictive way for the person to receive treatment and care for the person's mental illness.

A recommendation for assessment must be made within 7 days after the examination (s 39(2)).

Section 12 provides that a person is assessed as meeting treatment criteria when the following criteria are present:

a. *the person has a mental illness;*
b. *the person does not have capacity to consent to be treated;*
c. *because of the person's illness, the absence of involuntary treatment, or the absence of continued involuntary treatment, is likely to result in —*
   i. *imminent serious harm to the person or others; or*
   ii. *the person suffering serious mental or physical deterioration.*

Section 14 provides that a person has capacity to consent to treatment if the person:

a. *is capable of understanding, in general terms —*
   i. *that the person has an illness, or symptoms of an illness, that affects the person's mental health and wellbeing; and*
   ii. *the nature and purpose of the treatment for the illness; and*
   iii. *the benefits and risks of the treatment, and alternatives to the treatment; and*
   iv. *the consequences of not receiving the treatment; and*
b. *is capable of making a decision about the treatment and communicating the decision in some way.*

(2) a person may have capacity to consent even though the person decides not to receive treatment.

If an authorised doctor is satisfied that the person meets the treatment criteria, a **treatment authority** may be made (**s 48**). The category of treatment authority may be **inpatient treatment authority (ITA)** or a **community treatment authority (CTA)** (**s 51**). The determination of whether the treatment authority should be inpatient or community will depend on the person's circumstances, taking into account the person's treatment needs as well as the safety of the person and the safety of others (s 51(2) and (3)). Where a person is categorised as requiring an inpatient treatment authority, an authorised doctor may authorise limited community treatment for the person if considered appropriate (**s 52**). The phrase 'limited community treatment' is defined in Schedule 3 of the Act as being the treatment and care of a person in the community, including the grounds and buildings (other than an inpatient unit) of an authorised mental health unit, for a period of not more than 7 consecutive days.

A copy of a treatment authority made must be given to the person and its contents explained to the person. Also, within 7 days of the making of a treatment authority, the person's nominated support person and carers must be given a copy and the tribunal must be notified (**s 55**).

A treatment authority is required to be assessed by an authorised doctor every 3 months (**ss 59** and **205**). In undertaking such an assessment, the authorised doctor must determine whether the treatment criteria still apply and whether there is a less restrictive way for the patient to receive treatment and care (s 205). An authorised psychiatrist may revoke or amend a treatment authority. If a treatment authority is revoked, the tribunal must be notified (**s 207**).

Electroconvulsive Therapy

It is an offence to perform ECT on a person unless it is done in accordance with the provisions of the Act (**s 235**).

Sections 233–237 of the Act permit the administration of ECT on the basis of informed consent or in an emergency. For the purposes of ECT administration, informed consent is defined in section 233 as:

a. the person has capacity to give consent to the treatment; and

b. the consent is in writing signed by the person; and

c. the consent is given freely and voluntarily

A person is deemed to have capacity to consent to treatment if the person has the ability to:

a. understand the nature and effect of a decision relating to the treatment; and

b. make and communicate the decision.

A person is able to give informed consent in an advance care directive.

Section 236 permits the performance of ECT on a person who has given informed consent or on an adult who is unable to give informed consent where the tribunal has approved the treatment, or in the case of a minor where the tribunal has approved the treatment.

Section 237 permits the performance of ECT in any emergency subject to the approval of the tribunal, if it is considered necessary to save the patient's life or to prevent the patient suffering irreparable harm.

Non-Ablative Neurosurgical Procedure

The **Dictionary** at the end of the Act defines **non-ablative neurosurgical procedure** as 'a procedure on the brain, that does not involve deliberate damage to or removal of brain tissue, for the treatment of a mental illness'.

It is an offence to perform a non-ablative neurosurgical procedure on a person in order to treat the person's mental illness other than in accordance with the provisions of the Act (**s 238**). The specific conditions of chronic tic disorder, dystonia, epilepsy, Gilles de la Tourette syndrome, Parkinson disease or tremor are declared **not** to be a mental illness.

Section 239 permits the performance of a non-ablative neurosurgical procedure on a person where the person has given informed consent and the tribunal has approved it. An example of such a procedure would be deep brain stimulation.

Mechanical Restraint, Seclusion, Physical Restraint and Other Practices

The power to restrain patients in mental health facilities or to place a patient in seclusion can be a very contentious issue in the care of involuntary mentally ill patients.

The Act includes very detailed provisions concerning the circumstances in which they may be used and the observation, monitoring and recording of what must be done when they are used.

Methods of restraint and seclusion orders invariably involve nursing staff. Consequently, the provisions in the Act in relation to these matters together with established policies should be known by all nursing staff caring for involuntary patients in authorised mental health services in Queensland.

In addition to the provisions set out in the Act, **section 273** requires the Chief Psychiatrist to make a 'restraint, seclusion and other practices policy'. An authorised doctor, authorised mental health practitioner or administrator of an authorised mental health service must comply with the policy (s 273(2)).

Mechanical Restraint. **Section 244** of the Act defines **mechanical restraint** as the restraint of a person by the application of a device to the person's body, or a limb of the person, to restrict the person's movement.

Section 246 allows an authorised doctor or a health practitioner authorised by an authorised doctor to use mechanical restraint if the patient is in an authorised mental health service and if the following applies:

- the authorised mental health service is a high-security unit or a mental health service approved by the Chief Psychiatrist; and
- the device used is an approved device; and
- the Chief Psychiatrist has approved the use of mechanical restraint on the person; and
- the use of mechanical restraint has been authorised by an authorised doctor; and
- the use of mechanical restraint complies with the restraint policy; and
- a reduction and elimination plan for the patient has been approved; and
- the use of the mechanical restraint is with 'no more force than is necessary and reasonable' in the circumstances; and
- the patient is observed continuously while restrained.

Once restraint is authorised, **section 251** lists the obligations to be observed by the health practitioner in charge (that would almost invariably be a registered nurse) to ensure that the restraint is applied as authorised, that the patient's needs such as bedding and clothing, access to toilet facilities and sufficient food and drink are met and that relevant details in accordance with the policy relating to the use of mechanical restraint are recorded in the patient's clinical file.

Section 252 permits the health practitioner in charge of the unit to end the use of mechanical restraint if satisfied it is no longer necessary to protect the patient or others from physical harm.

Authorised Seclusion. **Section 254** defines **seclusion** as being 'the confinement of the patient at any time of the day or night, alone in a room or area from which free exit is prevented'. However, section 254(2) provides that the overnight confinement of a person in a high-security unit or other authorised mental health service for security purposes for a period of not more than 12 hours (between 8 pm and 8 am) is not seclusion.

Section 256 states that seclusion of a patient may be authorised at any time by an authorised doctor subject to the following provisions:

- the seclusion of the patient is authorised; and
- the seclusion complies with the relevant written direction given to the authorised mental health service; and
- the seclusion complies with the seclusions policy; and
- the seclusion complies with any reduction and elimination plan in place; and
- the seclusion is done with no more force than is reasonable and necessary; and
- while in seclusion, the patient is observed either continuously or at intervals of not more than 15 minutes.

Section 263 provides for a health practitioner in charge on an inpatient or other unit in an authorised mental health service to use seclusion in an emergency if there is no other reasonably practical way to protect the patient and others from physical harm. An authorised doctor must be notified, the seclusion cannot be more than 1 hour or up to 3 hours in any 24-hour period and the patient must be observed continuously during the seclusion period.

***Reduction and Elimination Plans.* Section 264** states that a 'reduction and elimination plan' is a written plan for a patient developed by an authorised doctor designed to provide for the reduction and elimination of either mechanical restraint or seclusion or both. Such a plan is to include strategies designed to reduce the use of mechanical restraint or seclusion on a patient and record how effective those strategies have been.

***Physical Restraint.* Section 268** defines 'physical restraint' of a patient as the use by a person of his or her body to restrict the patient's movement but does not include:

- the giving of physical support or assistance reasonably necessary to enable a person to carry out daily living activities; or to redirect the patient because he or she is disorientated; or
- physical restraint of the patient as required in urgent circumstances.

Section 270 permits the use of physical restraint to be authorised to:

- protect the patient or others from physical harm;
- provide treatment and care to the patient;
- prevent the patient from causing serious damage to property;
- prevent the patient from leaving an authorised mental health service.

***Medication of a Patient.* Sections 273–274** provide that medication of a patient includes sedation of the patient and that it is an offence under the Act to administer medication to a patient unless it is clinically necessary for the patient's treatment and care for a medical condition, which includes preventing imminent serious harm to the patient or others.

Treatments Prohibited by the Act

Sections 240 and **241** specifically prohibit the administration of insulin-induced coma therapy, deep sleep therapy or the performance of psychosurgery on a person.

4. Review of Care and Appeal Provisions Under the Act

The Act makes provision for the following:

- the appointment of inspectors;
- the Mental Health Review Tribunal;
- the Mental Health Court.

The setting up of the tribunal and the court with their respective jurisdictional roles is essentially complementary, with the role of the Mental Health Court being to hear and determine appeals from the tribunal, among other functions.

Appointment of Inspectors

Section 555 permits the Chief Psychiatrist to appoint persons as inspectors whose role is expressed in **section 556** as being to investigate, monitor and enforce compliance with the provisions of the Act. Inspectors are given wide-ranging powers under the Act — for example, the power to enter premises (**s 565**) and a general power including, for example, the power to search a place, confer with a patient alone, and inspect, examine or film any document (**s 577**).

Mental Health Review Tribunal

Section 705 details the role of the tribunal in reviewing treatment decisions and orders made in relation to both civil and forensic patients. The tribunal also reviews the fitness for trial of persons found by the Mental Health Court to be unfit for trial.

Section 413 requires the tribunal to conduct a review of the treatment authority for patients initially within 28 days after the initial order is made and thereafter every 6 months.

Section 421 provides that, when reviewing a treatment authority, the tribunal is to consider whether the treatment criteria no longer applies to the person or whether there is a less restrictive way for the person to receive treatment and care.

Section 423 provides that, when reviewing a treatment authority, the tribunal may either confirm or revoke the inpatient treatment order (ITO). If the tribunal confirms the order, it may direct that the category be changed from an inpatient to a community treatment authority having regard to the person's treatment and care needs and the safety of the person and others.

Schedule 2 allows a party to appeal against a decision of the tribunal to the Mental Health Court.

Mental Health Court

The court comprises a Supreme Court Judge sitting alone, assisted by two psychiatrists, or one in certain circumstances (**s 638**).

The role of the Mental Health Court, as provided in **section 639** includes:

a. *deciding appeals against decisions of the tribunal;*
b. *deciding references of the mental conditions of persons;*
c. *reviewing the detention of patients in authorised mental health services or the forensic disability service.*

Chief Psychiatrist

Section 298 provides for the appointment of a Chief Psychiatrist who is independent of the public service (**s 302**). **Section 301** details the powers and functions of the Chief Psychiatrist, which include, to the extent practicable, 'ensuring the protection of the rights of involuntary patients under this Act while balancing their rights with the rights of others'. In addition the Director, to the extent practicable, is to ensure that the 'involuntary examination, assessment, treatment, care and detention of persons under the Act complies with [the] Act'. In carrying out his or her functions, the Director reports to the Minister.

Section 301 also gives the Chief Psychiatrist the 'power to do all things necessary or convenient to be done in performing' his or her function. That power also includes an obligation to issue policies and practice guidelines about the treatment and care of patients (**s 305**) or investigate a matter or direct an inspector to investigate a matter relating to the treatment and care of a patient in any authorised mental health service concerning a patient's care and treatment (**s 308**).

SOUTH AUSTRALIA: *MENTAL HEALTH ACT 2009*

1. Objectives, Principles and Rights Under the Act

Section 6 sets out the objectives of the Act that include, for example, to aim to ensure that people with a severe mental illness receive a comprehensive range of services and retain their freedom, rights, dignity and self-respect as far as is consistent with their protection, the protection of the public and the proper delivery of services.

Section 7 establishes the guiding principles to be observed by the Minister, the tribunal, Chief Psychiatrist, health professionals and other persons and bodies in the administration of the Act and the discharge of their respective functions under the Act — for example, that mental health services should be designed to bring about the best therapeutic outcomes for patients, and, as far as possible, their recovery and participation in community life.

Section 47 states that a patient is entitled to have another person's support wherever practicable in exercising his or her rights under the Act. That other person may be the patient's parent or guardian, medical agent, relative, carer or friend who has been nominated by the patient.

Section 46 requires that a patient be given a written copy of an approved **statement of rights** informing the patient of his or her legal rights as well as a copy of any order made by the tribunal in relation to the patient. That information must be given in a language the patient understands and a copy must be given to the patient's support person.

Section 48 of the Act sets out a patient's rights to communicate with others outside a treatment centre, to receive visitors and to be afforded reasonable privacy in communicating with others.

Section 48A of the Act prohibits a person exercising a power or function under the Act from placing a **spit hood** on the head of a person. A maximum penalty of two years imprisonment is imposed for a breach of this provision.

Section 49 states that a person who has the oversight, care or control of a patient and who wilfully neglects the patient is guilty of an offence. The maximum penalty is $25 000 or 2 years imprisonment.

2. Relevant Definitions Under the Act

Section 3 contains the definitions of relevant words used in the Act. The definition of **mental illness** is expressed as 'any illness or disorder of the mind'.

The definition is extremely general in nature. Indeed, the absence of clarity in the definition leaves the judgment as to what is or is not mental illness and who is or is not suffering from mental illness largely up to the determination of the individual psychiatrist or medical practitioner, or to the courts if they are ever called upon to do so. Where a court had to make such a finding it would be guided by expert opinion evidence from psychiatrists and/or psychologists.

Schedule 1 at the end of the Act lists certain conduct, some 13 types in all, that **may not**, by itself, indicate mental illness — for example, that a person expresses, or refuses or fails to express, a particular opinion or belief as to politics or religion, or a particular philosophy, or sexual preference or orientation. Significantly, sub-clause (j) of Schedule 1 identifies that where a person 'has developmental disability of mind' it does not mean the person has a mental illness.

Section 3 of the Act also states that an 'approved treatment centre' and a 'limited treatment centre' are places approved as such by the Chief Psychiatrist, and also confirms that reference to the **tribunal** throughout the Act is a reference to the South Australian Civil and Administrative Tribunal.

Section 5A provides at the outset that, in the absence of any evidence or law of the state to the contrary, a person is presumed to have full decision-making capacity in respect of decisions about his or her healthcare and treatment. A person will be considered to have impaired decision-making capacity if the person is not capable of:

i. *understanding any information that may be relevant to the decision (including information relating to the consequences of making a particular decision); or*
ii. *retaining such information; or*
iii. *using such information in the course of making the decision; or*
iv. *communicating his or her decision in any manner.*

Also, if an advance care directive exists, the person must have satisfied any requirement in it that sets out when the person is to be considered to have impaired decision-making capacity.

Section 5A(3) provides circumstances where a person's decision-making capacity is not to be considered impaired — for example, merely because the person is not able to understand matters of a technical or trivial

nature; and that a person may fluctuate between having impaired decision-making capacity and full decision-making capacity.

Section 96 states that in determining a place to be an 'approved treatment centre', the Chief Psychiatrist may attach such conditions or limitations to the decision and may vary or revoke a determination made.

Similarly, in **section 97**, the Chief Psychiatrist may determine a place to be a 'limited treatment centre' and may vary or revoke such a determination. Where the expression 'treatment centre' is used in the Act it means an 'approved treatment centre' or a 'limited treatment centre'.

Section 94 provides that the Chief Psychiatrist may approve 'a specified person, or a person of a specified class' as an **authorised health professional**.

3. Admission, Detention, Care and Treatment of Persons Under the Act

Treatment and Care Plans

The Act provides for treatment and care plans for both voluntary and involuntary patients. Once approved, a treatment plan is designated as an **inpatient treatment order (ITO)** or a **community treatment order (CTO)**. There are three levels of ITO able to be made and two levels of CTO. The provisions relating to both are elaborated upon further in this section.

Voluntary Admission

Section 39(2) provides that a voluntary patient may be a voluntary community patient or a voluntary inpatient.

Section 8 provides that a person may be admitted as an inpatient to a treatment centre at his or her own request and may leave that treatment centre at any time unless an inpatient treatment order applies.

Section 9 requires that, as soon as practicable after admission, a voluntary inpatient must be given a written statement of rights. Also, a copy must be given to the patient's guardian, medical agent, relative, carer or friend.

Section 39 requires that a written treatment and care plan be formulated for a voluntary patient, preferably in consultation with the patient or guardian, medical agent, relative, carer or friend. The plan must describe the treatment and care that will be provided including rehabilitation and other services to be provided after discharge.

Involuntary Admission for Examination

Subject to a patient assistance request (**s 54A**) or a patient transport request (**s 55**), **sections 56** and **57** give power to an authorised officer and a police officer respectively to apprehend persons who appear to be suffering from a mental illness.

Where an authorised officer or a member of the police force has reasonable cause to believe that a person has a mental illness and the person has caused harm, or there is a significant risk of the person causing harm to himself or herself or to others, the authorised officer or police officer may enter any place to apprehend and restrain the person using such force as is reasonably necessary in the circumstances and have the person transported as soon as practicable to a treatment centre for examination.

Section 3 defines an authorised officer as a mental health clinician, an ambulance officer, a medical officer or flight nurse employed by the Royal Flying Doctor Service of Australia (Central or South Eastern Sections) or any other person approved by the Chief Psychiatrist.

Inpatient Treatment Orders

Once an examination occurs by a mental health clinician, a decision may be made to place the person on an ITO or CTO. The making of an inpatient treatment order (ITO) is the process by which a person may be involuntarily detained and treated in a treatment centre.

In the first instance, **section 20** provides that a person's refusal or failure to comply with a community treatment order (CTO) may be a relevant consideration in making an ITO.

Three levels of ITO may be made under the Act. In each case, the criteria for making an order are the same — that is:

- the person has a mental illness; and
- because of the illness, the person requires treatment for his or her own protection and the protection of others from harm (physical or mental); and
- the person has impaired decision-making capacity relating to appropriate treatment of the person's mental illness; and

- there is no less restrictive means of treatment other than an ITO of ensuring appropriate treatment of the person's mental illness.

In making or reviewing an ITO, irrespective of the level of the order being made or reviewed, consideration must be given as to whether the treatment is able to be given on a voluntary basis or by compliance with a CTO.

The three levels of ITO able to be made under the Act are summarised as follows:

1. **Section 21** provides that a **Level 1 ITO** may be made by a medical practitioner or an authorised mental health professional who, having examined the person, is of the opinion that the person fulfils the criteria for admission as an involuntary patient (as described above) and may order that the person be detained and treated as an involuntary patient.

   A Level 1 ITO is valid for 7 days. Once the order is made, the patient must then be examined by a psychiatrist or an authorised medical practitioner (though not the person who made the initial order) within 24 hours of the order being made, or as soon as practicable. Following that examination, the psychiatrist or authorised medical practitioner may confirm or revoke the Level 1 ITO or substitute it with a CTO.

2. **Section 25** provides that where a Level 1 ITO is made or confirmed by a psychiatrist or an authorised medical practitioner, they may, after a further examination of the patient and before the Level 1 order expires, make a further order, known as a **Level 2 ITO**.

   A Level 2 ITO expires after 42 days. During that time the psychiatrist or authorised medical practitioner may revoke the Level 2 ITO at any time and may substitute it with a CTO.

3. **Section 29** requires a **Level 3 ITO** to be made by the tribunal. In making the order, the tribunal must be satisfied that the person fulfils the criteria for admission as an involuntary patient (as described above). The tribunal may make an order even though a Level 2 or Level 3 ITO already applies to the person.

   An application for a Level 3 ITO may be made by the Public Advocate, the director of an approved treatment centre or an employee of an approved treatment centre authorised to do so. The tribunal may revoke or vary a Level 3 ITO at any time. If it revokes a Level 3 ITO it may substitute it with a Level 2 ITO. An application to revoke or vary a Level 3 ITO may be made by the Public Advocate, a medical practitioner, a mental health clinician, guardian, medical agent, relative, carer or friend of the patient, or any other person who the tribunal is satisfied has a proper interest in the patient's wellbeing.

A Level 3 ITO expires 6 months after it is made with respect to a child and 12 months for all other persons.

Where a patient is detained pursuant to a Level 1, Level 2 or Level 3 ITO, he or she may be given treatment authorised by a medical practitioner without consent.

Section 41 requires that a treatment and care plan must be in place when a patient is being detained and treated on a Level 2 or Level 3 ITO. The treatment plan must describe the treatment and care to be given including rehabilitation and other services on discharge. As far as is practicable, the patient should be consulted in the preparation and revision of a treatment and care plan as well as the patient's guardian, medical agent, relative, carer or friend.

Community Treatment Orders

There are two levels of CTO that may be made under the Act.

Section 10 allows a **Level 1 CTO** to be made by a medical practitioner or authorised mental health professional if the following criteria are met:

- the person has a mental illness; and
- because of the mental illness, the person requires treatment for his or her protection and the protection of others; and
- the person has impaired decision-making capacity relating to appropriate treatment of the person's mental illness; and
- there are facilities and services available for the appropriate treatment of the illness; and
- there is no less restrictive means available other than a CTO for treating the person's illness.

Section 10(2) requires that when a decision is made to make a Level 1 CTO, consideration must be given to having the person receive the treatment on a voluntary basis.

A Level 1 CTO must be in writing and expires 42 days after the order is made (**ss 10(3)** and **(4)**). If a Level 1 CTO is **not** made by a psychiatrist or an authorised medical practitioner, one of them must examine the patient within 24 hours of the order being made, or as soon as practicable. On completion of the examination, the psychiatrist or authorised medical practitioner may confirm or revoke the Level 1 CTO (**s 10(5)**) or substitute it with a level 1 ITO.

Section 11 provides that once a Level 1 CTO is confirmed or revoked by the psychiatrist or authorised medical practitioner, the Chief Psychiatrist must be notified in writing within 1 business day of the order being made or revoked. A copy of the order must be given to the patient as soon as practicable as well as a statement of rights in a language or manner the patient can comprehend. In addition, a copy must be given to the patient's guardian, medical agent, relative, carer or friend as appropriate (**s 12**).

Section 13 provides that, where a Level 1 CTO is made, treatment authorised by a psychiatrist or an authorised medical practitioner who has examined the patient may be given despite the patient's refusal to give consent, or absence of consent. Also, treatment may be given without authorisation in an emergency if a medical practitioner considers the treatment is needed for the patient's wellbeing and authorisation is not readily obtainable.

Section 16 provides that a **Level 2 CTO** may be made by the tribunal based on the same criteria required to be present in the making of a Level 1 CTO as detailed above. As with a Level 1 CTO, consideration must be given to the person receiving treatment on a voluntary basis. Section 16(4) provides that an application to the tribunal for a Level 2 CTO may be made by:

- the Public Advocate;
- a medical practitioner;
- a mental health clinician;
- the guardian, medical agent, relative, carer or friend of the person who is the subject of the application;
- any other person who the tribunal is satisfied has a proper interest in the patient's welfare.

A Level 2 CTO expires 6 months after it is made in relation to a child and after 12 months in all other cases (s16(5)).

Section 17 provides that the Chief Psychiatrist must be notified by the tribunal within 1 business day of the making, variation or revocation of a level 2 CTO.

Section 18 provides that, where a Level 2 CTO is made, treatment may be authorised by a psychiatrist or authorised medical practitioner who has examined the patient despite the patient's refusal to give consent, or the absence of consent, where treatment is required to be given urgently and it is not practicable to obtain authorisation from the tribunal.

Section 40 requires a treatment plan to be made where a Level 2 CTO is in place. The treatment plan must detail the treatment to be provided to the patient including rehabilitation and other services, whether on an involuntary basis or through the patient's voluntary participation. As far as is practicable, the patient's guardian, medical agent, relative, carer or friend is to be consulted in preparing and revising the treatment and care plan.

Prescribed Psychiatric Treatment Panel

Section 41A makes provision for the setting up of the Prescribed Psychiatric Treatment Panel (PPTP). The persons who are members of the Treatment Panel are specified in **section 41A(2)** and they include the Chief Psychiatrist and no more than eight other persons appointed by the Governor on the recommendation of the Minister, and must include at least one patient or former patient, one carer and former carer, one senior psychiatrist, one neurosurgeon, one legal practitioner and one person with credentials and experience in bioethics.

The functions of the PPTP are provided for in **section 41C** as follows:

a. *to conduct a review of the progress of a patient who has, in the course of any 12-month period, received three or more courses of ECT treatment;*
b. *to conduct a review of the progress of a patient to whom, in the course of any 12-month period, two or more courses of ECT have been administered without consent in reliance on section 42(6);*
c. *to authorise the carrying out of neurosurgery on a patient as a treatment for mental illness;*

d. *to carry out any other function conferred on the Panel under the Act.*

It is clear that the primary purpose of the PPTP is to generally oversee, review and, in the case of neurosurgery, approve the administration of ECT and neurosurgery to persons with a mental illness in South Australia.

Electroconvulsive Therapy

Section 42 allows for ECT to be undertaken on a voluntary or involuntary basis in accordance with the following criteria:

- ECT is permitted on a **voluntary** basis where:
  - the patient has a mental illness; *and*
  - ECT or a course of ECT has been authorised by a psychiatrist who has examined the patient; *and*
  - written consent is given by the patient or on behalf of the patient, *or* if the patient is under 16 years of age, by the tribunal on the application of a mental health practitioner or medical practitioner; *and*
  - in accordance with an advance care directive by a substitute decision-maker or by the tribunal where an application is made.

Any consent that is given is limited to a maximum of 12 doses of ECT given over a maximum period of 3 months. Any subsequent course of ECT requires further written consent.

- ECT may be given on an **involuntary** basis (without consent) if the patient has a mental illness of such a nature it is considered to be urgently required for the patient's wellbeing and it is not practicable to obtain consent. If that occurs, the Chief Psychiatrist must be notified in writing within 1 business day of the administration of the ECT. A failure to notify is considered an offence subject to a maximum penalty of $50 000 or 4 years imprisonment.

Neurosurgery

Section 3 defines neurosurgery as 'a leucotomy, amygdaloidotomy, hypothalamotomy, temporal lobectomy, cingulectomy, electrode implantation in the brain or any other brain surgery for the relief of mental illness by the elimination or stimulation of apparently normal brain tissues'.

Section 43 permits such surgery where:

- the patient has a mental illness; and
- the neurosurgery is authorised as treatment by the person who is to carry out the procedure *and* by two psychiatrists, one of whom is a senior psychiatrist, who have each separately examined the patient, and by the Prescribed Psychiatric Treatment Panel; and
- if the patient (from the age of 16 years) is capable of giving effective consent, he or she has given written consent; or
- if the patient is not capable of giving effective consent, consent has been given by the tribunal on application by a medical practitioner or mental health clinician.

The person who is to carry out the neurosurgery must notify the Chief Psychiatrist 14 days before the proposed neurosurgery is to be carried out. Also, a person who carries out the neurosurgery must provide a report to the Chief Psychiatrist within 3 months of carrying out the neurosurgery with details of the patient's progress including an independent report from a psychiatrist who has examined the patient.

A failure to abide by the above provisions is considered an offence with a maximum penalty of $50 000 or 4 years imprisonment.

Section 44 provides that 'other prescribed psychiatric treatments' (other than ECT or neurosurgery) that may be undertaken are to be provided for in the Regulations that accompany the Act.

Seclusion and Restraint

There is no specific provision in the Mental Health Act in relation to the use of seclusion and restraint as a part of mental health care. However, **section 90(b)** provides that one of the functions of the Chief Psychiatrist is 'to monitor the treatment of voluntary inpatients and involuntary inpatients and the use of restrictive practices in relation to such patients'.

Pursuant to that obligation, the Chief Psychiatrist has authorised the implementation of a detailed policy titled *Restraint and seclusion standard and observation in mental health services*.[10] The policy is mandatory

and applies to all clinical, medical, nursing, allied health, emergency, dental, mental health and pathology staff employed in the delivery of mental health services in South Australia.

The policy document is comprehensive and detailed. It includes specific objectives and definitions as well as role, responsibility and reporting requirements for all nursing staff in relation to the application of seclusion and restraint. All nursing staff involved in the mental health sector where seclusion and restraint are utilised from time to time in relation to the care of a patient should be very familiar with the contents of the policy and a copy of the policy should be readily accessible to all staff working in the mental health sector.

4. Review of Care and Appeal Provisions Under the Act

Civil and Administrative Tribunal

Section 79 provides that the tribunal must review CTOs and inpatient treatment orders made, specifically Level 1 and Level 2 CTOs and Level 1 and Level 3 ITOs. In carrying out its role, the tribunal may conduct any review it considers appropriate and in any manner it considers appropriate (s 79(2) and (3)).

Section 80 provides that in completing a review, the tribunal must revoke any ITO or CTO order if it is not satisfied there are proper grounds for it to remain in operation. In reviewing orders the tribunal may affirm, vary or revoke an order or make an order not being an ITO if it considers it should be made in relation to the person including a treatment and care plan (**s 81**).

Community Visitors

Section 50 of the Act permits the Governor to appoint people to the positions of Principal community visitor and Community visitor.

Section 51 states that the functions of Community visitors are to:

- visit and inspect treatment centres — **section 52** specifies that, every 2 months, two or more Community visitors must conduct such visits; and
- refer matters of concern relating to the organisation or delivery of mental health services or the care, treatment or control of patients to the Minister, Chief Psychiatrist or other appropriate body; and

- act as advocates for patients to assist in the resolution of issues relating to their care, treatment or control; and may
- make enquiries about the care and treatment of inpatients; and
- undertake any other functions assigned by the Act.

In visiting treatment centres, Community visitors must, as far as practicable, inspect all parts of the centre and make inquiries about care, treatment and control of patients being detained or treated. Following such inspections, a report must be made to the Principal community visitor.

Section 52 empowers Community visitors to visit treatment centres at any time of the day or night, with or without notice. A visit may be requested by a patient or by the patient's guardian, medical agent, relative, carer or friend who may also wish to speak to a Community visitor (**s 53**). Section 52A also empowers Community Visitors to visit community mental health centres.

Section 54 requires the Principal community visitor to report to the Minister on or before 30 September each year, and the report must be tabled in Parliament.

Appeals to the Supreme Court of South Australia

Section 83A provides that decisions of the tribunal (with minor exceptions) may be appealed to the Supreme Court of South Australia pursuant to the *Civil and Administrative Tribunal Act 2013* (SA).

TASMANIA: *MENTAL HEALTH ACT 2013*

1. Objectives, Principles and Rights Under the Act

Section 12 sets out the objects of the Act that include, for example, the objective 'to provide for the assessment, treatment and care of persons with mental illnesses' and 'to provide for such assessment, treatment and care to be given in the least restrictive setting consistent with clinical need, legal and judicial constraints, public safety and patient health, safety and welfare'.

Section 15 requires all persons exercising responsibilities under the Act to have regard to the **Mental Health Service Delivery Principles** that are detailed in **Schedule 1** at the end of the Act, for example, 'to respect, observe and promote the inherent rights, liberty, dignity, autonomy and self-respect of persons with a mental illness'.

Section 62 sets out the rights (from sub-paras (a) to (m)) that every **involuntary patient** has under the Act including the right to be given 'clear, accurate and timely information' about the rules governing his or her conduct in hospital and his or her diagnosis and treatment.

Section 129 provides that, whenever a person is admitted to or discharged from an approved facility, he or she is to be given a statement of rights in a form that has been approved by the Chief Psychiatrist. The statement, as well as any information given to the patient, must be in a language the patient understands using the assistance of an interpreter as required (**s 135**).

Section 214 imposes a criminal penalty on a person who intentionally ill-treats a person with a mental illness who is unable to take proper care of himself or herself. The penalty may be either financial or a term of imprisonment not exceeding 2 years, or both.

2. Relevant Definitions Under the Act

Section 3, titled Interpretation, contains the definition of key words and phrases used throughout the Act, but does not include the definition of mental illness. That definition and a number of other relevant words or phrases used in the Act are to be found in specific sections of the Act and will be referred to as necessary.

Section 4(1) provides that a person has a **mental illness** if he or she experiences, temporarily, repeatedly or continually:

- a serious impairment of thought (which may include delusions); *or*
- a serious impairment of mood, volition, perception or cognition; *and*
- nothing prevents the serious or permanent physiological, biochemical or psychological effects of alcohol use or drug-taking from being regarded as an indication that a person has a mental illness.

However, **section 4(2)** does list (from sub-paras (a) to (o)) a number of personal characteristics or behaviours that are not to be taken as an indication the person has a mental illness including, for example, by reason only of the person's:

- current or past expression of, or failure or refusal to express, a particular political opinion or belief; or
- current or past engagement in anti-social activity; or
- intellectual or physical disability; or
- acquired brain injury or dementia.

Section 3 defines **disability** as being 'any restriction or lack of ability to perform an activity in a normal manner (being a restriction or lack of ability arising from any absence, loss or abnormality of mental, psychological, physiological or anatomical structure or function)'.

Section 3 defines a **statement of rights** as 'a written statement that sets out and succinctly explains, in plain language, what rights a patient or prospective patient has in the particular circumstances under this Act in which he or she is required to be given such a statement'.

Section 3 defines a **support person** of a patient or a prospective patient as a person who provides a patient with ongoing care or support.

Section 139 provides for the appointment of **mental health officers** by the Chief Psychiatrist. Such persons would include ambulance officers and police officers.

Section 140 permits the Minister to approve hospitals, assessment centres or secure mental health units as premises for the purposes of the Act.

3. Admission, Detention, Care and Treatment of Persons Under the Act

Provision for a Single Treatment Order to Authorise Treatment in a Hospital or in the Community

When a person is treated and cared for under the mental health legislative provisions of a state or territory, a distinction is generally made between treatment orders that are identified as either inpatient treatment orders or community-based treatment orders. However, the Tasmanian Act makes no such distinction and simply makes provision for a single **treatment order** that enables treatment to be given in the most appropriate 'treatment setting' which includes 'an approved facility (other than a secure mental health unit

(SMHU)) or a premises or place specified in the order'. Such a provision would enable a treatment order to be made authorising treatment in a hospital, the community, or a combination of both.

Voluntary Patient and Voluntary Inpatient — Admission and Treatment

Section 3 defines a **voluntary patient** as a person who is not an involuntary patient or a forensic patient and a **voluntary inpatient** as a person who has been admitted to a facility voluntarily and is receiving treatment on the basis of informed consent.

Section 16(1) provides that the policy that governs the treatment of a voluntary patient is that the patient may be given treatment with informed consent either as a hospital inpatient or in the community and may be given special psychiatric treatment if it is authorised by the tribunal and informed consent has been given by the patient.

The meaning of **informed consent** is set out in **section 8** and essentially requires that, at the time of giving consent, the person has decision-making capacity, has been given detailed information as to the advantages and disadvantages of having the proposed treatment, has had the opportunity to consider the decision to be made and has freely and voluntarily given that consent.

Section 7 provides that an adult person is taken to have decision-making capacity unless the person:

- is unable to make the decision because of an impairment of, or disturbance in, the functioning of the mind or brain; and
- is unable to understand information relating to the decision, or unable to retain such information, or unable to weigh such information or unable to communicate the decision (either by speech, gesture or other means).

In relation to a child (a person defined in section 3 as a person under the age of 18 years), section 7(2) provides that a child is taken to have decision-making capacity if the child is sufficiently mature to make decisions and, despite any impairment or disturbance of the child's mind or brain, the child is able to understand information relevant to the decision, able to retain and weigh such information, and able to communicate the decision (by speech, gesture or other means). For both an adult and a child, understanding information relevant to the decision means the adult or child 'is able to understand the nature and consequences of the decision given in a way that is appropriate to his or her circumstances' (s 7(3)).

Information relevant to the decision is stated to be information on the consequences of making, deferring or failing to make the decision (s 7(4)).

Section 184 provides that the tribunal must review the status of a voluntary patient if he or she has been a voluntary patient for 6 continuous months. In doing so, the tribunal may affirm the patient's status or direct that an approved medical practitioner apply for a treatment order for the patient.

Involuntary Patients – Admission and Treatment

In the first instance, **section 16(2)** provides that the policy that governs the treatment of involuntary patients (other than forensic patients) is that such patients may be given treatment under the Act where:

- informed consent has been given; or
- the treatment is authorised by a treatment order; or
- the treatment is urgent and has been authorised as required.

Also, an involuntary patient may be given special psychiatric treatment if it is authorised by the tribunal and informed consent has been given where required.

Where circumstances require it, **section 17** permits a mental health officer or police officer to take a person into **protective custody** where it is reasonably believed the person has a mental illness and should be assessed and that the safety of the person or others is at risk if the person is not placed in protective custody. The person can then be transported to an authorised hospital for assessment.

Section 23 permits a medical practitioner, nurse, mental health officer, police officer, guardian, parent, support person or ambulance officer to apply to a medical practitioner for an **assessment order** if the applicant is satisfied the person has or might have a mental illness, and an attempt to have the person assessed with informed consent has failed or it would be futile or inappropriate to make such an attempt.

In making an assessment order, the medical practitioner who has examined the person must be satisfied that the patient meets the **assessment criteria**. **Section 25** provides that the assessment criteria are:

- the person has, or appears to have, a mental illness that requires or is likely to require treatment for the person's health or safety or the safety of others; and
- the person cannot be properly assessed regarding the mental illness or the making of a treatment order except under the authority of the assessment order; and
- the person does not have decision-making capacity.

Once an assessment order has been made, the patient must be independently assessed by another approved medical practitioner within 24 hours (**s 30**).

Section 27 confirms that the purpose of authorising an assessment order is to determine whether the person meets the assessment criteria and to determine whether the patient also meets the **treatment criteria** under the Act.

Section 40 provides that the **treatment criteria** in relation to a person are:

- the person has a mental illness; and
- without treatment the mental illness will, or is likely to, seriously harm the safety of the person or others; and
- the treatment will be appropriate and effective in terms of outcomes referred to in section 6(1); and
- the treatment cannot adequately be given except under a treatment order; and
- the person does not have decision-making capacity.

The steps referred to above are identified in **section 6(1)** as being the 'professional intervention' necessary to prevent or remedy mental illness; or to manage and alleviate, where possible, the effects of mental illness; or to reduce the risks the person with a mental illness may pose to themselves or others; or to monitor or evaluate a person's mental state.

If a person is assessed as meeting the treatment criteria, application can be made by an approved medical practitioner to the tribunal for the making of a **treatment order** (ss 36 and 37).

Section 42 provides that the effect of a **treatment order** is authority for the patient, without consent, to be given the treatment specified in the **treatment plan**, which may include the patient's admission and detention in an approved facility for the purposes of receiving the treatment proposed. The treatment order may also authorise the treatment to be given in a different treatment setting, such as the community. If a patient fails to comply with a treatment order, the order may be varied to reflect alternative treatment or a different treatment setting (**s 47**) and, where the patient's health or safety or the safety of others is in issue, the treating medical practitioner may have the patient involuntarily admitted to an approved facility (s 47A).

Section 44 provides that a treatment order continues in effect for such period (not exceeding 6 months) as the tribunal specifies in the order. The tribunal may renew a treatment order on the application of any approved medical practitioner (**s 48**). Also, the tribunal must review a treatment order within 60 days after it is made if it is in effect and it must further review the order within 180 days after it is made if it is still in effect. After the further review, the order is subject to review by the tribunal every 180 days for as long as it remains in effect (**s 181**).

Section 49 provides that a treatment order may be discharged by an approved medical practitioner or by the tribunal pursuant to section 181.

Section 51 requires that every involuntary patient is to have a **treatment plan** setting out an outline of the treatment the patient is to receive. **Section 53** provides that the treatment plan may be prepared by the medical practitioner involved in the patient's care who must consult the patient and may, with the patient's knowledge, consult such other persons as the medical practitioner considers appropriate in the circumstances.

Special Psychiatric Treatment

Section 122(1) of the Act permits special psychiatric treatment and defines it as:

  a. *psychosurgery; or*
  b. *any treatment that the regulations declare to be special psychiatric treatment.*

The section further elaborates on the types of procedures encompassed by the term 'psychosurgery' as being:

  a. *the use of surgery or intracerebral electrodes to create a lesion in a person's brain with the*

intention of permanently altering the person's thoughts, emotions or behaviour;
  b. *the use of intracerebral electrodes to stimulate a person's brain (without creating a lesion) with the intention of temporarily altering or influencing the person's thoughts, emotions or behaviour.*

Given the above definition, section 122 would appear to include the administration of ECT as there is no other specific reference in the Act to ECT treatment.

Section 123 confirms that the provisions relating to special psychiatric treatment apply 'to all patients and to all voluntary patients' under the Act.

Section 124 details the restriction in place in the giving of special psychiatric treatment to a patient, including the requirement for the tribunal to authorise the treatment beforehand and in writing and that informed consent has been given. The administration of special psychiatric treatment by a medical practitioner, nurse or other health practitioner without the requisite approval from the tribunal and the patient's informed consent constitutes an offence and is also deemed to be 'professional misconduct of the most serious kind'. The penalty is a fine or imprisonment for a term not exceeding 12 months.

Seclusion

Section 3 defines **seclusion** as 'the deliberate confinement of an involuntary patient or forensic patient, alone, in a room or area that the patient cannot freely exit'.

Section 56 permits seclusion to be implemented in an improved hospital in relation to an involuntary patient for a prescribed reason so long as it is implemented in accordance with the provisions of that section, which include that:

  ■ the seclusion is authorised in writing in accordance with the Chief Civil Psychiatrist (CCP) standing orders or clinical guidelines; and
  ■ the patient is clinically observed every 15 minutes by the nursing staff or as otherwise authorised; and
  ■ the patient is examined by a medical practitioner or approved nurse every 4 hours and by an approved medical practitioner at intervals not exceeding 12 hours; and

- the seclusion must not exceed 7 hours unless the patient has been examined by a medical practitioner and the extension is authorised by the CCP within those 7 hours; and
- the patient is provided with suitable clothing and bedding, adequate sustenance and toilet facilities with adequate ventilation and light and a means of summoning aid.

Restraint

Section 3 defines **restraint** as any form of chemical, mechanical or physical restraint. **Section 57** permits restraint in relation to an involuntary patient as long as it is done for a 'prescribed reason' and is implemented in accordance with the provisions of that section. The provisions for the authorisation, recording, observation and care to be provided to a patient where restraint is implemented are in similar terms to those applying to the implementation of seclusion.

Urgent circumstances treatment

Section 55 (for involuntary patients) and **section 87** (for forensic patients) permits treatment to be given in urgent circumstances without informed consent or the tribunal's authorisation if the relevant Chief Psychiatrist considers the treatment as being urgently needed and in the patient's best interests. The situations in which the proposed 'urgent circumstances' arise are set out in section 55(3):

- an approved medical practitioner has concluded that the patient has a mental illness that is generally in need of treatment; and
- the treatment is urgently needed for the patient's health or safety or the safety of others; and
- the treatment is likely to be effective and appropriate; and
- the need to achieve the treatment outcome would be compromised by waiting for authorisation by the tribunal; and
- the Chief Civil Psychiatrist agrees and is satisfied that attempts to administer the treatment with informed consent have failed or it would be futile to make such attempt.

Similar provisions apply with respect to forensic patients under section 87, except that reference is made to the Chief Forensic Psychiatrist where appropriate.

4. Review of Care and Appeal Provisions Under the Act

Official Visitors

Section 155 provides for the appointment of a Principal Official Visitor who, in turn, may appoint more Official visitors.

Section 157 sets out the functions of an Official visitor which are essentially to regularly visit approved facilities where patients are being cared for, to investigate complaints from patients and to ensure their rights are being protected. The Official visitor reports to the Principal Official Visitor. Complaints received by the Principal Official Visitor may be referred to the Health Complaints Commissioner or Ombudsman.

Chief Psychiatrists

Tasmania is the only state or territory that creates two positions of Chief Psychiatrist. That is, **sections 143** and **144** create the positions of Chief Civil Psychiatrist and Chief Forensic Psychiatrist respectively. Their powers and functions are identical as expressed in **section 146**. A Chief Psychiatrist has, in relation to prescribed matters, the power (under **section 147**) to intervene directly in the assessment, treatment and care of any patient under the Act relevant to his or her jurisdiction — that is, civil or forensic.

Section 147(8) states that, for the purposes of the section, 'prescribed matters' means:

a. *the use of seclusion;*
b. *the use of force;*
c. *the use of restraint;*
d. *the granting, refusal and control of leave of absence;*
e. *the giving or withholding of patient information;*
f. *the granting, denial and control of visiting, correspondence and telephone rights;*
g. *assessment and treatment generally;*
h. *matters prescribed by the regulations.*

Mental Health Review Tribunal

Section 167 establishes the Mental Health Review Tribunal. The functions of the tribunal are set out in **section 168(1)** as follows:

a. *to make, vary, renew and discharge treatment orders;*

b. to authorise the treatment of forensic patients;

c. to authorise special psychiatric treatment;

d. to determine applications for leave, from secure mental health units, for patients subject to restriction orders;

e. to carry out any further functions given to it under this or any other Act.

Appeals to the Supreme Court of Tasmania

Section 174 of the Act provides that any person who is a party to proceedings of the tribunal may appeal to the Supreme Court of Tasmania from any determination made in those proceedings on a question of law, as of right, or on any other question, with the leave of the Supreme Court.

VICTORIA: *MENTAL HEALTH ACT 2014*

1. Objectives, Principles and Rights Under the Act

Section 10 sets out the objectives of the Act, which include, for example, an objective to provide for the assessment of persons who appear to have a mental illness and the treatment of persons who have a mental illness. A further objective is for those persons to receive that assessment and treatment in the least restrictive way possible with the least possible restrictions on human rights and dignity.

Section 11(1) sets out the **mental health principles** that must apply to the provision of mental health services under the Act. The principles state, for example, that persons receiving mental health services should have their rights, dignity and autonomy respected and promoted and that Aboriginal persons receiving mental health services should have their distinct culture and identity recognised and responded to.

Section 12 provides that a **statement of rights** is an approved document that sets out a person's rights under the Act as well as information by which the person will be assessed or treated under the Act.

Section 13 requires that when a person is given a statement of rights the person must also receive an oral explanation of the statement. The statement of rights and oral explanation must be given in a way that the person comprehends and in a language the person understands.

Section 15 asserts an inpatient's right to communicate lawfully with any person particularly for the purpose of seeking legal advice or representation. **Section 14** provides that 'communicate' includes communication by letter, telephone or electronic communication as well as receiving visitors including legal representatives and nominated persons.

Section 19 provides for a person to make an **advance statement**, which is a document that sets out a person's preferences in relation to treatment in the event that the person becomes a patient.

Section 24 allows a person to nominate another person as a **nominated person** under the Act. The nomination has to be in writing, specifying the nominated person's details. The person nominated must sign a statement confirming his or her agreement to be a nominated person. **Section 23** states that the role of such a person is to provide support and represent the interests of the patient, to receive information and be consulted about the patient's treatment and to assist the patient to exercise any of his or her rights under the Act.

2. Relevant Definitions Under the Act

Section 3 includes definitions of key words and phrases used in the Act. Note, however, that the definitions of some words and phrases appear in specific sections of the Act.

Section 3 defines a **patient** as being:

a. a compulsory patient;

b. a security patient; or

c. a forensic patient.

Section 4(1) states that **mental illness** is a medical condition that is characterised by a 'significant disturbance of thought, mood, perception or memory'.

However, **section 4(2)** identifies a list (sub-paras (a) to (o)) of characteristics and beliefs that a person may hold and will not be considered to have a mental illness, such as that the person expresses, refuses or fails to express a particular political opinion or belief, or that the person engages in immoral or illegal conduct, or is intellectually disabled, or takes drugs or alcohol. Notwithstanding the above, **section 4(3)** states that nothing prevents the serious temporary or permanent physiological, biochemical or psychological effects of taking drugs or alcohol from being regarded as an indication that a person has a mental illness.

The Act distinguishes between **treatment** and **medical treatment**.

Section 6 states that, for the purposes of the Act, a person receives **treatment** for a mental illness if things are done in the course of exercising professional skills to remedy the person's mental illness **or** to alleviate the symptoms and reduce the ill effects of the mental illness. Treatment includes ECT and neurosurgery for mental illness.

Section 3 states that, where it is used in the *Mental Health Act*, the term '**medical treatment**' has the same meaning as it has in the *Medical Treatment Planning and Decisions Act 2016* but does **not** include treatment as defined in section 6 above. The *Medical Treatment Planning and Decisions Act* defines medical treatment as including treatment with physical or surgical therapy, treatment with prescription pharmaceuticals or approved medicinal cannabis product within the meaning of the *Access to Medicinal Cannabis Act 2016*, dental treatment and palliative care.

However, where a person who is a mental health patient requires medical treatment including neurosurgery for a mental illness, such treatment comes within the definition of treatment as stated in section 6 of the *Mental Health Act*.

3. Admission, Detention, Care and Treatment of Persons Under the Act

Voluntary Admission and Treatment Generally

The Act makes no specific mention of voluntary treatment and admission but provision is made for a person to receive treatment on the basis that they have the capacity to give informed consent.

Assuming a person were to meet the criteria set out in the Act as having the requisite capacity to give informed consent, the person could agree to be treated as a voluntary patient.

Section 68 provides that a person 'has the **capacity** to give informed consent' under the Act subject to the provisions of section 68(1), they being that the person:

a. *understands the information he or she is given that is relevant to the decision; and*
b. *is able to remember the information that is relevant to the decision; and*

c. *is able to use or weigh information that is relevant to the decision; and*
d. *is able to communicate the decision he or she makes by speech, gestures or any other means.*

Section 68(2) sets out a number of principles that are intended to provide guidance to a person who has to determine a person's capacity to give informed consent; for example, a person's capacity to give informed consent may change over time, and a decision that a person does not have capacity to give informed consent should not be based only on his or her age, appearance, condition or an aspect of his or her behaviour.

If a person were to meet the above provisions, he or she would be able to be treated as a voluntary patient, as long as the person has been given sufficient information to satisfy the provisions of informed consent as expressed in the Act. That is, **section 69(1)** states that a person gives **informed consent** if the person:

- has the capacity to give informed consent to the treatment or medical treatment proposed; and
- has been given adequate information to enable the person to make an informed decision; and
- has been given a reasonable opportunity to make the decision; and
- has given consent freely without undue pressure or coercion by any other person; and
- has not withdrawn or indicated any intention to withdraw consent.

Section 69(2) sets out the information that must be given to a person to ensure the person can make an informed decision about proposed treatment or medical treatment — for example, an explanation of the proposed treatment or medical treatment, including the type, method and duration of the proposed treatment or medical treatment, and an explanation of the advantages and disadvantages of the proposed treatment or medical treatment.

Admission and Treatment of Compulsory Patients

Unlike the other states and territories, the Victorian Mental Health Act does not use the expression 'involuntary' patient. Instead it uses the expression 'compulsory' patient.

Section 3 defines a **compulsory patient** as a person who is subject to:

a. *an assessment order; or*
b. *a court assessment order; or*
c. *a temporary treatment order; or*
d. *a treatment order.*

The first step to determine whether a person should be a 'compulsory patient' under the Act is to make an **assessment order**. **Section 28** provides that an assessment order is an order made by a registered medical practitioner or a mental health practitioner that enables a person who is subject to an assessment order to be compulsorily:

a. *examined by an authorised psychiatrist to determine whether treatment criteria apply to the person (community assessment order); or*
b. *taken to and detained in a designated mental health service and examined there by an authorised psychiatrist to determine whether the treatment criteria apply to the person (inpatient assessment order).*

To be made subject to an assessment order, **section 29** requires that the person meet the **assessment criteria**, which are:

- the person appears to have a mental illness; and
- because of that, the person appears to need immediate treatment to prevent serious deterioration in the person's mental or physical health or serious harm to the person or others; and
- if the person is subject to an assessment order, he or she can be assessed; and
- there is no less restrictive means reasonably available to enable that to be done.

Section 30 provides that, before a registered medical practitioner or mental health practitioner makes an **assessment order** in respect of a person, he or she must, to the extent that is reasonable, inform the person of the proposed examination **and** explain the reason for the examination. If the assessment criteria set out in section 29 above apply to the person, a practitioner may make the assessment order and, in doing so, specify whether it is to be a **community assessment order** or an **inpatient assessment order**.

If an **inpatient assessment order** is made, **section 33** provides the person must be taken to a designated mental health service as soon as practicable but not later than 72 hours after the order is made.

Section 38 provides that a person who is subject to an assessment order may not be given treatment unless the person gives informed consent to the treatment **or** a registered medical practitioner in a designated mental health service is satisfied that urgent treatment is necessary to prevent a serious deterioration in the person's mental or physical health or to prevent serious harm to the person or others.

On occasions where a person appears before a court charged with an offence where it is believed the person may have a mental illness, a **court assessment order** may be made. When such an order is made, **section 40** requires the person to be taken to a designated mental health service. When that occurs the person's family, nominated person, guardian or carer must be notified.

Section 41 provides that, after assessment by an authorised psychiatrist, a person on a **court assessment order** may be placed on a community assessment order or an inpatient assessment order.

After assessing a person subject to an assessment order or court assessment order, **section 45** of the Act allows an authorised psychiatrist to make a **temporary treatment order**.

A temporary treatment order enables the person to be treated compulsorily in the community (community temporary treatment order) or taken to, detained and treated in a designated mental health service (inpatient temporary treatment order).

Section 46 provides that an authorised psychiatrist may make a temporary treatment order if satisfied that the **treatment criteria** apply.

Section 45 states that the treatment criteria for a person to be made subject to a temporary treatment order or treatment order are:

- the person has a mental illness; and
- because of that, the person needs immediate treatment to prevent serious deterioration in the person's mental or physical health or serious harm to the person or others; and
- the immediate treatment will be provided to the person if he or she is subject to a temporary treatment order or treatment order; and

- there is no less restrictive means reasonably available to enable the person to receive immediate treatment.

Section 51 provides that the duration of a temporary treatment order, unless it is revoked or it expires, is 28 days. It may be extended by the tribunal pursuant to **section 192**.

Section 52 provides that a treatment order is an order made by the tribunal that enables a person to be treated compulsorily in the community or taken to and detained and treated in a designated mental health service. A treatment order will be designated as either a **community treatment order (CTO)** or an **inpatient treatment order (ITO)**.

Section 55 provides that, after receiving an application, the tribunal must hold a hearing and make a treatment order if it is satisfied that the treatment criteria as set out above apply to the person. A treatment order made by the tribunal allows a person to be compulsorily treated in the community on a CTO or taken to and detained and treated in a designated mental health service on an ITO.

Section 57 provides that, where the person is under the age of 18 years, the duration of a treatment order is 3 months, whether that is a community or an inpatient treatment order. Where the person is over 18 years, the duration of a community treatment order is 12 months and an inpatient treatment order is 6 months.

Electroconvulsive Therapy

Section 3 defines electroconvulsive therapy as being the application of electric current to specific areas of a person's head to produce a generalised seizure.

The Act allows for the administration of ECT subject to certain safeguards. Where it is considered necessary to administer ECT to a young person (under 18 years), **section 94** specifies that it is necessary to obtain the informed consent in writing of the young person **or** have it approved by the tribunal following an application by an authorised psychiatrist. Where the person is not a young person, **section 92** provides that ECT may be performed if the patient has given informed consent in writing **or** the tribunal has granted approval subject to an application being made.

Section 93 provides that where a patient who is not a young person and does not have the capacity to give informed consent to proposed ECT, the tribunal may grant approval subject to an application being made by an authorised psychiatrist.

Section 91 provides that the number of ECT treatments that may be given should not exceed 12 treatments over a period of 6 months.

Neurosurgery

Section 3 contains a definition of **neurosurgery for mental illness** as including any surgical technique or procedure by which one or more lesions are created in a person's brain, or the use of intracerebral electrodes to create lesions in the brain or to stimulate the person's brain without creating a lesion.

Sections 100 and **101** provide that the tribunal must hear and determine an application from a psychiatrist to perform neurosurgery for mental illness on a person. After hearing the application the tribunal may grant or refuse the application. **Section 102** provides that the tribunal must not grant an application unless it is satisfied the person has given informed consent in writing to the proposed neurosurgery and that the performance of the neurosurgery will benefit the person.

Restrictive Intervention

Section 3 defines 'restrictive intervention' as meaning **seclusion** or **bodily restraint**.

Section 105 provides that restrictive intervention may be used on a person receiving mental health services in a designated mental health service only after all reasonable and less restrictive options have been tried or considered and have been found to be unsuitable.

Section 107 requires an authorised psychiatrist to take reasonable steps to notify a number of persons as soon as practicable after restrictive intervention is commenced. The persons include the person's nominated person, guardian, and carer or parent if applicable.

Seclusion

Section 110 allows seclusion to be used in the treatment of a person in a designated mental health service if it is necessary to prevent imminent and serious harm to the person or others. **Section 111** requires it to be authorised by an authorised psychiatrist or, if an authorised psychiatrist is not immediately available, a registered medical practitioner or the senior registered nurse on duty (**s 111**).

Section 112 details the monitoring provisions that must be in place when seclusion is implemented including regular clinical observation not less than every 15 minutes and examination by an authorised psychiatrist or medical practitioner not less than every 4 hours.

Bodily Restraint

Section 113 allows bodily restraint to be used in the treatment of a person in a designated mental health service if it is necessary to prevent imminent and serious harm to the person or others or to administer treatment or medical treatment to the person. **Section 114** requires it to be authorised by an authorised psychiatrist or, if an authorised psychiatrist is not immediately available, by a registered medical practitioner or the senior registered nurse on duty.

Section 115 permits a registered nurse to approve the use of a bodily restraint (in the form of physical restraint only) on a person receiving mental health services in a designated mental health service if it is necessary as a matter of urgency to prevent imminent and serious harm to the person or another person and an authorised psychiatrist, a registered medical practitioner or the senior registered nurse on duty is not immediately available to authorise the use of bodily restraint on the person. In such circumstances, the registered nurse must seek the authorisation of an authorised psychiatrist, a registered medical practitioner or the senior registered nurse on duty as soon as practicable.

Section 116 details the monitoring provisions that must be in place when bodily restraint is used including that the person on whom bodily restraint is used 'must be under continuous observation by a registered nurse or registered medical practitioner'. Also, the bodily restraint must be clinically reviewed frequently but not less than every 15 minutes and the person must be examined by an authorised psychiatrist or medical practitioner not less than every 4 hours.

Medical Treatment

The definition of **medical treatment** as set out in the *Medical Treatment Planning and Decisions Act 2016* has been referred to earlier in relation to relevant definitions of terms used in the Act and the need to distinguish it from the definition of **treatment** — the latter being the term used to refer to a wide range of mental health treatments under the Act.

When used in the *Mental Health Act*, the term 'medical treatment' covers the range of medical or dental treatments for physical health-related conditions including the supply of pharmaceuticals that a person may need as part of his or her overall care and treatment under the Act. For example, a person may require surgery, or treatment and medication for diabetes or heart disease.

Section 74 provides that, if informed consent is able to be given, medical treatment may be administered. If informed consent is unable to be given, **section 75** provides the category of bodies or persons who must be appointed to give consent on behalf of the patient if the patient does not have capacity to give informed consent — for example, a person appointed by the Victorian Civil and Administrative Tribunal (VCAT) to make decisions on behalf of the person, or a person appointed under a guardianship order, or the authorised psychiatrist.

4. Review of Care and Appeal Provisions Under the Act

Chief Psychiatrist

Section 119 provides for the appointment of a Chief Psychiatrist. The functions of the Chief Psychiatrist are set out in **section 121**. Those functions include:

- to develop standards, guidelines and practice directions for the provision of mental health services and to publish or otherwise make available those standards, guidelines and practice directions;
- to assist mental health service providers to comply with the standards, guidelines and practice directions developed by the Chief Psychiatrist;
- to develop and provide information, training and education to promote improved quality and safety in the provision of mental health services.

Community Visitors

Section 214 provides for the appointment of Community Visitors under the Act.

Section 216 sets out the functions expected of a Community Visitor, which are essentially to visit any mental health service in Victoria for the purposes of inquiring into a number of aspects of that service including:

- the adequacy of services for persons receiving mental health services; *and*
- the appropriateness and standard of facilities provided for the accommodation, physical well-being and welfare of persons receiving mental health services; *and*
- the adequacy of opportunities and facilities for the recreation, occupation, education, training and recovery of persons receiving mental health services; *and*
- the extent to which persons receiving treatment are being given the best possible treatment appropriate to their needs in the least possible restrictive environment and least possible intrusive manner consistent with the effective giving of that treatment; *and*
- any failure to comply with the provisions of this Act; *and*
- any other matter that the Community Visitor considers appropriate having regard to the objectives and principles of the Act; *and*
- any complaint made to a Community Visitor by a person receiving treatment under the Act.

Section 217 provides Community Visitors with very wide powers to inspect any part of the premises to see any patient who is receiving treatment, unless the person receiving treatment requests otherwise, and can make any inquiries relating to admission, detention, care, treatment and control of people in the particular service. In addition, a Community Visitor may inspect any documents (other than clinical records) about a person's treatment as long as he or she has obtained the consent of the person.

Section 220 requires any member of staff to provide 'reasonable assistance' to a Community visitor in carrying out his or her functions.

Mental Health Complaints Commissioner

Section 226 establishes the position of Mental Health Complaints Commissioner. The functions of the Commissioner include to accept, assess, manage and investigate complaints relating to the providers of mental health services and to attempt to resolve the complaints using formal and informal dispute resolution mechanisms. Also, **section 228** requires the Commissioner to issue compliance notices, to review quality, safety and other issues arising out of complaints and to provide information and make recommendations to a number of agencies including mental health service providers, the Chief Psychiatrist and the NDIS Commission.

Mental Health Tribunal

Section 152 establishes the tribunal. Its functions are set out in **section 153** and include a requirement for it to hear and determine a number of matters including whether to:

- make a treatment order; or
- revoke a treatment order or temporary treatment order; or
- approve ECT or neurosurgery.

Victorian Civil and Administrative Tribunal (VCAT)

Section 201 provides that a person who was a party to proceedings before the Mental Health Tribunal may apply to VCAT for review of any determination made by that tribunal under the Act.

Supreme Court of Victoria

Section 197 also provides for application to be made to the Supreme Court of Victoria where a question of law arises in proceedings before the Mental Health Tribunal. That application may be made by the tribunal of its own motion or by any person who is a party to the proceedings.

WESTERN AUSTRALIA: *MENTAL HEALTH ACT 2014*

1. Objectives, Principles and Rights Under the Act

The **Long Title** at the commencement of the Act states that it is an Act:

- *to provide for the treatment, care, support and protection of people who have a mental illness; and*
- *to provide for the protection of the rights of people who have a mental illness; and*

- *to provide for the recognition of the role of carers and families in providing the best possible care and support to people who have a mental illness; and*
- *for related purposes.*

Section 7 sets out the matters a person must consider when making a decision as to what is in the best interests of a person receiving treatment under the Act. For example, regard must be had to the person's wishes as far as practicable as well as the views, where applicable, of the person's enduring guardian, parents, nominated person, carer or family member.

Section 8 requires that, in ascertaining a person's wishes, regard must be had to any treatment decision in an advance care directive made by the person and any term of an enduring power of attorney made by the person.

Section 10 sets out the objectives of the Act that include ensuring that people who have a mental illness are provided the best possible treatment and care with the least possible restriction of their freedom and the least possible interference with their rights and with respect for their dignity.

Section 11 provides that 'a person or body performing a function under this Act' must have regard to the *Charter of mental health care principles*. The Charter is set out in full as **Schedule 1** to the Act and is a rights-based set of principles. **Section 12** provides that a private psychiatric hostel must make every effort to comply with the Charter.

Section 244 requires the person responsible to ensure that the person is provided with an explanation of his or her rights under the Act, and **section 245** requires the same explanation to be given to the person's carer, close family member or other personal support person. **Section 246** sets out the categories of persons responsible for ensuring that the requisite explanation is provided including the person in charge of an authorised hospital, or the psychiatrist who makes a treatment order, or the psychiatrist who grants leave of absence.

Section 273 allows the person, including a child, to appoint a **nominated person**, and the role of such a person as provided in **section 263** is to assist the person to observe his or her rights under the Act and take that person's interests and wishes into account.

Section 189 requires that the provision of treatment under the Act to a patient who is of **Aboriginal or Torres Strait Islander** descent must be provided in collaboration with:

- Aboriginal or Torres Strait Islander mental health workers; and
- significant members of the patient's community, including elders and traditional healers.

Sections 253 and **254** provide significant criminal penalties where a staff member ill-treats or wilfully neglects a person and fails to report a suspected reportable incident. 'Reportable incident' is defined to include 'unlawful sexual contact' and 'unreasonable use of force' by a staff member (s 254).

2. Relevant Definitions Under the Act

Section 4, titled 'Terms used', contains the definition of particular key words used in the Act. Note, however, that the definition of some words and phrases appear in specific sections of the Act.

For example, **section 6(1)** states that a person has a mental illness if the person has a condition that:

a. *is characterised by a disturbance of thought, mood, volition, perception, orientation or memory; and*
b. *significantly impairs (temporarily or permanently) the person's judgment or behaviour.*

However, **section 6(2)** states that a person does not have a mental illness by reason only of one or more of a number of characteristics including, for example, that the person:

a. *holds, or refuses to hold, a particular religious, philosophical, or political belief or opinion;*
b. *is sexually promiscuous, or has a particular sexual preference;*
c. *engages in immoral or indecent conduct;*
d. *has an intellectual disability;*
e. *takes drugs or alcohol;*
f. *demonstrates anti-social behaviour.*

Critical to the delivery of care and treatment to a person with a mental health condition is the determination as to whether the person has the intellectual capacity at the relevant time to be able to make decisions about agreeing or otherwise to treatment proposed. Very often, when a person is acutely mentally ill, their intellectual capacity is impaired and the person is unable to make the necessary decisions about agreeing to have treatment that is best for them. When that happens, the person's decision-making capacity is impaired and a decision about treatment to be given has to be made on their behalf by somebody else (generally a mental health professional, carer, guardian, parent or support person) acting in the person's best interests.

One of the principles incorporated in the *Charter of mental health care principles* (schedule 1 of the Act — principle 5) is to 'involve people in decision-making and encouraging self-determination … including by recognising people's capacity to make their own decisions'. Hence, the determination of whether a person has decision-making capacity is necessary at the outset when decisions are being made by mental health professionals about recommended treatment to be given.

Section 15 provides that a person has decision-making capacity if the person:

- understands any information or advice about the decision that is required to be provided; and
- understands the matters involved in the decision; and
- understands the effect of the decision; and
- is able to weigh up the above three criteria for the purpose of making the decision; and
- is able to communicate the decision in some way.

Section 13 provides that, where an adult is shown not to have decision-making capacity, the person authorised by law to do so may make the decision on the adult's behalf.

Section 14 provides that a child is presumed not to have decision-making capacity 'unless the child is shown to have that capacity'. If the child does not have decision-making capacity, the child's parent or guardian is able to make the decision on the child's behalf. **Section 4** defines a child as a person under 18 years of age.

In addition to determining decision-making capacity, the Act requires that the person (or a person acting on his or her behalf) who agrees to have treatment has sufficient information to give an informed consent to the proposed treatment. **Section 17** provides that the patient may give informed consent to proposed treatment or, if the patient does not have decision-making capacity, the person who is authorised by law may consent on the patient's behalf. Any consent given must be freely and voluntarily given.

Section 18 provides that a person has the capacity to make a treatment decision if the person:

- understands the information required to be communicated to the person as set out in section 19; and
- understands the matters involved in making the treatment decision; and
- understands the effect of the treatment decision; and
- is able to weigh up the criteria referred to above in making the treatment decision; and
- is able to communicate the treatment decision in some way.

Section 19 details the information that must be given to a person prior to a person being asked to consent to proposed treatment being given. That is, the person must be provided with a clear explanation of the proposed treatment sufficient to enable the person to make a balanced judgment. Also the person must be given information about alternative treatments and why they are not being recommended and the risks inherent in the proposed treatment. The extent of the information given is to be such information that a reasonable person in the patient's position would want to know.

Section 4 defines a **mental health service** as including a hospital that provides treatment or care to persons who have or may have a mental illness, a community mental health service and any other service prescribed as such. It does not include a private psychiatric hostel or a declared place as defined in section 23 of the *Criminal Law (Mentally Impaired) Act 1996*.

Section 538 defines a **mental health practitioner** as one of the following persons with 'at least 3 years experience in the management of people who have a mental illness', they being:

a. *a psychologist;*
b. *a nurse whose name is entered on Division 1 of the Register of Nurses kept under the Health*

Practitioner Regulation National Law (Western Australia) as a registered nurse;

c. an occupational therapist;
d. a social worker.

Section 541 states that an **authorised hospital** is 'a public hospital, or part of a public hospital, in respect of which an order is in force'; or a private hospital whose licence is endorsed under section 26DA of the *Hospitals and Health Services Act 1927* (WA).

3. Admission, Detention, Care and Treatment of Persons Under the Act

Voluntary Patients and Voluntary Inpatients

Generally speaking, the main distinction between a voluntary and involuntary patient is that a voluntary patient is presumed to have decision-making capacity and is able to give and withhold consent to treatment whereas an involuntary patient does not.

Section 4 defines **voluntary patient** as a person to whom treatment is being or is proposed to be provided by a mental health service but who is not an 'involuntary patient' or a 'mentally impaired accused'. It would appear that this definition is designed to apply to those persons who consent to treatment as a voluntary patient in the community because a 'voluntary inpatient' is separately defined.

Section 4 defines **voluntary inpatient** as 'a voluntary patient who is admitted by a mental health service as an inpatient'.

Section 33 provides that, where a person is admitted as a voluntary inpatient by an authorised hospital, any community treatment order in place is suspended until he or she is discharged or an inpatient treatment order is made.

Section 34 provides that, where a voluntary inpatient wants to leave an authorised hospital against medical advice, the person in charge of the ward may order an **assessment** to be done and the person can be detained for up to 6 hours to enable the assessment examination to be done by a psychiatrist.

Section 36 provides that, where a voluntary patient is assessed by a medical practitioner or authorised mental health practitioner because of an order requested under section 34 (above), or during the course of the voluntary patient's inpatient treatment

in an authorised hospital and the practitioner believes the patient is in need of an involuntary patient order (as per the criteria under s 25), the practitioner may refer the voluntary inpatient for examination by a psychiatrist. If that occurs, the voluntary inpatient may be detained at the authorised hospital for up to 24 hours to enable the examination to be conducted.

Section 50 provides that, where it is practicable and appropriate to do so, the assessment of a person of Aboriginal or Torres Strait Islander descent must be conducted in collaboration with Aboriginal and Torres Strait Islander mental health workers and significant members of the person's community, including elders and traditional healers.

Section 55 provides that, once the assessment under section 36 has been undertaken, the psychiatrist may make an **inpatient treatment order** or a **community treatment order**. Alternatively, the person may be detained for a further examination or may be discharged.

Involuntary Patients and Admission

Section 21(1) defines an **involuntary patient** as a person who is under an involuntary treatment order. **Section 21(2)** states that an involuntary treatment order may be subject to an inpatient treatment order or a community treatment order.

Section 22 provides that an inpatient treatment order permits a person to be admitted by a hospital and detained to enable the person to be treated without informed consent having been given to the treatment provided. **Section 23** provides for a community treatment order to be given to a person in the community, also without informed consent being given.

Section 24 provides that only a psychiatrist may make an involuntary treatment order. In doing so, the psychiatrist must be satisfied that the criteria specified in **section 25** are satisfied and, if so, consider whether the objectives of the Act would be better achieved by making a community treatment order in respect of the person. An involuntary treatment order must be in force for as brief a period as practicable, be reviewed regularly and be revoked as soon as practicable after the person no longer meets the criteria for the order.

Section 25(1) provides the criteria that must be satisfied in order to make an involuntary treatment order are that:

a. the person has a mental illness for which the person is in need of treatment; and
b. because of the mental illness, there is:
   i. a significant risk to the health or safety of the person or to the safety of another person; or
   ii. a significant risk of serious harm to the person or another person; and
c. the person lacks capacity as required by section 18 to make a treatment decision for himself or herself; and
d. treatment in the community cannot reasonably be provided;
e. a less restrictive treatment environment would be inadequate for the person.

Section 25(2) sets out the criteria to be satisfied where a community treatment order may be made. They are in similar terms to those applying in relation to an inpatient treatment order except that the treatment required can reasonably be provided in the community.

Section 26 provides that a medical practitioner or authorised mental health practitioner may refer a person to a psychiatrist for an **examination** if they reasonably believe, having regard to the criteria in section 25 (above), the person is in need of an involuntary treatment order or, if they are under a community treatment order, an inpatient treatment order.

Section 29 allows a medical practitioner or authorised mental health practitioner to make a **transport order** to convey a person to an authorised hospital for examination.

Section 149 authorises a **transport officer** or, if considered necessary, a police officer (**s 149**) to apprehend and transport a person to the relevant hospital for examination. A transport order generally remains in force for 72 hours (**s 150**).

Sections 52 and **53** authorise the detention of a person who has been referred to an authorised hospital for examination pursuant to section 26 or section 36 (as above) for a period of up to 24 hours.

Section 55(1) provides that, once a psychiatrist has completed examining the person, the psychiatrist must make one of the following four orders:

a. *an inpatient treatment order authorising the person's detention at the authorised hospital for the period specified in the order in accordance with* **section 87(a) or (b)**;
b. *a community treatment order in respect of the person;*
c. *an order authorising the continuation of the person's detention at the authorised hospital to enable a further examination to be conducted by a psychiatrist;*
d. *an order that the person cannot be detained.*

Where the psychiatrist orders a continuation of the person's detention to enable a further examination to be done, **section 55(3)** permits the detention to continue for a further period not exceeding 72 hours to enable the examination to be conducted by another psychiatrist.

Where a decision is made to detain the person for a further examination, **section 72** permits the psychiatrist completing the examination to make one of the same orders as detailed above except for an order requiring the person to be subject to further examination.

Section 86 provides that the making of an inpatient treatment order is authority for the involuntary patient's admission as an inpatient to a specified hospital and subsequently any authorised hospital, and for the patient's detention there.

Section 87 provides that where an inpatient treatment order pursuant to section 55 is made, the period of detention cannot exceed 21 days for an adult and 14 days for a child.

Section 89 requires that a person detained on an inpatient treatment order must be examined within 7 days before the order ends. If it is considered necessary to continue to detain the person, a **continuation order** may be made to further detain the person. When such an order is made, the detention period must not exceed 3 months when the person is an adult and 28 days when the person is a child.

Once an involuntary treatment order is made it is subject to review by the tribunal. **Section 386** provides that the tribunal must undertake an initial review within 35 days of the order being made where the person is an adult involuntary patient. If the involuntary patient is a child the review must be within 10 days of the order being made.

Community Treatment Orders

Section 114 provides that a psychiatrist cannot make a community treatment order unless satisfied as to the following:

- the treatment of a person in the community would not be inconsistent with the need for safe and proper care to be given; and
- suitable arrangements can be made for the care and treatment of the person in the community including arrangements for a psychiatrist to be the supervising psychiatrist and arrangements for a medical practitioner or mental health practitioner to be the practitioner under the order. The supervising psychiatrist can also be the person's treating practitioner.

Section 115 sets out the details that must be included in a community treatment order including the names of the supervising practitioner, medical practitioner or mental health practitioner and the patient's address details. Section 115(2) provides that the period of time a community treatment order can remain in force must not exceed 3 months from the date on which it is made.

Section 121 permits the supervising psychiatrist to make a **continuation order** further extending a community treatment for a period not exceeding 3 months.

Where an involuntary community patient fails to comply with the provisions of a community treatment order, **section 127** authorises the supervising psychiatrist to issue a breach order giving notice to the patient of the order and the details of the patient's non-compliance. If the person still fails to comply, he or she may be transported to and detained at an authorised mental health service and, if considered necessary, an inpatient treatment order made (**ss 128–131**).

Electroconvulsive Therapy

Section 192 defines ECT as being treatment involving the application of electric current to specific areas of the person's head to produce a generalised seizure that is modified by general anaesthesia and the administration of a muscle-relaxing agent.

ECT is permitted under the Act **except** in relation to a child under 14 years of age where it is prohibited (**s 194**).

Section 195 provides that, where a child is over 14 years and under 18 years of age and is a voluntary patient, a medical practitioner may perform ECT subject to informed consent being given, and approved by the Mental Health Tribunal.

Section 196 permits ECT to be administered to a child over 14 years and under 18 years of age who is an involuntary patient or is a mentally impaired accused person required to be detained in an authorised hospital subject to the approval of the Mental Health Tribunal, and **section 198** permits ECT to be given to an adult involuntary patient or mentally impaired accused person on the same terms.

Section 197 permits ECT to be administered to an adult voluntary patient subject to informed consent being given by the patient and that the ECT is performed at an approved mental health service. The criteria required to be satisfied as to informed consent are detailed above when dealing with relevant definitions of words or phrases used in the Act.

Emergency Psychiatric Treatment

Section 202(1) makes provision for a person to be treated in emergency circumstances if it is considered necessary:

a. *to save the person's life; or*
b. *to prevent the person from behaving in a way that is likely to result in serious physical injury to the person or another person.*

However, **section 202(2)** states that emergency psychiatric treatment does not include ECT, psychosurgery, deep sleep or insulin coma or insulin sub-coma therapy.

Section 203 permits emergency psychiatric treatment to be given to a person without informed consent being given.

Psychosurgery

Section 205 of the Act defines psychosurgery as treatment involving:

a. *the use of a surgical technique or procedure or intracerebral electrodes to create in a person's*

brain a lesion intended (whether alone or in combination with one or more lesions created at the same or other times) to alter permanently:
 i. the person's thoughts or emotions; or
 ii. the person's behaviour other than behaviour secondary to a paroxysmal cerebral dysrhythmia;

or

b. the use of intracerebral electrodes to stimulate a person's brain creating a lesion with the intention that the stimulation (whether alone or in combination with other such stimulation at the same or other times) will influence or alter temporarily:
 i. the person's thoughts or emotions; or
 ii. the person's behaviour other than behaviour secondary to a paroxysmal cerebral dysrhythmia.

Section 207 prohibits psychosurgery on a child under 16 years of age.

Section 208 permits psychosurgery to be performed by a neurosurgeon on an adult or a child who is 16 years or over but under 18 years of age subject to the patient giving informed consent and approval by the Mental Health Tribunal.

Treatment Prohibited by the Act

Section 210 provides that deep sleep therapy, insulin coma therapy and insulin sub-coma therapy are all prohibited treatments under the Act.

Seclusion

Section 212(1) defines seclusion as 'the confinement of a person who is being provided with treatment or care at an authorised hospital by leaving the person at any time of the day or night alone in a room or area from which it is not within the person's control to leave'.

Section 212(2) provides that it is not seclusion merely because the person is alone in a room that he or she is unable to leave because of frailty, illness or mental or physical disability.

Section 213 states that a **seclusion order** must be authorised and **section 214** authorises a medical practitioner or mental health practitioner at an authorised hospital, or the person in charge of a ward at an authorised hospital, to orally authorise the seclusion of a patient admitted or referred to the authorised hospital

for examination. **Section 215** makes similar provisions with respect to written seclusion orders.

Section 216 provides that the criteria for authorising seclusion must be to prevent the person from:

- physically injuring himself or herself or another person; or
- persistently causing serious damage to property; and
- there is no less restrictive way of preventing the injury or damage.

Section 222 details the requirements that must be observed by 'the person in charge of the ward', a 'mental health practitioner or a nurse' when a person is in seclusion. They include that:

- the person must be observed every 15 minutes and a record made of that observation; and
- a medical practitioner must examine the person every 2 hours and record the results of that examination; and
- the person must be provided with adequate bedding, clothing, food and drink and access to toilet facilities.

Restraint

Section 227(1) defines bodily restraint as the physical or mechanical restraint of a person who is being provided with treatment or care at an authorised hospital. **Sections 227(2)** and **(3)** define physical restraint as the restraint of a person by the application of bodily force to the person's body to restrict the person's movement and state that a person is not being physically restrained merely because the person is being provided with physical support or assistance to enable the person to carry out daily living activities or to redirect the person because the person is disorientated.

Section 229 requires bodily restraint to be authorised either orally or in writing as a bodily restraint order.

Section 230 permits a medical practitioner, a mental health practitioner or the person in charge of a ward at an authorised hospital to orally authorise the use of bodily restraint on a patient at an authorised hospital or a person referred to an authorised hospital for examination. **Section 231** makes similar provisions with respect to bodily restraint orders.

Section 232 sets out the criteria that must be present to authorise bodily restraint, they being that the person needs to be restrained to:

- provide the person with treatment; or
- prevent the person from physically injuring himself or herself or others; or
- prevent the person from persistently causing serious damage to property; and
- there is no less restrictive way of providing treatment or preventing injury or damage; and
- the use of bodily restraint is unlikely to pose a significant risk to the person's health.

Section 238 sets out the requirements that must be observed by the 'person in charge of the ward' or a 'nurse' or 'mental health practitioner' when bodily restraint is used. They are:

- a medical practitioner or nurse must be in physical attendance on the person at all times and record all observations made; and
- a medical practitioner must examine the person at least every 30 minutes and record that in the appropriate form; and
- the patient must be provided with bedding and appropriate clothing, sufficient food and drink, access to toilet facilities and any other care appropriate to the person's needs.

4. Review of Care and Appeal Provisions Under the Act

Chief Psychiatrist

Section 508 provides for the appointment by the Governor of a psychiatrist as Chief Psychiatrist.

The responsibilities of the Chief Psychiatrist are extensive and wide-ranging. Overall, **section 515** states the Chief Psychiatrist is responsible for overseeing the treatment and care of:

- all voluntary patients being provided with treatment or care by a mental health service;
- all involuntary patients;
- all mentally impaired accused persons required to be detained at an authorised hospital;
- all persons referred for an examination to be conducted by a psychiatrist at an authorised hospital or other place.

Section 515(2) states that the Chief Psychiatrist must discharge that responsibility by publishing standards for treatment and care as required under **section 547(2)** of the Act.

Section 547 requires the Chief Psychiatrist to publish guidelines for a range of purposes (sub-paras (a)–(h)) including, for example, guidelines on making decisions about whether or not a person is in need of an inpatient treatment order or a community treatment order, the performance of electroconvulsive therapy, and ensuring compliance with the Act by mental health services and specifically for the treatment and care to be provided by mental health services to the persons specified in section 515(1) (as listed above).

Chief Mental Health Advocate and Mental Health Advocates Generally

Section 349 creates the position of Chief Mental Health Advocate appointed by the Minister. **Section 351** details the functions of the Chief Mental Health Advocate including ensuring that identified persons are visited or otherwise contacted as required, and promoting compliance with the *Charter of mental health care principles* by mental health services.

Section 350 provides for the appointment of persons as mental health advocates.

Section 352 sets out the functions of a mental health advocate, which is to inquire into or investigate any matter relating to the condition of mental health services or any identified person and to assist the person to enforce his or her rights under the Act and to access legal services as required.

Section 353 confers such powers on a mental health advocate as are considered 'necessary or convenient' to allow the advocate to perform his or her functions under the Act.

Mental Health Review Tribunal

Section 380 established the Mental Health Tribunal. The role and function of the tribunal is wide-ranging and includes:

- reviewing involuntary treatment orders;
- declaring the validity of treatment orders;
- reviewing the admission of long-term voluntary inpatients;
- approving ECT and psychosurgery.

State Administrative Tribunal

Section 494 permits a person to apply to the State Administrative Tribunal for a review of a decision made by the Mental Health Tribunal about the person where the person is dissatisfied with that decision. Also, any other person whom the State Administrative Tribunal considers has sufficient interest in the matter may, with leave of the State Administrative Tribunal, apply for a review of a decision made by the Mental Health Tribunal.

Supreme Court of Western Australia

Section 503 allows a person, without leave, to appeal a decision or order of the State Administrative Tribunal to the Supreme Court of Western Australia.

CONCLUSION

For nurses working in the field of mental health, the relevant legislation imposes quite specific additional professional and legal obligations that would be encompassed within the duty and standard of care that is owed to a patient or client in the delivery of one's professional services. In determining the standard of care expected of a nurse working in mental health, any obligations arising under the legislation would be considered relevant to determining what was considered competent professional practice in the delivery of a particular treatment.

For example, in relation to seclusion and restraint, the obligations imposed under the legislation would be considered, as well as any practice guidelines or policies in place to determine whether what was done or not done on a particular occasion fell below the expected standard.

Given the above, a thorough working knowledge of the relevant mental health legislation as it applies to the day-to-day practice of a nurse working in mental health care is essential.

CHAPTER 10 REVIEW QUESTIONS

Following your reading of **Chapter 10**, consider these questions in reaching the objectives of this chapter. Guidance on which part of the chapter will assist you in answering the questions can be found at http://evolve.elsevier.com/AU/Staunton/law/. You may, of course, consider other sources as part of your considerations.

1. What are the objectives of the mental health legislation in your state or territory?

2. Are the words 'mental illness' defined in the mental health legislation of your state or territory? If so, what are the definitions?

3. Does the mental health legislation of your state or territory provide for voluntary and involuntary admission of a person to a mental health facility for care and treatment? If so, what is the difference between a voluntary and an involuntary admission?

4. What are the specific provisions in the legislation of your state or territory requiring a person receiving mental health care to be given a statement of their rights?

5. If you were caring for a patient in a mental health unit who required restraint or seclusion to be implemented, what steps would you need to take?

ENDNOTES

1. *Mental Health and Cognitive Impairment Forensic Provisions Act 2020* (NSW); *Criminal Law (Forensic Procedures) Act 2007* (SA); *Criminal Justice (Mental Impairment) Act 1999* (Tas); *Crimes (Mental Impairment and Unfitness to be Tried) Act 1997* (Vic).

2. *Mental Health Act 2015* (ACT); *Mental Health Act 2016* (Qld); *Mental Health Act 2014* (WA).

3. Inquest into the death of Miriam Merten, Coroner's Court of NSW, 7 September 2016.

4. *Health Care Complaints Commission v Borthistle* [2017] NSWCATOD 56, at 85.

5. New South Wales Mental Health Drug and Alcohol Office, *The Mental Health Act (2007) guide book*, 4th ed, p 97 (lSBN 0 7313 2900 7).
6. Ibid, p 6.
7. Ibid, p 56.
8. Ibid, p 60.
9. Ibid, p 61.

10. South Australia: Restraint and seclusion in mental health services policy guideline. Policy document: DO 382: issued May 2015: Updated 1 July 2021 Version 1:1 issued 28 May 2021: Compliance from 1 July 2021: Chief Psychiatrist: Restraint and seclusion standard: issued by the Chief Psychiatrist pursuant to s 90 of the *Mental Health Act 2009*.

11

CORONIAL JURISDICTION

LEARNING OBJECTIVES

In this chapter, you will:

- understand the role of the Coroner's Court as part of Australia's legal system
- learn the role and function of a coroner
- learn what deaths are 'reportable deaths' for the purposes of the *Coroners Acts* in each state and territory, and the procedures that must be followed
- understand the issues to be addressed where a coroner's inquest follows the death of a patient in a hospital or healthcare setting
- learn the recommendations and findings that may follow a coroner's inquest particularly in relation to your professional registration as a nurse or midwife
- gain an awareness of the right to legal representation at an inquest and of the procedures if you are required to give evidence at a coroner's inquest.

INTRODUCTION

If a registered or enrolled nurse or midwife is to become caught up in any aspect of the legal system, the Coroner's Court is the most likely place for that to occur. That is, if a nurse or midwife was involved in caring for a patient who subsequently died, the circumstances of that death may require a coroner's inquest to be held. Such a legal process would generally require the nurse or midwife to give evidence at the inquest which would, among other matters, consider the facts and circumstances of the care given, and by whom, leading to the patient's death in order to determine the manner and cause of that person's death. As well, the outcome of a coronial inquest may have significant professional implications for a nurse or midwife, and the findings of a coroner's inquest may be the springboard for a person or party to commence civil or criminal proceedings involving the nurse or midwife. For those reasons, a knowledge and understanding of the coronial jurisdiction is important to all practising nurses and midwives.

THE ROLE OF THE CORONER IN AUSTRALIA'S LEGAL SYSTEM

Coroners have been in existence for many hundreds of years and their presence in our legal system is part of the legacy we inherited from the English common law system.

All of the states and territories have legislation dealing with the role and function of coroners, and the title of the Acts is the same — the *Coroners Act*.[1]

The role of a coroner historically began as the process developed to inquire into and detect unlawful homicide; that is, when a person died in unusual, unexpected, violent or unnatural circumstances, it was necessary to inquire into the manner and cause of death to ensure that no 'foul play' went undetected. That role has expanded somewhat to include provision for coroners to make specific recommendations designed to enhance public health and safety.

THE CORONER'S COURT STRUCTURE IN AUSTRALIA

The coronial court structure varies a little from state to state and territory to territory, generally depending on the size and coronial workload of the jurisdiction. All states appoint a person to the position of State Coroner, and the territories appoint a Territory Coroner. In all jurisdictions, except Victoria, the person appointed as State or Territory Coroner is a magistrate. In Victoria, the person appointed is a County Court judge.

The State or Territory Coroner is responsible for overseeing and coordinating the coronial services of the state or territory. In carrying out their functions and as the workload demands it, the State Coroner is assisted by additional magistrates appointed as deputy coroners, either on a full-time or on an as-required basis.

In the capital cities of the larger states, because of the volume of work they are required to perform, coroner's courts are separate courts. Where that is not the case, particularly in regional cities and country towns, the local court house is used as the venue for coroner's inquests.

In an inquest the coroner may be assisted by a lawyer generally referred to as 'counsel assisting the coroner'. The task of that person, with the assistance of the police officers who have investigated the death of the person concerned, is to produce evidence, including calling witnesses considered relevant, to enable the coroner to determine those matters that he or she is required to determine.

The Role and Function of a Coroner

The primary task of a coroner is to:

- confirm that death occurred;
- confirm the identity of the deceased;
- state the date, place, manner and cause of death;
- where relevant, determine the cause of fires or explosions; and
- make recommendation in relation to matters arising in connection with an inquest or inquiry including recommendations concerning public health and safety and the investigation or review of matters by persons or bodies.

Reportable Deaths as Defined by the *Coroners Act*

Obviously, a coronial inquest is not required into the death of every person. For the coroner to have the power to investigate a person's death, the death must be a 'reportable death' as defined by the *Coroners Act* of the state or territory. The police usually notify the coroner of such a death, once the death is reported to them.

What constitutes a 'reportable death' varies from state to state and territory to territory. In general terms, a death must be reported to a coroner in circumstances where:

- the person died unexpectedly and the cause of death is unknown;
- the person died under suspicious or unusual circumstances;
- the person died in a violent or unnatural manner;
- the person died during the process or as a result of being administered an anaesthetic;
- the person was 'held in care', or temporarily absent from a mental health facility, or in custody immediately before he or she died;
- a doctor has been unable to sign a death certificate giving the cause of death; or
- the identity of the person who has died is not known.

In relation to the death of a person in a hospital or healthcare setting, the obligation to report such a death to a coroner will depend on the circumstances of the death. Each state and territory provides for such circumstances but in slightly different wording.

Who Notifies the Coroner of a Reportable Death?

All states and territories make provision that any person who has reasonable grounds to believe that a reportable death has not been reported must report it to a police officer or coroner as soon as possible. A failure to do so is considered an offence subject to financial penalty and, in the case of the Australian Capital Territory and South Australia, potential imprisonment.[2]

Reportable Death Provisions in Relation to Healthcare Procedures

In **New South Wales**, section 6 of the *Coroners Act*, among other provisions, says that a person's death is reportable 'where the person's death was not the reasonably expected outcome of a health-related procedure carried out in relation to the person'. A 'health-related procedure' is defined as 'a medical, surgical, dental or other health-related procedure (including the administration of an anaesthetic, sedative or other drug)'.

In **Victoria**, section 4 of the Act refers to a death that occurs 'during a medical procedure' and where 'a registered medical practitioner would not, immediately before the procedure was undertaken, have reasonably expected the death' **or** following a medical procedure 'where the death may be causally related to the medical procedure'. A similar provision is to be found in section 10AA of the **Queensland** Act, although expressed in more detail and wider terms.

In **South Australia**, section 3(g) also defines a reportable death as being a death that 'occurs during or as a result, or within 24 hours, of the carrying out of a surgical procedure or an invasive medical or diagnostic procedure or the administration of an anaesthetic for the purposes of carrying out such a procedure'.

The **Northern Territory** (s 12) and **Western Australia** (s 3) Acts refer to a death that occurs 'during an anaesthetic' or 'as a result of an anaesthetic and is not due to natural causes'.

The **Tasmanian** Act (s 3) uses similar wording, referring to a death that occurs 'during a medical procedure' or where a death 'does not appear to be due to natural causes'.

The **Australian Capital Territory** Act does not define 'reportable death' but section 13 requires that a coroner 'must' hold an inquest into the manner and cause of a person's death where (among other provisions) the person 'dies after having undergone' 'an operation of a medical, surgical, dental or similar nature or an invasive medical or diagnostic procedure'.

All states and territories require a death to be reported where the person dies while in police custody or control, or while in gaol, where the person is being cared for within the relevant mental health provisions of the state or territory, or where the person is a child or young person in care.

Victoria also makes provision for an inquest to be held in relation to a reviewable death. Section 5(1) of the Victorian Act provides that the death of a child is a reviewable death if 'the deceased child is the second or subsequent child of the deceased's child's parent to have died' and where the child's body is in Victoria, or the death occurred in Victoria, or the cause of death occurred in Victoria, or the child ordinarily resided in Victoria.

Section 5(2) provides that the death of a child is not reviewable if the death occurs in a hospital, and the child was born at a hospital and had always been an inpatient of a hospital, and the death is not a reportable death.

Deaths Occurring Under the Provisions of Voluntary Assisted Dying Legislation

Where voluntary assisted dying legislation is in place, provision is made in either the *Coroners Act* of that state or in the voluntary assisted dying legislation that excludes a death occurring in accordance with the voluntary assisted dying legislation from being a 'reportable death' for the purposes of the *Coroners Act*.[3]

Notifying Reportable Deaths that Occur in the Healthcare Environment

For reportable deaths of persons in a hospital or healthcare setting, the relevant hospital management or healthcare authority must notify the police, who, in turn, submit the notification of that death to the Coroner's Office.

If a person dies in a hospital or nursing home in circumstances that would render that death reportable and the authorities fail to notify the police, a member of staff or a relative of the deceased could report that death to the police. The police would then investigate that report and notify the coroner if satisfied it was a reportable death.

There may be occasions in small or isolated rural hospitals and healthcare services, or nursing homes, where the registered nurse or midwife may have to notify the local police. In such circumstances, it is to be expected that a clear protocol is in place clarifying who is responsible for notifying the police. If in doubt, inquiries should be made of the hospital or healthcare management in the first instance. However, if, in the circumstances, that is not possible, the medical officer certifying the death, or the registered nurse or midwife present at the time of death, may have to notify the local police.

In circumstances where a nurse or midwife believes the person has died under suspicious or unusual circumstances and that the manner and cause of death have not been correctly recorded, the nurse or midwife is under a legal obligation to report the death to the local police. Should such a situation arise, the nurse or midwife should, in the first instance, raise his or her concerns with the medical officer who certified the death. If notification is made independently of the healthcare authority and/or medical officer concerned, it is advisable that the nurse or midwife is able to objectively detail the facts and circumstances relied upon that caused him or her to notify the police.

The Procedure Following Notification of a Reportable Death

Once a death has been reported to police, the coroner will receive a report submitted by the police detailing their investigation into the person's death together with any accompanying statements. An autopsy may be undertaken as well.

All documentation received from the police, together with additional scientific forensic tests such as toxicology and post-mortem results, will be considered by the coroner to determine whether a coronial inquest needs to be held or whether the coroner is able to make the formal findings as to the person's death without the need to call witnesses and receive further evidence. The decision to dispense with a formal coronial inquest is open to a coroner, who will formally certify the death of the person and the formal findings to be made based on the documentary material received.

A CORONER'S COURT INQUEST

Criminal Proceedings Following a Coroner's Inquest

It is important to bear in mind that the coroner may come to the view that the person died as a result of a criminal act committed by a known or unknown person or persons. In such circumstances, it is not the task of the coroner to formally charge anyone with a criminal offence or determine a person's guilt or innocence — a coroner does not conduct criminal trials. If a coroner concludes that a person met his or her death as a result of a criminal act, the coroner must refer the matter to the prosecuting authorities for their consideration and action.

Civil Proceedings Following a Coroner's Inquest

While the coroner may conclude that no criminal act caused the person's death, he or she may also conclude

that the actions (or inactions) of a person or persons or an organisation were significantly deficient in a number of areas and contributed to the person's death.

Although such a view may emerge from the evidence, the coroner has no power to determine the outcome of potential civil litigation on behalf of the relatives of the deceased.

If the relatives of the deceased believe, based on the evidence produced at the inquest, that somebody's negligent act (a civil wrong) has caused the death of their relative, they must pursue their action in the appropriate civil court depending on the amount of monetary compensation being sought.

Coroner's Inquests for Deaths in a Hospital or Healthcare Setting

A coroner is generally somewhat cautious in deciding to dispense with an inquest arising out of a person's death in a hospital or healthcare setting, even if there are no suspicious circumstances.

The main reason for such caution is that, on many occasions, the relatives of the deceased want to know what happened, particularly if the person's death was unexpected and not directly attributable to whatever had necessitated the patient's being in hospital. In such a situation the coroner will generally determine to have an inquest so that the relatives of the deceased have the opportunity to discover the facts that led to the patient's death and to reassure themselves that all that could have been done was done. In all states and territories, provision is made for the next of kin of the deceased person to request an inquest if the circumstances leading to the person's death are not fully known or if the next of kin are unhappy about the circumstances leading to the person's death.

It is possible for criminal charges to be laid against a nurse or midwife following a coroner's inquest. Admittedly it would be relatively rare for such an outcome to occur — but it could happen, and has happened.

In New South Wales, in two separate coronial inquests in 1993 and 1994 respectively, the coroner found that the evidence disclosed that the actions of the nurse concerned were sufficient to warrant the circumstances of each matter being referred to the prosecuting authorities to determine whether criminal charges should be laid. Both cases involved serious medication errors resulting in the death of a patient. These are examined in **Case examples 11.1** and **11.2**.

Coroner's inquest into the death of Clinton Norwood[4]

In this case, a newly graduated registered nurse employed to work in the intensive care unit of a major public teaching hospital in Sydney injected Dilantin oral suspension into the central venous line instead of down the nasogastric tube of a patient in his care. As a result the patient had a cardiac arrest and died.

The coroner's inquest determined that the circumstances that led to the patient's death amounted to criminal negligence and referred the matter to the Director of Public Prosecutions. The nurse was subsequently charged with manslaughter. A jury acquitted the nurse of that charge.

Coroner's inquest into the death of Sara Slapp[5]

In this case, a registered nurse significantly overdosed a patient with methotrexate, causing death. This was despite the clearly written instructions in the patient's notes as well as evidence given which acknowledged that the dose administered was far in excess of what would reasonably be expected to be given. In the inquiry into this patient's death the coroner found that:

The breach of the duty of care by certain persons was not merely a breach which called for compensation, but the evidence clearly establishes there has been evidence which amounts to recklessness and gross negligence.[6]

In considering all the evidence, as well as the coroner's findings, the prosecuting authorities ultimately decided not to lay any criminal charges against the nurse concerned.

Findings and Recommendations Arising from a Coroner's Inquest

At the conclusion of an inquest, in addition to determining the manner and cause of death as required, the coroner may comment critically about the circumstances leading to the death of the deceased and make certain recommendations about steps that should be taken to prevent similar circumstances arising again.

The recommendations made are usually directed to the government of the day or the organisation responsible for overseeing the actions that led to the person's death. A good example where a specific recommendation was made following a coroner's inquest is set out in **Case example 11.3**.

A coroner's inquest was held in Sydney into the death of an elderly patient who had died as a result of burns received from suddenly turning on the hot water tap while showering in hospital. She was in a wheelchair and had been wheeled into the shower by one of the nursing staff members who then left her to attend to another patient. The sudden rush of scalding water so shocked the patient that she was unable to turn the tap off before help arrived and she sustained severe burns from which she later died.

In giving his findings as to the manner and cause of death, which was as a result of severe burns sustained while showering, the coroner also made certain recommendations concerning the temperature of hot water in hospitals and nursing homes. He recommended that the temperature of the hot water should be thermostatically controlled to prevent such occurrences.

The coroner's recommendation was forwarded to the appropriate state government department and, as a result, hospitals and nursing homes in New South Wales were directed to ensure that the temperature of hot water provided for patient use was such that sustained exposure would not cause severe burns.

Provisions in the *Coroners Act* for Recommendations to Be Made

All states and territories have provisions in their respective *Coroners Acts* for a coroner to make recommendations or comments arising from an inquest.[7]

New South Wales provides for recommendations to be made concerning 'matters relating to public health or safety'; so also do the **Australian Capital Territory**, the **Northern Territory**, **Queensland**, **Tasmania**, **Victoria** and **Western Australia**.

South Australia provides for recommendations on matters that 'might ... prevent, or reduce the likelihood of, recurrence' of a 'similar' event that would embrace public health or safety issues. Queensland has a similar provision in addition to 'public health or safety'.

Both **Queensland** (s 48(4)) and **Western Australia** (s 50) provide for a coroner to refer a matter arising from an inquest to a 'disciplinary body of a trade or profession'. Such an express provision clearly refers to the registration authority relating to nurses and midwives.

A reference received from a coroner to such an authority would provide the basis for an inquiry to be made into whether the nurse or midwife involved should undergo a disciplinary process that may lead to a charge of professional misconduct and, if established, the potential loss of professional registration.

While the other states and territories do not have the express provision for a coroner to refer matters to a 'disciplinary body of a trade or profession', it is clear that a reference to the relevant professional registration authority can and has been made by a coroner in the other states under the catch-all provision of 'public health or safety'.

The role and powers of the registration authorities governing nurses and midwives in relation to disciplinary proceedings is detailed in **Chapter 4**. Also, in **Chapter 7** in particular are the outcomes of a number of coronial inquests where the coroner has been critical of nurses or midwives. The facts and circumstances of some of those inquests have formed the basis for ongoing civil litigation by the family of the deceased seeking compensation for civil negligence by the staff concerned.[8]

Responsibility of State and Territory Health Authorities to Act on the Coroner's Recommendations

State and territory health departments have a responsibility to act on recommendations made by a coroner that are relevant to the administration and delivery of health services.

Where a coroner hands down a report identifying the manner and cause of a person's death that includes critical reference to aspects of care given in a hospital or healthcare facility, as well as recommendations intended to be implemented to address the deficiencies identified, that report will be sent to the Attorney-General and/or the Minister for Health of the state or territory.

As a matter of procedure, upon receipt of a coroner's report and recommendations, the minister responsible is required to act on the report and recommendations, and advise the State Coroner accordingly within a set time frame — usually between 3 and 6 months. The actions undertaken by the minister may include:

- referring the whole or parts of the matter to others for investigation and reporting back — for example, to the Chief Health Officer, the body for investigating healthcare complaints, or relevant public health branches;
- initiating one or more of the following actions:
  - the development and promulgation of new policy;
  - remedial action or a change of procedure within the healthcare system;
  - professional disciplinary action against identified health professionals.

THE RELEVANCE OF A CORONER'S INQUEST FOR NURSES AND MIDWIVES

In addition to determining the manner and cause of death, evidence given before a Coroner's Court inquest may form the basis of disciplinary charges against a health professional in addition to any civil or criminal liability that may arise. For this reason, if required to give evidence at an inquest, nurses and midwives should be particularly mindful of the power of a coroner's inquest and findings to impact on their professional registration and should familiarise themselves with the procedures that arise when an inquest is to be held.

Legal Representation at the Inquest

In all states and territories, any person who is required to give evidence at a coroner's inquest is deemed to have 'sufficient interest' in the inquiry to permit them to have legal representation.

If the staff members of a hospital, nursing home or healthcare-related entity are involved in an inquest, the employer will usually ensure that, if necessary, they are represented by the legal representative of that entity.

If that is not done, or if conflict arises, legal representation is generally provided for nurses or midwives if they are a member of the relevant nursing and midwifery association in each state and territory.[9]

If such legal representation is not provided or available, it may be possible to apply for state-funded legal aid if it is available, or the nurse or midwife may have to obtain and pay for his or her own legal representation. Given the cost of legal services, it is to be hoped such a situation never arises.

For those nurses and midwives who are members of their state or territory association, preliminary advice should be obtained to assist in responding to the coroner's inquiries and disciplinary inquiries generally.

The Right to Remain Silent

Nurses and midwives have the right to refuse to answer any questions from a police officer or others in authority which may lead to a criminal charge against them — that is, incriminate them. All members of the community have this right. Although such an outcome to a coroner's inquest for nursing staff is rare, it is important to remember that right and, as a general rule, make no statement, written or otherwise, until legal advice is obtained.

Giving a Statement to a Police Officer

In some cases, the first inkling a nurse or midwife will have that they are required to give evidence at an inquest is when they are approached by a police officer requesting a statement as to their recollection of events at the time of the person's death — sometimes many months after the death occurred.

The fact that a police officer requests a statement in such a situation does not mean that a criminal offence is suspected. It is just that one of the routine tasks of police officers is to obtain the necessary statements for the coroner that they, in turn, refer to the coroner for his or her consideration once their inquiries are completed.

When a request for a statement is made by a police officer, it is advisable to indicate that you will agree to provide whatever relevant information can be clearly recalled that may assist the coroner in his or her inquiry as to the manner and cause of death. A refusal to cooperate or appear at the inquest will normally result in the issue of a subpoena compelling attendance. However, it is wise, even as a precautionary measure, to seek legal advice concerning any statement to be made or provided to the police if the events surrounding the patient's death are likely to prompt any expressions of concern.

It is perfectly proper and legally permissible to decline to give any statement immediately but to indicate a willingness to do so after legal advice has been obtained. The guiding principle in this respect should always be that, if in any doubt, seek advice. With hindsight, it may prove to have been unnecessary, but it is better to err on the side of abundant caution in such situations.

Preparatory Steps for an Inquest

This section outlines the preparatory steps that may be taken by nurses and midwives when an inquest is to be held or is likely to be held.

Preparing a Statement for the Police

As a matter of policy, where possible, staff should be informed by the administration or the patient's doctor if an inquest is likely to arise following a patient's death. This will allow the staff involved to obtain legal advice as necessary and prepare a draft statement at the time of the patient's death rather than relying on their memory many months after the event.

With some inquests, staff may be asked for statements many years after the patient's death when they generally, and not surprisingly, have little or no recollection of the patient, let alone the events surrounding the patient's death. At the time of notification the police will usually take the minor preliminary details and return some time later for any statements that may be required.

In some situations the police may make their inquiries immediately after they are notified, in which case, depending on the circumstances surrounding the patient's death, it may be appropriate to give the police whatever information is required at the time. However, if there are concerns regarding the circumstances surrounding the patient's death, arrangements should be made to give a statement at a later time after legal advice has been obtained.

Making and Retaining a Draft Statement or Notes

If it appears that a patient or client's death is reportable and that a statement may be required by the police, it is advisable to prepare a draft statement or notes setting out the relevant details as soon as possible after the person's death while they are fresh in one's memory. That draft statement or notes should be retained until a formal statement is called for.

A draft statement or notes should not be handed over to the police or relevant authorities until any necessary legal advice is obtained and a formal statement prepared.

When a formal statement is requested by the police or hospital administration, the draft statement or notes made at the time of the patient's death will assist in writing such a statement. Once again, should any particular concern be felt or expressed, it is advisable to seek legal advice before submitting the formal statement.

Before handing over a formal statement, a copy should always be taken and retained.

Access to the Deceased Person's Medical Records

It is advisable to obtain access to the deceased person's medical records at the time of preparing a formal statement, especially where a statement is requested some considerable time after the person's death when the particular patient may have long been forgotten, and no draft statement or notes were made at the time.

In such circumstances, the medical records would help refresh one's memory about past care and treatment given to the patient or client. Such access does not always help recall specific details, but it does allow identification of one's handwriting of any entries made at the time.

In an inquest into the death of a person who has been a patient or client of a hospital or healthcare service and who has died in circumstances related to the person's care or treatment received, his or her medical records will be very carefully scrutinised to ascertain whether there is any information contained within them that may assist the coroner to determine the manner and cause of death.

If the person's relatives are legally represented at the inquest, they will also have access to those records and may wish to cross-examine the health professionals about entries made by them.

Accordingly, it is important for nurses and midwives to ensure that entries made in a patient or client records are accurate, contemporaneous and objectively factual. Refer to **Chapter 9** for assistance in such matters.

The Body of the Deceased

Where it is known at the time of a person's death that a coroner's inquest will be held, the body of the deceased should be left as it is at the time of death. As a general rule, all drainage tubes, intravenous lines, in-dwelling catheters, nasogastric tubes, cardiac-monitoring pads, sutures, dressings and so forth should remain in position. Obviously some of those lines will have to be disconnected externally and capped or sealed. The body should then be transported to the morgue in the normal manner and in due course, if considered necessary, arrangements will be made for a post-mortem to be conducted.

Guidelines for the Purposes of Giving Statements

Box 11.1 contains an extract of guidelines to follow when giving statements for coroner's inquests and other disciplinary matters.[10] Although these guidelines are prepared by the New South Wales Nurses and Midwives' Association, the extracts reproduced here are of sufficient general application to nurses and midwives in all states and territories.

The Association has formulated a number of guidelines that it recommends to members faced with the prospect of an interview in relation to any situation described as a 'disciplinary/fact-finding interview' by any investigating body or officer.

CONCLUSION

For health professionals, including nurses and midwives, the holding of a coronial inquest into the manner and cause of a person's death is not an isolated occurrence. That is partly because of the very role of the healthcare system in caring for people who, for diverse reasons, are seriously ill and where death is an outcome. Also, hospitals and other healthcare environments are fraught with risks to patients. Mistakes made by health professionals entrusted with a person's care can sometimes have catastrophic consequences for that person and result in their death. In

BOX 11.1
NSW NURSES AND MIDWIVES' ASSOCIATION GUIDELINES[11]

1. When you contact the Association, please try to provide as much information about the request as possible. This could include:
   a. What the request is — e.g. a statement, interview or response?
   b. Who the request is from — e.g. your employer, the police, the HCCC or the NMC?
   c. Any date of interview or date that the statement or response is requested by.
2. If you are asked to attend an interview, this request must be in writing. The request should include the reason for the interview, any allegations (if applicable), who will be conducting the interview, your right to bring a support person and the date, time and location of the interview.
3. You must be given reasonable written notice of the date and time for an interview. What is reasonable will depend on your roster as well as your ability to obtain advice and a support person prior to the interview.
4. You have the right to view relevant healthcare records in order to refresh your memory prior to providing any information; however, it is important that you do not access any records yourself. These records should be provided to you by the person making the request.
5. Before attending an interview, the person interviewing you should tell you:
   a. you have the right to have a support person;
   b. anything you say as well as the transcript of the interview can become evidence in any court or tribunal hearing; and
   c. you have the right to refuse to be audio or video recorded.
6. If, during an interview, additional concerns are raised, the interview should be stopped immediately and you should be given written notice of those additional concerns.
7. Interviews must be conducted in a fair, impartial and respectful manner. If you feel that an interviewer is acting in an intimidating or inappropriate way, the interview should be stopped immediately.
8. If you agree to being recorded, you should be provided with a copy of the recording and the transcript as soon as it is available. You may be asked to sign the transcript or a record of interview. You should only do this if you have read it carefully and are satisfied that it is an accurate recording of the interview.
9. Members who participate in investigations and inquiries must be treated with respect. This includes ensuring that processes and communications are conducted in a fair, transparent and efficient manner. The Association is committed to ensuring that members are well supported during these processes.
10. Being involved in an investigation can be very stressful. It is important that members are aware of the support services available to them. Most employers provide access to counselling through an Employee Assistance Program (EAP) or you can talk to your general practitioner about seeking a Mental Health Care Plan. Nurses and midwives can also access counselling through Nurse & Midwife Support on 1800 667 877.

such circumstances, a coroner's inquest will almost invariably follow.

For those reasons, nurses and midwives need to know the role and function of a coroner's inquest and the steps they should take if required to provide evidence before one. Given the potential outcome for one's professional registration, let alone any other outcomes, such knowledge is essential.

CHAPTER 11 REVIEW QUESTIONS

Following your reading of **Chapter 11**, consider these questions in reaching the objectives of this chapter. Guidance on which part of the chapter will assist you in answering the questions can be found at http://evolve.elsevier.com/AU/Staunton/law/. You may, of course, consider other sources as part of your considerations.

1. What is the role and purpose of the Coroner's Court?

2. Under what circumstances is a death reportable to a coroner in your state or territory?

3. In what way may a coroner's inquest become relevant for a nurse or midwife?

4. In a hospital, nursing home or any other health-care setting, who is generally responsible for notifying police in the event of a reportable death?

5. If a nurse or midwife is asked to provide a statement to the police in relation to a coroner's inquest, should he or she agree to do so or refuse?

6. Would a nurse or midwife who is required to give evidence at an inquest be entitled to legal representation at an inquest? Who else is entitled to be represented?

7. Apart from determining the manner and cause of death, what else may be the outcome of a coronial inquest?

ENDNOTES

1. *Coroners Act 1997* (ACT); *Coroners Act 2009* (NSW); *Coroners Act (NT)*; *Coroners Act 2003* (Qld); *Coroners Act 2003* (SA); *Coroners Act 1995* (Tas); *Coroners Act 2008* (Vic); *Coroners Act 1996* (WA).

2. *Coroners Act 1997* (ACT) s 77; *Coroners Act 2009* (NSW) s 35; *Coroners Act (NT)* s 12; *Coroners Act 2003* (Qld) s 7; *Coroners Act 2003* (SA) s 28; *Coroners Act 1995* (Tas) s 19; *Coroners Act 2008* (Vic) ss 10 and 12; *Coroners Act 1996* (WA) s 17.

3. *Voluntary Assisted Dying Act 2022* (NSW) s 29 excludes a death under the VAD Act from being a suicide under the Crimes Act; *Coroners Act 2008* (Vic) s 4(3) excludes a death occurring 'in accordance' with the VAD Act 2017; *Coroners Act 2003* (Qld) s 8(5); *Voluntary Assisted Dying Act 2021* (SA) s 6 and s 84 require a medical practitioner to notify the coroner when a death has occurred pursuant to the VAD legislation; *End-of-Life Choices (Voluntary Assisted Dying) Act 2021* (Tas) s 93(2); *Coroners Act (WA) 1996* s 3A. As at June 2023 the territories are yet to enact voluntary assisted dying legislation.

4. Coroner's inquest into the death of Clinton Norwood, Westmead Coroner's Court, February 1994.

5. Coroner's inquest into the death of Sara Slapp, Westmead Coroner's Court, July 1993.

6. Ibid.

7. *Coroners Act 1997* (ACT) s 57; *Coroners Act 2009* (NSW) s 82; *Coroners Act (NT)* ss 27 and 35; *Coroners Act 2003* (Qld) s 46; *Coroners Act 2003* (SA) s 25; *Coroners Act 1995* (Tas) s 30; *Coroners Act 2008* (Vic) s 72; *Coroners Act 1996* (WA) s 25.

8. See Chapter 7, for example: Coroner's inquest into the death of Samara Lea Hoy, Southport Coroner's Court, Feb–Jun 2010; *McCabe v Auburn District Hospital* (SC (NSW), Grove J, No. 11551 of 1982, 31 May 1989, unreported); Coroner's inquest into the death of Bodhi Eastlake-McClure, NSW Coroner's Court, 7 August 2014.

9. The NSW Nurses and Midwives' Association; the Queensland Nurses and Midwives Union; and, in all other states and territories, the state or territory branch of the Australian Nursing and Midwifery Federation.

10. Ibid.

11. The full text of the guidelines can be found on the Association's website in the members-only section: http://www.nswnma.asn.au.

12

HUMAN TISSUE TRANSPLANTATION

INTRODUCTION

This chapter focuses on the law and some practicalities relating to human tissue transplantation and research. It also briefly explores issues surrounding assisted reproductive technology and donation of reproductive tissue. This is a highly specialised area of law and ethics, as the scientific developments often overtake the law. For this reason, only broad topics are covered. However, many useful references and websites for further reading are provided for interested nurses and midwives.

HISTORY AND BACKGROUND OF HUMAN TISSUE TRANSPLANTATION AND RESEARCH

Human tissue transplantation has been a growing part of medical and scientific development for many years.

In his book *The body as property*, Russell Scott recounts that, more than 2000 years ago, Indian surgeons were transplanting human skin in the operation of rhinoplasty.[1] Blood transfusions have long been commonplace, and the nineteenth century saw the first transplantation of certain body parts, such as teeth and bone. The twentieth century, and more particularly the last 60 years, has seen enormous developments in the field of human tissue transplantation. The first successful kidney transplant was performed in 1954 and the first successful transplant of a human heart took place in December 1967, in South Africa, but on that first occasion the recipient died 18 days later. However, a heart transplant performed in the United States only 10 months later kept the recipient alive for over 8 years.[2] Since that time the list of tissue — regenerative and non-regenerative, and even human and non-human — that has been transplanted with varying degrees of success has grown considerably.

In the first years of the COVID-19 pandemic, there was a slump in organ donation, but according to the *Australian Organ and Tissue Donation and Transplantation Authority (OTA) Report*, this mostly picked up again in 2022, with an increase of 57 kidney donations to 713 in 2022, 7 liver donations to 260 in 2022, 5 more heart donations to 117 in 2022 and 10 more pancreas donations to 47 in 2022, but 29 fewer lung donations, down to 142 in 2022. Kidneys made up more than half of organs transplanted, followed by livers, lungs and heart.[3] However, there was a 17% decrease in tissue donors (2748) compared with 2021 (3307).[4]

In global terms, Australia lags well behind many other resource-rich nations in its donation rates per head of population. **Figure 12.1**[5] demonstrates Australia's position in a world table of deceased organ donor rates.

Much of this debate is beyond the scope of an undergraduate textbook and some aspects of the debate, particularly those relating to the use of human genetic material in research, will be mentioned only briefly, with further references supplied for the interested reader. Some of the controversy in the past has related to the retention and use of human tissue after death and the conduct of post-mortem examinations,

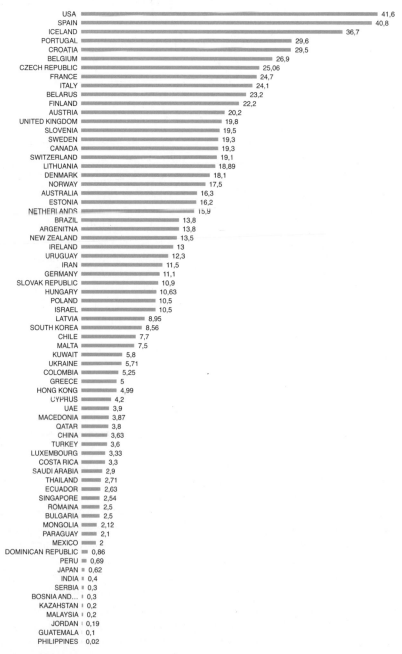

Figure 12.1 ■ International deceased organ donor rates 2021. Source: https://www.irodat.org/img/database/grafics/2021_01_worldwide-actual-deceased-organ-donors.png.

another topic not directly related to the regular work of nurses or midwives. However, this latter subject has been a matter of much concern among the general public, so it will be discussed in slightly more detail as nurses (and sometimes midwives) may find themselves required to answer questions by anxious patients and (more probably) relatives.

As a matter of careful practice, specific questions about any matter relating to the use of human tissue should be referred to the appropriate treating medical practitioner, but this area of law has developed so rapidly that undergraduate nurses and midwives now do need to be aware of it. Another area where the law has developed rapidly in recent years is the development of assisted reproductive technologies, which is discussed briefly later in this chapter.

Classifications of Human Tissue

Human tissue is classified in two ways for the legal consideration of its use in transplantation: namely, regenerative and non-regenerative tissue. Regenerative tissue is the tissue that can be replaced in the body by the normal process of growth and repair. Non-regenerative tissue is all other tissue. The lists in **Table 12.1** provide an example of the wide range of regenerative and non-regenerative tissues currently being transplanted in one form or another.

TABLE 12.1
Classification of Tissue for Transplant Purposes[6]

Regenerative Tissue	Non-Regenerative Tissue
Blood	Blood vessels
Bone marrow	Bone and cartilage
Skin	Corneas
Semen	Ear tissue (ossicles, tympanic membrane)
	Fascia
	Heart
	Hormone-producing glands (pituitary, thyroid, etc.)
	Intestines
	Kidneys
	Liver
	Lung
	Pancreatic tissue

THE DEVELOPMENT OF LAW IN RELATION TO THE USE OF HUMAN TISSUE

The subject of human tissue transplantation inevitably highlights legal and ethical issues. As is often the case, the law has had to move fast to respond to these issues, which often develop far more speedily than the law itself. In addition, established common law principles are clearly inadequate for coping with the complexities of the issues. Common law principles have for many years recognised only a limited right to deal with a person's body after death — usually only for the purposes of burial. Legislation in relation to the functions of the coroner established the right to conduct postmortems, and permission to do so could also be given by the surviving spouse or relative (see **Chapter 11**). Common law limitations prohibited the use of dead bodies and the retention of body organs for research purposes and teaching anatomy. Accordingly, it was necessary for parliaments to allow such procedures by passing the appropriate legislation, known as the *Anatomy Act* in most states and territories.

The common law had also never permitted the removal of body parts or organs from a living person. Such a principle rested largely on the belief that the removal of a body part or organ from a living person, even with the person's consent, was not of benefit to that person and technically constituted the criminal offence of maim. In addition, the increasing amount of tissue transplantation, particularly kidney transplants, highlighted the fact that the state of the law was not sufficient to deal with the legal problems that arose. Those problems included the issue of consent generally, the removal of tissue from living persons and the need to make specific provisions concerning children.

The need for parliaments to legislate in this area was first recognised in Australia in 1976, when the then Commonwealth Attorney-General, Mr R J Ellicott, referred the whole matter of human tissue transplantation to the Australian Law Reform Commission under wide-ranging terms of reference. The commission produced its report in 1977, entitled *Human tissue transplants*.[7] One of the main features of the report was the proposed draft legislation, which was set out in Appendix 4 to the report. It was intended that the draft legislation, presented to the Commonwealth

Government in 1977, would be used as a model by all Australian states and territories in relation to this subject. The subject of tissue transplantation is an area within which the states and territories have power to legislate and hence the Commonwealth Government could not impose the draft legislation on the states or territories — it could only put it forward as a suggested model. The Commonwealth Government used the draft legislation proposed by the Australian Law Reform Commission as the basis for the *Transplantation and Anatomy Act 1978* in the Australian Capital Territory.

Following that lead, all states and territories have now introduced legislation based on the Commonwealth's proposed draft legislation.[8] The legislation deals with such matters as:

- the donation of tissue by living persons, particularly with reference to children and the issue of consent (blood donations are dealt with separately);
- the donation of tissue after death;
- the donation of tissue for anatomical purposes;
- issues arising in relation to post-mortem examinations;
- a prohibition of trading in tissue;
- a definition of death.

The even more complex legal issues arising from in-vitro fertilisation and embryo transplants were not dealt with in the legislation, and have required further legislation by most jurisdictions in recent years; some of these statutes are included in the list above.[8] This is discussed further later in this chapter.

The legislation varies to some extent between the states and territories, but there is a significant degree of commonality between them, largely because they have adopted the draft legislation of the Australian Law Reform Commission. This particular piece of legislation is of importance to all hospitals and health professionals. It is of greatest significance to nursing and medical staff in intensive care and high-dependency units, because the majority of organs for transplantation still tend to come from patients who die from severe trauma, particularly as a result of motor vehicle accidents. However, donation after circulatory determination of death (DCDD) is increasing, and the Australian Government Organ and Tissue Authority

(OTA) has developed a best practice guideline for donation after circulatory determination of death that provides information to enable both health professionals and the public to understand how this process works in practice.[9]

Each of the states and territories has adopted the parts or sections of the proposed draft legislation that they have considered relevant or necessary for their purposes. However, not all matters mentioned above have been dealt with. As an example, South Australia and Western Australia have not adopted the proposed definition of death. Also, in New South Wales there is a separate statute in relation to donations for anatomical purposes or schools of anatomy in the *Anatomy Act 1977,* in addition to the New South Wales *Human Tissue Act 1983*.

The Federal Government is undertaking a national review of organ and tissue donation in conjunction with the OTA and the National Health and Medical Research Council (NHMRC).[10] This work is currently ongoing and the work of both the OTA and NHMRC will be referred to in more detail in the chapter. The provisions of the various statutes are set out in **Table 12.2** and are discussed in the following section.

The Requirement for Consent in Live Donations

In situations where tissue is to be donated from a living person, the requirement for valid consent is critical, as donating tissue carries with it a degree of risk due to the donor's being alive. However, this risk becomes even more significant if the tissue removed will not regenerate. The requirements for consent to remove non-regenerative tissue for donation are quite rigorous, and understandably so, particularly where children are concerned. In 2007 the National Health and Medical Research Council (NHMRC) endorsed the guidelines entitled *Organ and tissue donation by living donors: guidelines for ethical practice for health professionals*.[11] The document points out that, at the time of writing, in Australia, 40% of kidney donations were from living donors. However, more recent data show that this percentage has dropped in recent years, particularly during the COVID-19 pandemic.[12]

These guidelines are currently under review, along with the entire suite of NHMRC guidance in relation to organ donation and transplantation.[13] The original

TABLE 12.2
State and Territory Provisions for Blood and Tissue Donation

State or Territory Legislation	Tissue Donation by Live Adults	Tissue Donation by Live Children	Blood Donations	Donation of Tissue After Death	Tissue Donation for Anatomical Purposes	Post-Mortem Examination	Trading in Tissue	Definition of Death
Transplantation and Anatomy Act 1978 (ACT)	Section 8 regenerative tissue; section 9 non-regenerative tissue	Section 12 c/f parent and guardian; section 13 regenerative tissue — only to family or relative; section 14 non-regenerative tissue — many restrictions	Section 20 adults; section 21 children	Sections 27–31	Sections 36–41	Sections 32–35	Prohibited under section 44, subject to Minister's authorisation in special circumstances	Section 45
Human Tissue Act 1983 (NSW)	Section 7 regenerative tissue; section 8 non-regenerative tissue	Section 10 regenerative tissue only and only to parent, brother or sister (many requirements)	Section 19 adults; section 20 children (with child's consent); section 20A (without child's consent to parent, brother or sister)	Sections 23–27A; section 27A refers to Director-General's capacity to make guidelines for removal of tissue after death — where deceased person consented but family objected	See provisions of *Anatomy Act 1977* (NSW) sections 8–9 (including sections 8A, 8B, 8C)	Sections 28–31C	Prohibited under section 32, subject to authorisation by Minister under section 32(4)	Section 33
Transplantation and Anatomy Act 1979 (NT)	Section 8 regenerative and non-regenerative tissue	No provision for children	Section 14 adults; no provision for children	Sections 18–22	Sections 22A–22D	Section 20 coronial consent to removal of tissue; sections 19–23 of *Coroners Act* (NT) coronial consent to autopsy	Unauthorised trading prohibited under sections 22E–22F, subject to authorisation by Minister in special circumstances under section 22F	Section 23
Transplantation and Anatomy Act 1979 (Qld)	Section 10 regenerative tissue; section 11 non-regenerative tissue	Sections 12B–12E regenerative only	Section 17 adults; section 18 children	Sections 22–25	Sections 31–36; sections 37–38 refer to the establishment and inspection of schools of anatomy	Sections 26–30	Unauthorised trading prohibited under sections 40–42, subject to authorisation by Minister under section 40(2)	Section 45

Continued on following page

TABLE 12.2

State and Territory Provisions for Blood and Tissue Donation (*Continued*)

State or Territory Legislation	Tissue Donation by Live Adults	Tissue Donation by Live Children	Blood Donations	Donation of Tissue After Death	Tissue Donation for Anatomical Purposes	Post-Mortem Examination	Trading in Tissue	Definition of Death
Transplantation and Anatomy Act 1983 (SA)	Section 9 regenerative tissue; section 10 non-regenerative tissue	Section 12 general prohibition; section 13 only for regenerative tissue	Section 18 adults; section 19 children (as defined in section 17A)	Sections 21–24	Sections 29–32; sections 33–34 refer to schools of anatomy	Sections 25–28A; section 28A refers to conducting a post-mortem with regard for dignity of deceased	Prohibited under section 35, subject to authorisation by Minister in special circumstances under section 35(6)	Not defined
Human Tissue Act 1985 (Tas)	Section 7 regenerative tissue; section 8 non-regenerative tissue	Section 12 regenerative tissue only	Section 18 adults; section 19 children (as defined in section 17A)	Sections 23–26	Tissue donation for anatomical purposes; see *Anatomical Examination Act 2006* (Tas)	Non-coronial post-mortems; sections 26A–26F; coronial post-mortems; sections 35–38 *Coroners Act 1995* (Tas)	Section 27 prohibited subject to exception (special circumstances with Minister's approval)	Section 27A
Human Tissue Act 1982 (Vic)	Section 7 regenerative tissue; section 8 non-regenerative tissue	Section 14 non-regenerative tissue expressly prohibited; section 15 regenerative tissue only	Section 21 adults; section 22 children (as defined in section 20A)	Sections 24A–27	Sections 32–34; sections 35–37 cover schools of anatomy	Non-coronial post-mortems; sections 28–31; coronial post-mortems; sections 22–27 *Coroners Act 2008* (Vic)	Sections 38–40 prohibited subject to authorisation by Minister where desirable by reason of special circumstances (excludes sperm and ova)	Section 41
Human Tissue and Transplant Act 1982 (WA)	Section 8 regenerative tissue; section 9 non-regenerative tissue	Section 13: regenerative tissue can be donated to family or relative	Section 18 adults; section 19 children	Sections 21A–24A	*Anatomy Act 1930* (WA)	Sections 25–28	Prohibited under sections 29–30, subject to authorisation of Minister under section 29(4a)–(4b)	Not defined

and revised guidelines themselves embody a set of principles, which are a valuable guide to health professionals when addressing the issues and concerns of living donors. The original principles are set out in **Box 12.1**, but it will be important to revisit these when the new guidelines are released.

For nurses and midwives who are interested in this topic, the NHMRC website (www.nhmrc.gov.au) contains excellent advice for people in the community who are contemplating donation. The booklet *Making a decision about living organ and tissue donation*[15] also contains a set of principles for the benefit of the public. They are as follows:

- **Living donation must be altruistic.** Altruism means that the donor is thinking only about the other person and is not expecting to receive rewards.
- **The decision to donate must be free and voluntary.** People should not be forced or influenced by emotional pressures or promises of rewards like money.
- **Both donors and recipients must be fully informed.** Donors and recipients need clear information so that they can understand what the risks are and what might happen in the future.

- **Everyone involved in the decision-making process must be treated with respect and care.** Whether a donation goes ahead or not, the donor assessment and transplant teams follow the ethical principles outlined in this booklet and work towards the best possible results for the donor and recipient.
- **Cultural issues must be considered in planning programs and working with families.** Translators are important to give information to people whose first language is not English. The health professionals involved need to understand and be sensitive to the ways in which culture and beliefs can influence decisions about donation.[16]

Adults

The requirement to obtain consent for the removal of regenerative tissue is similar for all statutes, but the extent of detail differs. For example, in the *Transplantation and Anatomy Act 1978* (ACT), section 8 merely states that:

A person may give his or her written consent to the removal from his or her body of specified regenerative tissue (other than blood) —
a. for the purpose of the transplantation of the tissue to the body of another living person; or

---

BOX 12.1
PRINCIPLES IN THE NHMRC'S ORGAN AND TISSUE DONATION BY LIVING DONORS: GUIDELINES FOR ETHICAL PRACTICE FOR HEALTH PROFESSIONALS[14]

(a) Whether the donor and recipient are related or unrelated, living organ and tissue donation is an act of altruism and human solidarity that potentially benefits those in medical need and ultimately society as a whole.

(b) Respect for all those involved should be demonstrated through:
- decision-making processes that ensure that both donors and recipients are fully informed about potential risks and about alternatives to transplantation;
- ensuring that decisions about donation are free of coercion of any kind including undue emotional pressures or any material incentives such as money or in-kind rewards.

(c) In assessing whether to proceed with donation, the autonomy and welfare of the donor take precedence over the needs of the recipient to receive an organ or tissue.

(d) Living donation should take place only when there are minimal risks of short and long-term harm to the donor, with no clinically significant loss of a bodily function, and a high likelihood of a successful outcome for the recipient.

(e) For those who cannot make informed decisions (for example, young children or other dependent persons) to be considered as potential living donors there must be: minimal risks to the donor; no alternative donors available; and the prospective recipient must be a close relative of the child or dependent adult. There must be an independent judgement that the donation is in the overall best interests of the potential donor.

(f) Conflicts of interest should be minimised through the use of independent and separate assessment, advice and advocacy for potential donors.

b. for use for other therapeutic purposes or for medical or scientific purposes.

In contrast, section 9 of the *Transplantation and Anatomy Act 1983* (SA) has quite detailed provisions, stating that:

1. A person who —
  a. is not a child; and
  b. in the light of medical advice furnished to him understands the nature and effect of the removal, may, by writing signed by him otherwise than in the presence of any members of his family, consent to the removal from his body of regenerative tissue, other than blood, specified in the consent —
  c. for the purpose of the transplantation of the tissue to the body of another living person; or
  d. for use for other therapeutic purposes or for medical or scientific purposes.
2. A person who has given a consent referred to in subsection (1) may, at any time before the removal of the regenerative tissue to which the consent applies, revoke, either orally or in writing, his consent to the removal.

While not every statute specifies the need for the nature and effect of the removal to be explained to the person, as has been discussed in **Chapter 6**, those requirements are part of the common law in relation to consent to treatment. All statutes require the consent to be in writing.

Under all statutes there is a further requirement for a 24-hour 'cooling-off period' before any non-regenerative tissue can be donated and a specification that the time of consent shall be recorded. Some statutes also offer the option of a medical practitioner issuing a certificate in relation to consent — for example, section 10 of the *Transplantation and Anatomy Act 1978* (ACT).

Children

Obviously, removal of tissue from children carries additional complex ethical problems, particularly because children are not legally able to make the decision, which means that someone else has to do so on their behalf. Living donation of regenerative tissue from children is permitted only in strict circumstances and living donation of non-regenerative tissue is permitted only in the Australian Capital Territory and then under the most stringent circumstances, as discussed below.

The NHMRC guidelines contain unequivocal advice for ethical decision-making on behalf of children and dependent adults. This advice is set out in **Box 12.2**.

Probably as a result of the ethical complexity of this issue, the requirements for children differ considerably between jurisdictions. Some Acts make a clear distinction between parents and guardians for the purposes of giving consent within the legislation — for example, section 12 of the *Transplantation and Anatomy Act 1978* (ACT). Most Acts limit the possible recipients of regenerative tissue from children to a range of family members as follows:

- family members or relatives of the child, unspecified (ACT, Tas, WA);
- brothers and sisters (NSW, Qld, Vic);
- a parent, undefined (Qld, Vic);
- a parent whether biological, step or adoptive (NSW);
- a parent includes a step-parent, a person who is regarded as a parent of the child under either Aboriginal tradition or Island custom or the cultural traditions of their community and another person having or exercising parental responsibility for the child, whether or not the person is the legal guardian of the child (Qld); and
- unspecified, but must be specified in the consent (SA).

In most cases the requirements are extremely onerous.

Only the Australian Capital Territory makes provision for the removal of non-regenerative tissue from a child for transplantation, and this is in contrast to the NHMRC's advice (see **Box 12.2**). The Northern Territory legislation is silent on the matter, whereas other jurisdictions, such as Victoria, expressly prohibit the removal of non-regenerative tissue from a child.

Removal of Blood: Adults

Consent to the removal of blood from adults is relatively non-controversial. Section 18 of the *Human Tissue and Transplant Act 1982* (WA) states:

A person who —
a. has attained the age of 18 years; and
b. is of sound mind,

may consent to the removal of blood from his body for transfusion to another person or for use of the blood or of any of its constituents for other therapeutic purposes or for medical or scientific purposes.

Most of the statutes have a similar format.

Removal of Blood: Children

With the exception of the Northern Territory legislation, which is silent on the matter, all statutes allow for a parent to give consent to the removal of blood from a child, usually with some provision for a medical practitioner to provide an assurance that the removal will not be harmful to the child and, in most cases, with the agreement of the child. Section 20A of the *Human Tissue Act 1983* (NSW) makes specific provision for where the child is too young to be able to agree. This provision is unusual and so is set out in full:

Section 20A Consent to removal of blood from child if child unable to agree

A parent or guardian of a child who is under the age of 16 years may consent in writing to the removal of blood from the child's body without the consent of the child for the purpose of using the blood in the treatment of the child's parent (being the biological parent, step-parent or adoptive parent), brother or sister, but that consent is only effective if—

(a) a medical practitioner (other than the medical practitioner responsible for treating the child's parent, brother or sister) certifies in writing that, in the opinion of the medical practitioner —

　　(i) the child is unable to understand the nature and effect of the removal of blood from the child's body, and

　　(ii) any risk to the child's health (including psychological and emotional health) caused by the removal of the blood is minimal, and

(b) a medical practitioner certifies in writing that the parent, brother or sister is likely to die or suffer serious damage to his or her health unless blood removed from the child is used in the treatment.

Donation of Tissue After Death

In the past, prior to artificial ventilation or perfusion, if the heart and/or lungs failed, then adequate tissue perfusion would automatically cease. Although the individual cells of the body would continue to function until the remaining cellular oxygen supply was used up, there would have been nothing more that could be done to save a person's life. The person would have been dead, and clinically recognisably dead. Thus death could be defined as and determined by the failure of tissue perfusion, or what was commonly referred to as 'cardiac death'.

However, today, with the introduction of chemical and electrical cardiac stimulation, increased knowledge of cellular physiology and artificial ventilation, tissue perfusion need not necessarily cease. So tissue perfusion may be prolonged, if not indefinitely then at least for considerably longer than might previously have been anticipated.[18]

This understanding that a person may not independently be able to sustain circulation or respiration and yet might be kept perfused by artificial, scientific means required death to be redefined. Death no longer necessarily occurred when a patient stopped breathing or their heart stopped beating — the brain would have to have suffered tissue anoxia for death to occur. As long ago as 1968 a committee of the Harvard Medical School published a set of criteria for determining when death had occurred, which recommended that death should be understood in terms of a 'permanently non-functioning brain'.[19] It has been necessary to clarify this situation in law to enable perfused organs to be removed from patients who were recognised to be brain dead. As Windeyer J observed in *Mount Isa Mines Ltd v Pusey*, 'Law march[es] with medicine but in the rear and limping a little'.[20]

All the statutes except the *Transplantation and Anatomy Act 1983* (SA) and the *Human Tissue and Transplant Act 1982* (WA) provide a definition of death that includes a definition of brain death. All the statutes use similar if not identical language. For example, section 27A of the Tasmanian *Human Tissue Act 1985* states:

> For the purposes of the law of Tasmania, a person has died when there has occurred —
> a. irreversible cessation of all function of the brain of the person; or
> b. irreversible cessation of circulation of blood in the body of the person.

The mechanisms for the determination of brain death may also be included in the legislation. Alternatively, a specific protocol should be established in line with accepted international medical practice.

The question of when brain death has occurred and how it should be diagnosed continues to be a topic of controversy.[21] The Australian and New Zealand Intensive Care Society (ANZICS) has undertaken excellent work and released the fourth version of their *Statement on death and organ donation* in 2021.[22] The Statement begins with a table of 29 recommendations that contain the key elements of the process, legal and ethical issues, best practice and care of the patient and family. There are also changes in the sections on neurological and circulatory determination of death.

ANZICS states that the main purposes of the statement are:

- to provide a standard for intensivists and other health professionals in relation to the determination of death and the conduct of organ and tissue donation, including donation after circulatory determination of death; and
- to provide assurance to the Australian and New Zealand communities that determination of death and the conduct of organ and tissue donation are undertaken with diligence, integrity, respect and compassion, and in accordance with available medical evidence and societal expectations.[23]

The NHMRC produced a set of guidelines in 2016 (currently under review) entitled *Ethical guidelines for organ transplantation from deceased donors*[24] that identifies the key principles applying to all healthcare delivery and then applies these principles specifically to organ donation after death. Because these are so valuable, the key points are set out in **Box 12.3**.

ONGOING DIFFICULTIES WITH ORGAN DONATION

Although tissue transplantation is extremely successful, there are still difficulties in relation to the availability of organs, particularly in relation to donation after death. All statutes allow for the donation of tissue after death. Under section 26 of the *Human Tissue Act 1982* (Vic), where a person has died in hospital or where the body has been brought to the hospital, a designated officer may authorise the removal of tissue for transplantation or other scientific, medical or therapeutic purposes where:

- the deceased person had, at any time, in writing, or during his last illness, orally in the presence of two witnesses, expressed the wish for, or consented to, the removal after his death of tissue from his body for such a purpose or use;
- the senior available next of kin of the deceased person makes it known to the designated officer that he consents to the removal of tissue from the

body of the deceased person for such a purpose or use; or

■ the designated officer, after making such inquiries as are reasonable in the circumstances, is unable to ascertain the existence or whereabouts of the next of kin of the deceased person and has no reason to believe that the deceased person had expressed an objection to the removal after his death of tissue from his body for such a purpose or use.

BOX 12.3

APPLICATION OF ETHICAL PRINCIPLES AND VALUES TO ORGAN TRANSPLANTATION[25]

2.2.1. Donation of organs is an act of altruism, solidarity and community reciprocity that provides significant benefits to those in medical need.

Transplantation practices should be motivated by the needs of the recipient and the need to ensure the appropriate use of scarce health resources.

2.2.2. Processes and policies for determining a person's eligibility for transplantation and for allocating donated organs must be just, equitable and respectful of the inherent dignity and of the equal and inalienable rights of all persons.

2.2.3. Decision-making about transplantation must recognise and respect the autonomy of the recipient. As for all medical procedures, consent must be given before transplantation can proceed. The process of seeking and receiving consent should be sensitive to an individual's particular set of values, preferences and beliefs that may affect decision-making.

2.2.4. The allocation and transplantation of organs must be undertaken in a manner that protects recipients from harm. Organ transplantation should only be undertaken when it is believed that it provides a benefit to the recipient.

2.2.5. The process of allocating and transplanting organs should acknowledge both the needs and wellbeing of the recipient and the necessity to achieve the best outcome for the community as a whole.

2.2.6. The organisation and implementation of transplantation activities, as well as their clinical results, must be transparent and open to scrutiny, while ensuring that the personal anonymity and privacy of donors and recipients are always protected. Criteria used for decision-making about eligibility of potential recipients and suitability and allocation of organs for transplantation must be transparent and made publicly available.

Back in 2008 the Australian Government announced a national reform program to implement a world's best practice approach to organ and tissue donation for transplantation, which was endorsed by the Council of Australian Governments. The aim continues to be to improve access to life-transforming transplants for Australians through a sustained increase in the donation of organs and tissues by implementing a nationally coordinated approach. Evidence from comparable countries has demonstrated that the focus on clinical practice reform improves organ donation and transplantation rates and thus the Organ and Tissue Authority (OTA) works as an independent statutory body to achieve these aims under the title of DonateLife.[24] The current 2022–27 Strategic Plan has as its purpose 'To save and improve the lives of more Australians through organ and tissue donation and transplantation'.[27] The goals and objectives are to build support through having more people say yes to donation, to optimise opportunities so that donation and transplantation services deliver the best outcomes, and to enhance systems to enable quality outcomes through information, technology and resources.[28] Since 2008 there have been major changes in Australia's organ and tissue donation infrastructure, most notably with the establishment of specialist medical and nursing staff in this area in key hospitals across Australia.

Post-Mortem Examinations

Over the past few years, there have been a number of serious incidents relating to the conduct of post-mortem examinations and the retention and/or disposal of human tissue following post-mortem examinations.[29]

The events and subsequent inquiry into the practices at the Institute of Forensic Medicine in Glebe, Sydney, led to the passing of the *Human Tissue and Anatomy Legislation Amendment Bill 2003*, which made changes to the *Human Tissue Act 1983* (NSW), the *Anatomy Act 1977* (NSW) and the *Coroners Act 1980* (NSW). The Bill was described as follows:

> *These amendments protect the rights of individuals to control what happens to their bodies after their death. They also protect the rights of families to be informed of, and to give consent to, procedures that are undertaken on the bodies of family members who have died. The bill balances this respect for*

individuals' rights with the recognition that society has some legitimate interest in the use of human tissue, which should not be contingent on an individual's consent. Accordingly, the bill protects the use of tissue for coronial purposes for the investigation of crime and the proper functioning of the judicial system. The bill recognises the importance of medical teaching and research and allows these important interests to be advanced without offending the values of the general community. The bill represents a balance between the benefits that accrue from access to human tissue for therapeutic purposes, research, education and training on the one hand and respect for diverse cultural, religious and individual values and personal autonomy on the other hand.[30]

South Australia[31] and Western Australia[32] also undertook reviews into forensic practices, as did the NHMRC Australian Health Ethics Committee. In 2002 the Australian Health Ministers' Advisory Council Subcommittee on Autopsy Practice issued *The national code of ethical autopsy practice*.[33] This code has resulted in several states and territories amending their legislation in relation to autopsy (or post-mortem examination as it is most often called), and most states have issued revised policy documents to meet the requirements of the code.

While the conduct of post-mortem examinations is unlikely to be part of the experience of undergraduate nursing or midwifery students, or indeed the majority of practising nurses and midwives, post-mortems and the rights of patients and their relatives in relation to their bodies or the bodies of their loved ones are critical and worrying issues, and nurses and midwives may need to reassure patients and relatives about the changes that have been put in place since the events referred to above occurred.

Assisted Reproductive Technology and Donation of Reproductive Tissue

Another area of law that has seen extraordinarily rapid developments is that of assisted reproductive technology (ART). ART is defined as 'The application of laboratory or clinical techniques to gametes and/or embryos for the purposes of reproduction'.[34] Again, this is a highly specialised area of healthcare, and it is unlikely that most undergraduate students will work in this area, although it may be of interest to midwives, particularly in antenatal care.

ART is becoming far more common and is likely to increase as the demographic age of women having their first child increases, thus it is highly likely that nurses and midwives will encounter parents and children who have been involved in this technology in some way.[35]

The National Perinatal Epidemiology and Statistics Unit of the University of NSW reported that, in 2020:

There were 95 699 ART treatment cycles performed in Australian and New Zealand ART Units in 2020 (87 206 and 8493 respectively), representing an increase of 7.6% in Australia and 7.8% in New Zealand from 2019. This equates to 16.5 cycles per 1000 women of reproductive age (15–44 years) in Australia, compared with 8.3 cycles per 1000 women of reproductive age in New Zealand.

Women used their own oocytes or embryos (autologous cycles) in approximately 95% (90 529) of fresh and/or thaw cycles. These cycles were undertaken by 46 846 women, with more cycles per woman in Australia (2.0 cycles per woman) than in New Zealand (1.7 cycles per woman). Thawed embryos and oocytes were transferred in 37.1% of autologous cycles. There were 3642 cycles where all oocytes or embryos were frozen for medical or non-medical fertility preservation, and 238 surrogacy gestational carrier cycles. More than 8% of cycles performed in 2020 underwent preimplantation genetic testing (PGT).[36]

There is a robust framework for the conduct of ART in Australia. This framework consists of:

- Commonwealth legislation: *Prohibition of Human Cloning for Reproduction Act 2002* and *Research Involving Human Embryos Act 2002*;
- state and territory legislation — there is legislation in most states that seeks to regulate at least some aspects of ART:
  - the ACT *Human Cloning and Embryo Research Act 2004*;
  - the New South Wales *Assisted Reproductive Technology Act 2007*;

- the Queensland *Research Involving Human Embryos and Prohibition of Human Cloning for Reproduction Act 2003*;
- the South Australian *Assisted Reproductive Treatment Act 1988*;
- the Tasmanian *Human Cloning for Reproduction and Other Prohibited Practices Act 2003* and *Human Embryonic Research Regulation Act 2003*;
- the Victorian *Assisted Reproductive Treatment Act 2008* and Assisted Reproductive Treatment Regulations 2019;
- the Western Australian *Human Reproductive Technology Act 1991*.

Each of these pieces of legislation established a state regulatory body that issues licences to clinics that provide ART services. When there are anomalies between the state Acts and the guidelines, the legislation takes precedence:

- NHMRC guidelines, including the ART guidelines, the national protocol and the *National Statement on Ethical Conduct in Human Research (2007 — all sections are regularly updated)*
- accreditation of ART clinics by the Reproductive Technology Accreditation Committee (RTAC) of the Fertility Society of Australia.

The ART framework underpins the regulation of ART practice within Australia. RTAC accreditation is the basis of a nationally consistent approach for overseeing ART clinical practice. RTAC accreditation requires ART treatment centres to comply with laws and guidelines concerning the practice of ART. The ART guidelines are included in this requirement.[37]

The NHMRC *Ethical guidelines on the use of assisted reproductive technology in clinical practice and research* (the ART guidelines) were issued in 2004 and updated in 2007 to reflect amendments to the *Research Involving Human Embryos Act 2002* (Cth) and the *Prohibition of Human Cloning for Reproduction Act 2002* (Cth). Further revised guidelines were issued in 2017. The ART guidelines address both clinical and research aspects of assisted reproductive technology. The ART guidelines are primarily intended for ART clinicians, clinic nurses, embryologists, counsellors and administrators, researchers, Human Research Ethics Committees and governments.[38] Current reproductive technologies include the following.

Ovulation Induction

A series of hormone injections will be given to the woman to stimulate egg growth and ovulation. If ovulation can be successfully induced, conception may occur naturally.

Artificial Insemination

Artificial insemination is used in cases where the male has a low sperm count or a high number of abnormal sperm or the woman has sperm antibodies present in her cervical mucus. Sperm is treated in the laboratory to increase the chances of fertilisation. Large numbers of sperm are then inserted directly into the uterus for easy access to the fallopian tubes.

IVF (In-Vitro Fertilisation)

In-vitro fertilisation (IVF) is a procedure used to overcome a range of fertility issues, by which an egg and sperm are joined together outside the body, in a specialised laboratory. The fertilised egg (embryo) is allowed to grow in a protected environment for some days before being transferred into the woman's uterus, increasing the chance that a pregnancy will occur.[39]

GIFT (Gamete Intrafallopian Transfer)

Gamete intrafallopian transfer (GIFT) involves ovarian stimulation, monitoring and egg collection. The process then differs from traditional IVF in that the collected egg and sperm are placed in the woman's fallopian tube, allowing fertilisation to take place within the body.[40]

ZIFT (Zygote Intrafallopian Transfer)

ZIFT is a procedure similar to GIFT, but the egg is fertilised in the laboratory. Then the fertilised egg (zygote) is transferred into the fallopian tubes by a laparoscopic procedure.[41]

ICSI (Intracytoplasmic Sperm Injection)

Intracytoplasmic sperm injection (ICSI) is performed as an additional part of an IVF treatment cycle where a single sperm is injected into each egg to assist fertilisation using very fine micro-manipulation equipment.

In most cases, ICSI can be used to overcome severe male infertility.[42]

Epididymal and Testicular Sperm Extraction

Sperm are removed from the epididymis or directly from the testis using a needle. Fertilisation is performed by ICSI (see above). This treatment is used in cases of male infertility (azoospermia) and spermatic cord abnormalities. Usually enough sperm can be collected so that samples can be frozen for later use if required.

Freezing of Sperm and Embryos

If more embryos are produced through IVF than are needed for transfer into the woman's uterus, the extra embryos can be frozen. The stored embryos can be used later if the woman fails to become pregnant or if the couple wishes to have more children through IVF at a later date.

There is a limit to the number of years that embryos can be stored frozen and laws governing this may differ in each state and territory. Similarly, sperm can be frozen for use in subsequent IVF cycles or as insurance against infertility due to procedures such as cancer therapies, vasectomy or prolonged absence from a partner (such as men in military service may experience). Sperm can also be frozen and kept in sperm donor banks.

Donor Eggs, Embryos and Sperm

For women who have ovarian failure, men who do not produce sperm, or couples whose eggs fail to fertilise, the use of donor eggs, embryos or sperm may be an option. Older women may also wish to use donor eggs from younger women to overcome the problems of ageing.[43]

Although the use of ART has been increasing since the first Australian IVF baby was born in 1980, there is still concern about the lack of accurate data on success rates in terms of live, healthy births and the overly optimistic attitude the community seems to have towards ART as a complete and infallible solution for infertility.[44] The development of these techniques has raised a range of ethical and legal challenges over time, including the need to determine parentage, the question of payment for donors and surrogates, and even more potentially controversial issues such as cloning.

CONCLUSION

This chapter has examined the provisions of the various pieces of legislation dealing with human tissue transplantation and explored some of the ethical and clinical dilemmas inherent in the developments of these technologies. In addition, the chapter has briefly examined the law relating to assisted reproductive technologies and some of the current issues in relation to post-mortem practice in Australia. The chapter has provided a wide range of guidance documents and resources with further information on these complex and developing areas, as there is no doubt that these issues will prove to be challenges for law and ethics in the future and will require serious thought as readers progress in their nursing and midwifery careers.

CHAPTER 12 REVIEW QUESTIONS

Following your reading of **Chapter 12**, consider these questions in reaching the objectives of this chapter. Guidance on which part of the chapter will assist you in answering the questions can be found at http://evolve.elsevier.com/AU/Staunton/law/. You may, of course, consider other sources as part of your considerations.

1. Human tissue transplantation and research is developing rapidly. How could the law keep up with these developments?

2. Cultural issues are critical in planning transplant programs and working with families. What sorts of issues need to be considered when having discussions about organ donation and transplantation (at any time)?

3. Why do you think Australia has such ongoing difficulties with organ donation?

ENDNOTES

1. Scott R, *The body as property*, Allen Lane, London, 1981.
2. Health Resources and Service Administration, *Donation and transplant history*, 2022, https://www.organdonor.gov/learn/history.
3. Australian Government, *Australian Organ and Tissue Donation and Transplantation Authority (OTA) Activity Report*, 2023, https://www.donatelife.gov.au/sites/default/files/2023-02/OTA%202022%20Donation%20and%20Transplantation%20Activity%20Report.pdf p 13.
4. Ibid, p 29.
5. International Registry in Organ Donation and Transplantation, 'Database' tab, Organ donation activity charts worldwide actual deceased organ donors 2021 (PMP), https://www.irodat.org/img/database/grafics/2021_01_worldwide-actual-deceased-organ-donors.png.
6. Australian Government, 2023, op. cit.
7. Australian Law Reform Commission, *Human tissue transplants (ALRC report 7)*, AGPS, Canberra, 1977, https://www.alrc.gov.au/publication/human-tissue-transplants-alrc-report-7/.
8. *Transplantation and Anatomy Act 1978* (ACT); *Anatomy Act 1977* (NSW); *Human Tissue Act 1983* (NSW); *Human Cloning for Reproduction and Other Prohibited Practices Act 2003* (NSW); *Transplantation and Anatomy Act 1979* (NT); *Human Tissue Act 1985* (Tas); *Transplantation and Anatomy Act 1979* (Qld); *Transplantation and Anatomy Act 1983* (SA); *Human Embryonic Research Regulation Act 2003* (Tas); *Human Cloning for Reproduction and Other Prohibited Practices Act 2003* (Tas); *Human Tissue Act 1982* (Vic); *Human Tissue and Transplant Act 1982* (WA); *Human Reproductive Technology Act 1991* (WA).
9. Australian Government Organ and Tissue Authority, *Best practice guideline for donation after circulatory determination of death (DCDD)*, 2021, https://www.donatelife.gov.au/for-healthcare-workers/clinical-guidelines-and-protocols/national-guideline-donation-after-circulatory-death.
10. Australian Government Department of Health and Aged Care, *What we're doing about organ and tissue donation*, 2022, https://www.health.gov.au/topics/organ-and-tissue-donation/what-were-doing-about-organ-and-tissue-donation.
11. National Health and Medical Research Council (NHMRC), *Organ and tissue donation by living donors: guidelines for ethical practice for health professionals*, 2007, https://www.nhmrc.gov.au/about-us/publications/organ-and-tissue-donation-living-donors.
12. Australian Government Organ and Tissue Authority, *Australian Donation and Transplantation Activity Report*, 2022, https://www.donatelife.gov.au/sites/default/files/2023-02/OTA%202022%20Donation%20and%20Transplantation%20Activity%20Report.pdf.
13. NHMRC, *Ethical guidelines for organ and tissue donation and transplantation*, 2023, https://www.nhmrc.gov.au/research-policy/ethics/ethical-guidelines-organ-and-tissue-donation-and-transplantation.
14. NHMRC, *Organ and tissue donation by living donors: guidelines for ethical practice for health professionals*, 2007, https://www.nhmrc.gov.au/about-us/publications/organ-and-tissue-donation-living-donors p 6.
15. NHMRC, *Making a decision about living organ and tissue donation*, 2007, https://www.nhmrc.gov.au/about-us/publications/making-decision-about-living-organ-and-tissue-donation#block-views-block-file-attachments-content-block-1.
16. Ibid, p 5.
17. NHMRC, *Organ and tissue donation by living donors: guidelines for ethical practice for health professionals*, 2007, https://www.nhmrc.gov.au/about-us/publications/organ-and-tissue-donation-living-donors p 27.
18. Gardner D, Charlesworth M, Rubino A and Madden S, 'The rise of organ donation after circulatory death: a narrative review', (2020) *Anaesthesia* 75(9):1215–22, https://pubmed.ncbi.nlm.nih.gov/32430909/.
19. Ad Hoc Committee of the Harvard Medical School to examine the definition of brain death: a definition of irreversible coma, (1968) *Journal of the American Medical Association* 205:337–40.
20. *Mount Isa Mines Ltd v Pusey* (1970) 125 CLR 383 at 395.
21. See, for example, Morrison W and Kirschen M, 'A taxonomy of objections to brain death determination', (2022) *Neurocritical Care* 37(2):369–71. doi: 10.1007/s12028-022-01580-6; Schwartz A, 'Issues with the determination of brain death: the case for religious and moral exceptions', (2020), Law School Student Scholarship, 1106, https://scholarship.shu.edu/student_scholarship/1106.
22. Australian and New Zealand Intensive Care Society (ANZICS), *Statement on death and organ donation edition 4.1*, 2021, https://www.anzics.com.au/wp-content/uploads/2022/04/ANZICS-Statement-on-Death-and-Organ-Donation.pdf.
23. Ibid, p 9.
24. NHMRC, *Ethical guidelines for organ transplantation from deceased donors*, 2016, https://www.nhmrc.gov.au/about-us/publications/ethical-guidelines-organ-transplantation-deceased-donors#block-views-block-file-attachments-content-block-1, pp 4–5.
25. Ibid.
26. Australian Government, Organ and Tissue Authority, *About us*, https://www.donatelife.gov.au/about-us.
27. Australian Government, Organ and Tissue Authority, *Strategy 2022–2027*, https://www.donatelife.gov.au/sites/default/files/2022-08/OTA%20Strategy%202022-2027.pdf.
28. Ibid.
29. A number of older reports give examples of misuse such as Redfern M, QC, *The report of the Royal Liverpool Children's inquiry*, House of Commons, London, 2001; Walker B, *Report into post-mortem and anatomical examination practices of the Institute of Forensic Medicine*, New South Wales Government, Sydney, 2002.

30. Burton C (Parliamentary Secretary), *Hansard extract*, New South Wales Legislative Assembly, 28 May 2003 (article 5), https://www.parliament.nsw.gov.au/Hansard/Pages/HansardResult.aspx#/docid/HANSARD-1323879322-29703.

31. Selway B M, QC, *Report into the retention of body parts after post-mortems [sic]*, Solicitor General South Australia, 6 August 2001, (unpublished) cited in The Royal College of Pathologists of Australasia, *Policy: autopsies and the use of tissues removed from autopsies*, Approval Date: July 1993, Revised: November 2011, no. 1 of 1993, https://www.rcpa.edu.au/Library/College-Policies/Policies/Autopsies-and-the-Use-of-Tissues-Removed-from-Auto.

32. Kucera B (Minister for Health), Western Australian Government, *Hansard*, 2001, p 4495. See also *Hansard*, Thursday 13 April 2006 per The Hon. Giz Watson, https://www.parliament.wa.gov.au/Hansard/hansard.nsf/0/5e37c473bce55c63c82575700014703e/$FILE/A36%20S1%2020011017%20p4494c-4495a.pdf.

33. Australian Health Ministers' Advisory Council, Subcommittee on Autopsy Practice, *The national code of ethical autopsy practice*, South Australian Department of Human Services, Adelaide, 2002.

34 NHMRC (2017, updated 2023), *Ethical guidelines on the use of Assisted reproductive technology (ART)*, https://www.nhmrc.gov.au/about-us/publications/art#block-views-block-file-attachments-content-block-1, p 2.

35. Pettersson M, Bladh M, Nedstrand E, Svanberg A, Lampic C and Sydsjo G, 'Maternal advanced age, single parenthood, and ART increase the risk of child morbidity up to five years of age', (2022) *BMC Pediatrics* 22(1):39. doi: 10.1186/s12887-021-03103-2.

36. National Perinatal Epidemiology and Statistics Unit, *Assisted reproductive technology in Australia and New Zealand 2020*, University of New South Wales, Sydney, 2022 https://npesu.unsw.edu.au/surveillance/assisted-reproductive-technology-australia-and-new-zealand-2020

37. NHMRC, *Ethical guidelines for assisted reproductive technology (ART)*, 2017, https://www.nhmrc.gov.au/about-us/publications/art.

38. Ibid.

39. IVF Australia, *What is IVF?*, 2023, https://www.ivf.com.au/treatments/fertility-treatments/ivf-treatment.

40. Queensland Fertility Group, *What is GIFT?*, 2023, https://www.qfg.com.au/tests-treatments/fertility-treatments/gift-treatment#:~:text=With%20GIFT%2C%20instead%20of%20the,partner's%20sperm%2C%20using%20a%20laparoscope.

41. Szmelskyj I and Szmelskyj A, 'The fundamentals of ART', 2015, https://www.sciencedirect.com/topics/medicine-and-dentistry/zygote-intrafallopian-transfer.

42. IVF Australia, *What is ICSI?*, 2023, https://www.ivf.com.au/treatments/fertility-treatments/icsi-treatment.

43. Taebe M, Bahrahmi R, Bagheri-Lankarani N and Shahriari M, 'Ethical challenges of embryo donation in embryo donors and recipients, (2018) *Iranian Journal of Nursing and Midwifery Research* 23(1):36–39. https://www.ncbi.nlm.nih.gov/pmc/articles/PMC5769183/

44. Simoni M, Mu L and Collins S, 'Women's career priority is associated with attitudes towards family planning and ethical acceptance of reproductive technologies', (2017) *Human Reproduction* 32(10):2069–75.

INDEX